Pills, Power, and Policy

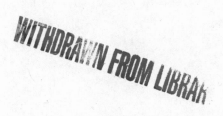

CALIFORNIA/MILBANK BOOKS ON HEALTH AND THE PUBLIC

Pills, Power, and Policy

*The Struggle for Drug Reform in Cold War America
and Its Consequences*

DOMINIQUE A. TOBBELL

University of California Press

BERKELEY　　LOS ANGELES　　LONDON

Milbank Memorial Fund

NEW YORK

University of California Press, one of the most distinguished university presses in the United States, enriches lives around the world by advancing scholarship in the humanities, social sciences, and natural sciences. Its activities are supported by the UC Press Foundation and by philanthropic contributions from individuals and institutions. For more information, visit www.ucpress.edu.

The Milbank Memorial Fund is an endowed operating foundation that engages in nonpartisan analysis, study, research, and communication on significant issues in health policy. In the Fund's own publications, in reports, films, or books it publishes with other organizations, and in articles it commissions for publication by other organizations, the Fund endeavors to maintain the highest standards for accuracy and fairness. Statements by individual authors, however, do not necessarily reflect opinions or factual determinations of the Fund. For more information, visit www.milbank.org.

University of California Press
Berkeley and Los Angeles, California

University of California Press, Ltd.
London, England

Library of Congress Cataloging-in-Publication Data

Tobbell, Dominique A., 1978–.
  Pills, power, and policy : the struggle for drug reform in cold war America and its consequences / Dominique A. Tobbell.
     p. cm.
  Includes bibliographical references and index.
  ISBN 978–0-520–27113–5 (cloth : alk. paper)
  ISBN 978–0-520–27114–2 (pbk. : alk. paper)
  1. Drugs—Research—United States—History—20th century.
2. Pharmaceutical industry—United States—History—20th
century.   I. Title.   II. Series: California/Milbank books on health and the public.
  [DNLM: 1. Drug Industry—history—United States.   2. Economics, Pharmaceutical—United States.   3. History, 20th Century—United States.   QV 711 AA1]
  RS122.T59 2012
  338.4'76151—dc22

                                                            2011014878

Manufactured in the United States of America

20 19 18 17 16 15 14 13 12
10 9 8 7 6 5 4 3 2 1

In keeping with a commitment to support environmentally responsible and sustainable printing practices, UC Press has printed this book on 50-pound Enterprise, a 30% post-consumer-waste, recycled, deinked fiber that is processed chlorine-free. It is acid-free and meets all ANSI/ NISO (Z 39.48) requirements.

To my teachers

Contents

Foreword

The Milbank Memorial Fund is an endowed operating foundation that works to improve health by helping decision makers in the public and private sectors acquire and use the best available evidence to inform policy for health care and population health. The Fund has engaged in nonpartisan analysis, study, research, and communication since its inception in 1905.

Pills, Power, and Policy: The Struggle for Drug Reform in Cold War America and Its Consequences by Dominique Tobbell is the twenty-third book in the series of California/Milbank Books on Health and the Public. The publishing partnership between the Fund and the University of California Press encourages the synthesis and communication of findings from research and experience that could contribute to more effective health policy.

In *Pills, Power, and Policy*, Tobbell examines how complex relationships forged with key players in the medical community by the pharmaceutical industry since the Second World War contributed to the industry's growth and created a political backing that would support it in the face of governmental reform efforts, while simultaneously influencing both academic research and pharmaceutical policy. Tobbell describes how both the criticisms raised against the pharmaceutical industry and the industry's defense have endured and are remarkably similar today. Tobbell also reveals how not only the industry but also Congress, the FDA, universities, medical schools, physicians, and researchers have all had a political, social, and financial interest in maintaining the status quo in pharmaceutical policy.

Tobbell's rich history of pharmaceutical politics will provide compelling reading to scholars and students of political science, the history of medicine and of business, pharmacology, and clinical epidemiology, and informed instruction to policymakers grappling with the current crisis in drug development and regulation.

Carmen Hooker Odom
President, Milbank Memorial Fund

Samuel L. Milbank
Chairman, Milbank Memorial Fund

Acknowledgments

I was in my final year of high school in England when I decided I wanted to write a book that would help advance the public's understanding of science. In the years since then, I have benefited enormously from the guidance, encouragement, and mentorship of inspirational teachers who have nurtured this commitment, influenced my intellectual development, and helped make that book a reality. It is to these teachers, particularly my high school biology teacher, Joy Hopkinson, that I dedicate this book.

In writing this book I benefited greatly from the knowledge and assistance of archivists at the University of Pennsylvania Archives, the University of Rochester Archives, the Archives Center of the National Museum of American History, the National Academies Archives, the Othmer Library of Chemical History at the Chemical Heritage Foundation, the National Archives in College Park, the Library of Congress, and the National Library of Medicine. Special thanks go to Jeffrey Sturchio for granting me access to the Merck Archives. I am grateful for the financial support I received from the Thouron Award, the Lemelson Center for the Study of Invention and Innovation, the American Institute for the History of Pharmacy, the Chemical Heritage Foundation, the Rovensky Fellowship, and the Miller Center of Public Affairs.

I received incredible support from my teachers and colleagues at the University of Pennsylvania. Ruth Schwartz Cowan gave me a seemingly endless supply of guidance, critical feedback, and warm support. Rosemary Stevens has been an inspiring mentor throughout my career, and her scholarship has served as a model of how to balance rigorous historical research with critical policy analysis. Susan Lindee, Robert Kohler, Robby Aronowitz, Sarah Igo, Tom Sugrue, and Walter Licht taught me to think critically and ask difficult questions. Beyond Penn, Louis Galambos's insights and support indelibly influenced this project, particularly in its early stages. From the beginning, Arthur Daemmrich challenged me to tackle tough questions and conceptualize my work beyond history. I am also thankful to Daniel Carpenter, who generously shared with me his knowledge of the Food and Drug Administration and his astute analysis of the pharmaceutical enterprise. As I transformed this work from dissertation to book, Daniel M. Fox generously provided me with invaluable advice, critical feedback, and encouragement that helped make this a better book. Friends and colleagues read and commented on portions of the manuscript and generously contributed their insights. Many thanks are due to Rebecca Kluchin, Corinna Schlombs, Emily Pawley, and Hilary Smith. Beth Linker deserves special thanks not only for serving as an invaluable sounding board and engaged reader but also for coming up with the title.

As I completed this book, I was very fortunate to have been surrounded by supportive and thoughtful colleagues in the Program in the History of Science, Technology, and Medicine and the Wangensteen Historical Library of Biology and Medicine at the University of Minnesota. I cannot imagine having had a more supportive chair than Jennifer Gunn, who could, within a matter of minutes of listening, help me crystallize my argument and dislodge my writer's block. Jole Shackelford, Mary Thomas, Susan Jones, Sally Gregory Kohlstedt, Lois Hendrickson, and Elaine Challacombe have also been especially kind and supportive. I have also benefited greatly from the support and insights of a number of scholars. Among these are Margot Canaday, Angela Creager, Patricia D'Antonio, Julie Fairman, Jeremy Greene, Greg Higby, Scott Keefer, Wendy Kline, Pamela Laird, Harry Marks, John McDonough, Kim Phillips-Fein, Scott Podolsky, Viviane Quirke, Nicolas Rasmussen, Leo Slater, Elaine Stroud, John Swann, Andrea Tone, Elizabeth Siegel Watkins, Jean Whelan, and Julian Zelizer. I am very fortunate to have had the guidance and support of my editor at the University of California Press, Hannah Love, who has been generous with her time and insights. I'm also grateful to Marilyn Schwartz, managing editor at the Press, and to my wonderful copyeditor, Madeleine B. Adams, who did a masterful job ensuring the accuracy of my prose and my footnotes. I am thankful to the external reviewers for the Press, and to the Milbank Memorial Fund for copublishing this book.

I am grateful to my friends who provided welcome relief from the writing process, and to my furry family members, Taka, Turtle, and Ben, who made even the most challenging of writing days bearable with their endlessly goofy and loving ways. Finally, thanks are due to Danny Muñoz-

Hutchinson for being a continual source of warmth, support, love, and laughter.

. . .

Some of the material presented in this book has previously appeared elsewhere. I thank the editors of the respective journals for their permission to reuse this material: "Who's Winning the Human Race? Cold War as Pharmaceutical Political Strategy," *Journal of the History of Medicine and Allied Sciences* 64, no. 4 (2009): 429–473 (chapter 4) and "Allied against Reform: Pharmaceutical Industry–Academic Physician Relations in the United States, 1945–1970," *Bulletin of the History of* Medicine 82, no. 4 (2008): 878–912 (chapters 5 and 6).

Introduction

Pharmaceutical Politics, Then and Now

Since the early 2000s, barely a week has gone by without the pharmaceutical industry being in the news. Of particular concern has been whether pharmaceutical companies charge too much for prescription drugs, withhold negative clinical trial data, and produce too many so-called me-too drugs—drugs with similar chemical properties and more or less identical therapeutic functions. Equally alarming have been questions about whether physicians and researchers who receive money and gifts from drug companies act in the best interest of patients and whether the federal Food and Drug Administration (FDA) has been captured by the industry it's charged to regulate.[1] Yet these concerns are not new. As early as the 1950s, critics berated the industry for its profit levels, its marketing strategies, the high cost of drugs, the abundance of me-too drugs, and drug safety problems.

The 1960s and 1970s, in particular, were decades of crisis for the American pharmaceutical industry as it confronted a pharmaceutical reform movement which had as its goal the passage of legislation that would increase the government's control over drug development, distribution, and therapeutic practice and would reduce prescription drug prices. This reform movement brought together congressional Democrats committed to protecting the economic interests of consumers and organizations dedicated to increasing Americans' access to affordable health care. It also included state welfare agencies and hospital groups struggling to balance their budgets amidst rising costs, and a growing number of physicians who accused pharmaceutical firms of spending far more on misleading and excessive marketing than on research, needlessly driving up the costs of prescription drugs. *Pills, Power, and Policy* examines the history of this reform effort and the emergence of a politically powerful pharmaceutical industry that fought against it.[2]

In the decades following World War II, the pharmaceutical industry developed extensive research and administrative networks with academic researchers, medical schools, and government officials. These relationships underpinned the innovativeness and growth of the U.S. pharmaceutical industry and formed the basis of the industry's political support after the war.[3] In particular, the shared interests of academic researchers and the pharmaceutical industry and the industry's responsiveness to the needs of the biomedical community led the pharmaceutical industry, organized medicine, and certain leading academic physicians to join forces against pharmaceutical reformers in the 1960s and 1970s. By describing the history of this pharmaceutical-medical alliance, *Pills, Power, and Policy* documents the economic and intellectual influence of pharmaceutical industry interests on research universities and medical schools in the second half of the twentieth century.

Pills, Power, and Policy, then, is about scientific and political coalition building in post–World War II America and the enduring influence of an industry-academic complex on pharmaceutical policy. It is also about pharmaceutical politics in the twenty-first century. The criticisms brought by consumer and patient groups, the press, and Congress against the pharmaceutical industry and the substance and character of the pharmaceutical industry's defense have remained remarkably consistent over the past six decades. By exposing these continuities, *Pills, Power, and Policy* makes clear that that the current crisis in drug development and regulation—and the contemporary character of pharmaceutical politics—are the result not just of drug companies but of Congress, the FDA, universities, medical schools, physicians, and researchers, who since the 1950s have been politically, socially, and financially invested in maintaining the status quo in pharmaceutical policy.

CONTINUITIES IN PHARMACEUTICAL POLITICS

In November 2009, AARP (formerly the American Association for Retired Persons) reported that prescription drug prices had increased 9 percent during the previous twelve months, the highest annual increase in drug prices since 1992. AARP and other industry critics accused drug firms of substantially raising their prices in response to the Obama administration's promise to reduce prescription drug spending as part of their effort to overhaul the health care system.[4] They also accused pharmaceutical firms of spending far more on marketing than on research, thereby inflating the cost of prescription drugs.[5] Fifty years earlier, AARP had raised similar concerns about prescription drug prices. On December 11, 1959, the president of AARP, Ethel Andrus, testified before Congress that senior citizens were struggling with high prescription drug prices, "their monthly costs for drugs prescribed for treatment" leaving "them little to live on."[6] The following day, Frank J. Wilson, the president of the National Association of Retired Civil Employees, testified that "senior citizens are reminded almost daily of astounding new drugs and remedies to relieve their aches and pains and prolong life, only to find that these miracle drugs are denied them because of the exorbitant prices attached to them." Wilson described "the financial hardships of [the association's] members, who are forced to live on small or moderate annuities, in buying drugs," and called on Congress to give "very serious consideration ... [to s]ome method of control of drug prices."[7]

Today, the pharmaceutical industry defends the prices it charges for prescription drugs—and the profit margins at which it operates—on the grounds that pharmaceutical research and development are extremely expensive because of the time and labor required to bring a drug to market and the high rate of failure in pharmaceutical innovation. The industry notes, for example, that a firm may spend millions of dollars developing a drug, only to see it fail in clinical trials, and may never see a return on its research investment. Similarly, the industry points out that the highly competitive nature of the pharmaceutical economy means that a new drug may become obsolete within a few years of reaching the market if a new, superior drug is subsequently introduced. In such cases, a firm may never sell enough of its drug to recoup the expense of bringing that drug to market. Prescription drug prices, the industry maintains, thus reflect the high cost and high risk of drug development, while the industry's high profit margins are necessary to sustain its continued intensive investment in research and to compensate for the risks inherent in pharmaceutical innovation.[8]

The pharmaceutical industry's defense of prescription drug prices has changed little over the past fifty years. In 1960, for example, Austin Smith, president of the Pharmaceutical Manufacturers Association (PMA, the industry trade association), testified before Congress that prescription drug prices reflected the "investment of vast sums of money in [research] endeavors which involve great risk." One of those risks was that of product obsolescence; as Smith continued, "competition forces each company as a matter of economic survival to dedicate itself to" developing increasingly efficacious drugs, thereby "obsoleting its own products." Because of the high rate of product obsolescence and the high risk of failure in pharmaceutical innovation, it was necessary for firms to operate at high profit margins. After all, he noted, "the pharmaceutical industry, now seeking cures for heart disease, cancer, and even the common cold, can hope to find them only if it can maintain reasonably profitable operation." Smith also reminded Congress that prescription drugs not only reduced human suffering but also "put people back to work more quickly" than older, less effective treatments and thus "lessen[ed] the drain on the community and on the family budget."[9]

Industry critics—today and fifty years ago—have challenged the drug industry's explanation, blaming high prescription drug prices instead on the large sums of money pharmaceutical companies spend on marketing their products. In response, the pharmaceutical industry has justified its marketing expenditures by claiming that its marketing activities constitute a critical source of physician and (since the arrival of direct-to-consumer advertising in 1997) patient education. In 1960, for example, Austin Smith assured Congress that pharmaceutical firms played a vital role in supplying "medical information ... concerning new drugs, to doctors." As evidence, he cited the fact that the majority of private practitioners "gain their information on what's new in the therapeutic field" from drug advertisements and their interactions with the pharmaceutical sales representatives who visited them in their offices. Rather than being a needless expense, Smith maintained, pharmaceutical marketing was a necessary activity that brought substantial benefits to physicians and patients.[10]

The continuities in pharmaceutical politics extend beyond the topic of prescription drug prices and drug development costs. One of the most serious issues confronting pharmaceutical consumers in the early twenty-first century is whether pharmaceutical companies withhold negative clinical trial data and obfuscate the risks of pharmaceutical consumption by overzealously marketing their drugs. In February 2010, for example, GlaxoSmithKline came under scrutiny for withholding negative clinical data on its diabetes drug Avandia. The *New York Times* reported that for eleven years the company had withheld from the FDA clinical findings that Avandia significantly increased patients' risk of cardiovascular disease. Since 1999, GlaxoSmithKline had marketed Avandia as a diabetes drug that *reduced* cardiovascular risk in patients.[11] Since its release, Avandia had been among the company's most heavily marketed and highest selling prescription drugs.[12]

Once again though, these concerns are not new. In 1953, for example, Parke-Davis & Co. was sued by the parents of several children who died from the rare blood disease aplastic anemia after taking its antibiotic Chloromycetin (chloramphenicol). In those suits, the parents (two of whom were physicians) accused Parke-Davis & Co. of continuing to manufacture and advertise the drug as "completely nontoxic," with "no evidence of intolerance" and "entirely free of troublesome reactions," despite knowing that in "many instances" use of Chloromycetin caused "aplastic anemia and other serious blood disorders, frequently resulting in death."[13] Seven years later, two former pharmaceutical sales representatives testifying before Congress accused companies of promoting potentially dangerous drugs "in such a fashion as to lull the physician concerning the hazards involved."[14] These former sales representatives joined with several physicians in accusing Parke-Davis, in particular, of "watering down" warnings in its promotional materials about Chloromycetin's hazards.[15]

Today, industry observers are also concerned about whether physicians and researchers receiving money and gifts from drug companies act in the best interest of patients. In 2007, Senator Charles Grassley (R-IA), the ranking Republican on the Senate Finance Committee, launched an investigation into the financial relationships between pharmaceutical and medical device manufacturers and academic researchers and physicians. Over the next three years, Grassley exposed several instances of financial conflicts of interest between manufacturers and prominent physicians at some of the country's leading research universities.[16] Yet, the relationships uncovered by Grassley have a far longer and far more complex history than most contemporary observers appreciate.

Beginning in the interwar years and intensifying after World War II, pharmaceutical firms developed extensive intellectual, financial, and political relationships with academic researchers, physicians, and their institutions.[17] Research-based drug companies like Merck, Pfizer, Parke-Davis, and Smith, Kline & French (a predecessor of GlaxoSmithKline) relied on academic researchers, serving as collaborators and consultants, to develop and maintain innovative research programs. In partnering with academic researchers, drug firms gained access to the work being done in academic laboratories and the invaluable insights of those working at the forefront of biomedical research. In return, the academic researchers who worked with drug firms received critical research funding and the opportunity to have their research translated into new therapeutic agents. After World War II, academic researchers and their institutions drew on these networks when they asked drug firms for help in solving their own problems, the most important of which were a perceived crisis in biomedical labor and the increasing authority of the federal government over medical education and practice—issues that proved equally troubling to drug firms. Thus, the tangled relationships among pharmaceutical firms, physicians, academic researchers, and their institutions developed out of shared needs and mutual interests.

Recently, industry observers expressed concerns about the pharmaceutical industry's relationship with the FDA, questioning whether the agency has been captured by the industry it's charged to regulate, and thus whether the FDA's ability to monitor drug safety has been compromised.[18] In 2007, for example, the Institute of Medicine found that the FDA's dependence on the user fees paid by drug firms that wanted to expedite the approval process had resulted in the agency's resources being disproportionately focused on premarket approval rather than on long-term postmarketing surveillance of drug safety.[19] The prestigious advisory body also criticized the agency's practice of allowing outside experts who have financial ties to drug firms to serve on its advisory committees. These are the very same committees that make decisions about which drugs should be approved and which drugs should be withdrawn from the market.[20] The FDA and Congress have since introduced measures intended to limit the industry's hold over the regulatory system. In March 2007, the FDA enacted new rules barring researchers who receive more than fifty thousand dollars from a company or a competitor of a company whose product is being discussed from serving on the FDA's advisory committees.[21] And in October 2007, Congress amended the Federal Food, Drug, and Cosmetic Act to include a provision restricting the number of conflict-of-interest waivers permitted on each FDA advisory committee. These waivers allow experts with otherwise "disqualifying financial interest" in the industry to serve on FDA advisory committees.[22]

These measures, however, represent only partial solutions to a problem that has plagued the drug regulatory system for several decades. In 1962, for example, Congress passed new drug regulations that expanded the FDA's regulatory authority over drug development. Congress failed to grant the FDA the necessary funds to secure the labor and resources needed to fulfill the agency's new regulatory burden. Left without the resources to perform its new regulatory functions, the agency called on pharmaceutical experts from academia—the majority of whom had ties with drug companies—to perform some of that regulatory work. In doing so, Congress and the FDA all but invited pharmaceutical companies into the center of the regulatory process.

Pharmaceutical reformers have, over the course of the past fifty years, made numerous attempts to introduce significant reforms into the pharmaceutical economy in the hope of reducing prescription drug prices and limiting the pharmaceutical industry's influence on the regulatory system. In 2003, for example, when Congress finally added a prescription drug benefit to Medicare, it looked as though major economic reform of the pharmaceutical industry would be forthcoming. Ceding to pharmaceutical industry pressure, however, Congress failed to include a provision that would allow the federal government to negotiate with pharmaceutical firms the prices it would pay for prescription drugs; a measure that, many reformers argued, would lead to an overall reduction in drug prices.[23] During the 1960s and 1970s, pharmaceutical reformers had similarly pushed for legislation they hoped would increase competition in the industry and force a reduction in prescription drug prices. These reform measures included reducing the patent term on prescription drugs, establishing a federal center of drug development that would conduct all preclinical and clinical testing of drugs, and making it mandatory for physicians to prescribe by generic-name only. Yet then, as now, pharmaceutical reformers confronted staunch opposition from the pharmaceutical industry, which—together with its medical allies—mobilized a series of powerful arguments against pharmaceutical reform.

Since the late 1950s, the pharmaceutical industry has argued that any effort to increase the government's control over the pharmaceutical industry would put America on the path to socialized medicine—a situation that, the industry and the medical profession have warned, every American should fear.[24] The industry has also maintained that increasing government regulation of the pharmaceutical industry would hinder drug innovation in the United States. In the early 1970s, for example, the clinical pharmacologists Louis Lasagna and William Wardell introduced the notion of a "drug lag."[25] They argued that as a direct result of federal drug regulations passed in 1962, the U.S. pharmaceutical industry had made significantly fewer pharmaceutical innovations, fewer new drug applications had been filed with the FDA, and even fewer new drug applications had been approved. Moreover, many new drugs were available to patients in European countries several years before they were available to patients in the United States. This, the industry argued, was evidence that greater government regulation of the industry threatened not only the public's health but also signaled the demise of America's technological superiority and economic strength by hindering pharmaceutical innovation. The pharmaceutical industry and its supporters mobilized the same arguments as

Congress debated the passage of Medicare Part D and specifically whether to allow the government to negotiate prescription drug prices.[26]

Pills, Power, and Policy takes as its subject these continuities in pharmaceutical politics, identifying the origins of the pharmaceutical critique and the industry's defense of it. In doing so, this book explains why, despite a sustained attack on the pharmaceutical industry's practices, significant reform of the pharmaceutical economy has up to now been elusive. Only by understanding the history of pharmaceutical politics and the complex relationships that developed among pharmaceutical firms, physicians, researchers, medical schools, and universities after World War II can policymakers begin to untangle the current crisis in drug development and regulation and recommend policy solutions that avoid the pitfalls of earlier reform efforts.

WHY HISTORY MATTERS

Much has already been written on the influence of government and corporate interests on the development of American universities in the second half of the twentieth century, particularly in the sciences, engineering, and medicine. The now-familiar narrative goes as follows: As research universities competed for federal and industry dollars during and after the war, they became service institutions, offering services to their patrons in exchange for research money. The universities' reward structures shifted to reflect this change. Faculty were no longer valued for their teaching but instead for their ability to secure grant money and generate patents and publications. At the same time, universities' emphasis on the capitalization of knowledge transformed research universities into drivers of regional economic development.[27] In this way, scientists and federal agencies co-opted one another in the postwar expansion of scientific research and technological innovation, and in the making of federal science policy.[28]

Pills, Power, and Policy adds to this narrative, revealing the extent to which the industry's co-opting of scientists, physicians, and government officials in the making of pharmaceutical policy was mutually conceived and mutually beneficial. In the decades after the war, physicians, researchers, and their academic institutions shared very real intellectual, political, and economic stakes with drug firms that led them to join the drug industry in opposing significant legislative reform of pharmaceutical policy. The central role of physicians and researchers within the pharmaceutical enterprise, in turn, proved critical in structuring the drug industry's relationship with the federal government. Because the government regarded academic physicians and researchers as credible experts—and interpreted academics' relations with drug firms as providing researchers with critical knowledge and insights into drug development—it routinely sought their help with the writing of pharmaceutical regulations and policy.

In this regard, the pharmaceutical industry's strategies served as a model for other industries eager to secure the guidance, expertise, and credibility of academic researchers as they fought against public criticism and expanding government regulation. The tobacco industry, for example, long recognized for its tactics of suppressing scientific evidence of the dangerous health effects of cigarette smoking, in the mid-1960s looked to the pharmaceutical industry for lessons on how to combat the burgeoning legislative attack on smoking.[29] In the first instance, the tobacco industry looked to emulate the drug industry's strategy of aligning with academic researchers able to undermine the scientific legitimacy of proposed regulatory reforms. For decades, the industry trade association, the Tobacco Institute, recruited prominent academic researchers as allies in undermining the scientific link between smoking and lung cancer and offering up scientific evidence of the supposed health benefits of its products. From the late 1950s through the 1970s, for example, the tobacco industry funded the research of Hans Selye, a leading stress researcher. During these decades, Selye provided the tobacco industry with research findings that the industry then used in litigation to argue against a causal link between smoking and cancer and heart disease. Moreover, Selye provided the tobacco industry with "expert evidence" that smoking actually had a significant health benefit by reducing stress. The tobacco industry went so far as to conceive of cigarettes as an over-the-counter remedy for stress.[30]

The tobacco industry also looked to the pharmaceutical industry for lessons on how to develop better public relations. In 1967, the Tobacco Institute hired William Kloepfer as its vice-president for public relations. Kloepfer was instrumental in the expansion of the pharmaceutical industry's public relations and public affairs capacities, having served as the PMA's public relations director since 1959. As such, Kloepfer brought with him to the Tobacco Institute "a particular appreciation for both the opportunities and limitations of research and scientific literature, as well as a knowledge of the Washington scene."[31] In short order, the Tobacco Institute was implementing some of the PMA's public relations strategies. In 1970, for example, the Tobacco Institute looked to "develop a counterpart cigarette industry activity" to the PMA's Speakers Bureau program, which throughout the 1960s had trained and used field personnel to communicate the pharmaceutical industry's public relations messages before local community groups and civic organizations.[32]

The Tobacco Institute's recruitment of a central figure in the pharmaceutical industry's politicization was part of an explicit effort by the tobacco industry to build alliances "with folks at other associations—primarily those representing highly regulated industries" so as to "share 'war stories' depicting either nonsensical or overly expensive regulatory efforts." The tobacco industry saw the pharmaceutical industry as its most natural ally "because of their heavy involvement with the FDA" and their success at preventing the enactment of tighter government regulation of its products and practices.[33] Moreover, like the pharmaceutical industry, the tobacco industry had a significant stake in winning the support of physicians and pharmacists in its efforts to sell the public on the beneficial health effects of smoking.[34] That the tobacco industry explicitly modeled its research and political strategies on those of the pharmaceutical industry is suggestive of the broad influence of the pharmaceutical industry–academic medicine complex model. Though the pharmaceutical industry was not the only science-based industry in the mid-twentieth century to confront government efforts to increase regulation of its activities and its products, it was, arguably, the most successful at undermining those regulatory reform efforts.[35]

The academic side of the pharmaceutical-medical complex also bore emulation. The academic researchers who received financial support from the pharmaceutical industry and whose careers clearly benefited from such relations, served as examples to their colleagues who, in the highly competitive entrepreneurial culture of the postwar university, were eager to secure sustained research support. That corporate support served pharmaceutical researchers so well and, until very recently, evoked little ethical conflict may have encouraged the likes of Hans Selye to follow suit and pursue the patronage of other corporate groups. In documenting the complex history of the relationships between pharmaceutical firms, academic researchers, and physicians, *Pills, Power, and Policy* offers a new chapter in the story of how corporate interests came to influence American universities and dominate American health care policy after World War II.[36] And in doing so, this book offers new insights to policymakers on how to begin unraveling those interests.

PART I

Forging Pharmaceutical Relations

1 Knowledgeable Relations

The Building of a Pharmaceutical Research Network

There have been many miracles in medicine during the last few decades, but when an historian of the 2000's comes to write the medical chronicle of the 1900's, he may, I submit, find that at least one major cause of these miracles was the inauguration of close, effective cooperation between science and industry, with pharmaceutical firms serving as a link between academic scientist, clinical investigator and the practicing physician.
> —FRANCIS BOYER, director and former chairman and president, Smith, Kline & French, 1968[1]

Between 1930 and the early 1950s, the American pharmaceutical industry underwent a transformation. Due to changes in the research and regulatory environments, the industry went from being one dominated by small and medium-sized companies specializing in the bulk manufacture of fine chemicals or the wholesale manufacture of pharmaceuticals to one dominated by several large, fully integrated companies, with extensive research facilities, growing medical departments, and significant marketing capability. This transformation did not come about smoothly; it required the concerted efforts of industrial and academic researchers, corporate managers, and government officials. Moreover, the changes taking place in the pharmaceutical industry depended on the circulation of research knowledge between industry and academia, and of administrative knowledge between governmental and academic science administrators and corporate executives.

This chapter explores the circulation of pharmaceutical knowledge—research and administrative—throughout a network composed of people and institutions from the drug industry, academia, and the government, and shows how critical these networks—and the knowledge moving throughout them—were to the success and growth of individual firms and the industry at large in the decade after World War II. These very same networks would later form the basis of the American drug industry's resistance to the pharmaceutical reform movement of the 1960s and 1970s.

THE AMERICAN DRUG INDUSTRY
IN THE POSTWAR DECADE

At the end of World War II, the American pharmaceutical industry consisted of two types of core companies. First, there were the manufacturers of fine chemicals, Merck and Pfizer the largest and most important among them. They bulk manufactured the chemical intermediates and the active pharmaceutical agents in drug production—the so-called fine chemicals—and sold them to the second type of core firm, the "old-line pharmaceutical companies." Included among this group were Abbott Laboratories, Parke-Davis & Co., Smith, Kline & French, Squibb, Upjohn, and Eli Lilly. These firms were integrated producers and wholesalers of pharmaceutical products, which purchased pharmaceutically active compounds from fine chemical manufacturers, packaged them as drugs, and sold them under their own trade names to physicians, pharmacists, and hospitals. Because of their emphasis on the marketing of drugs, the old-line pharmaceutical companies maintained small staffs of detail men who were responsible for selling the companies' drugs to pharmacists, physicians, and hospitals. In contrast, because they did not commercialize their own drug products, the fine chemical manufacturers tended to lack any significant marketing organization.[2]

In the immediate postwar years, however, more and more of the old-line pharmaceutical firms began integrating backward into the production of their own fine chemicals, undermining the sales base of fine chemical manufacturers like Pfizer and Merck. At the same time, Pfizer and Merck were producing an increasing number of innovative pharmaceutical compounds but these were not as profitable as they could have been because the firms lacked the capability to effectively market those drugs themselves. Instead, when they developed new drugs, Pfizer and Merck still sold the active ingredients to other pharmaceutical companies, which packaged and marketed them under their own trade names.[3] As a result, in the early 1950s both companies began to integrate forward into making their own finished products. Pfizer did so by building up its own marketing organization, whereas Merck merged with Sharp & Dohme, a pharmaceutical firm with a well-established sales and distribution system.[4]

Research was, clearly, the foundation of innovation. During the interwar years, the leading American pharmaceutical companies had already made research part of their competitive strategy, establishing their own in-house research laboratories and forging collaborative relationships with academic biomedical, chemical, and clinical researchers.[5] Through these collaborative efforts, several research-based drug firms had developed synthetic hormones and vitamins as new therapeutic agents; in 1935, a pharmacologist at the German company I.G. Farbenindustrie discovered a new anti-infective agent, sulfanilamide, while screening dyestuffs for antimicrobial activity.[6] Following this discovery, industrial and academic researchers began routinely screening chemical and natural compounds for antimicrobial activity, which led to the isolation of hundreds of different sulfa drugs and antibiotic agents, including penicillin in 1940. The development of the sulfa drugs and penicillin launched what medical historians have termed a "therapeutic revolution."[7] For the first time, physicians now had access to an array of drugs that could actually cure their patients of infectious diseases rather than simply relieving their symptoms, as older drugs had done.

By the early 1940s, in order to extend their research capacities, most of the core pharmaceutical firms in the United States had developed elaborate research networks with the biomedical community through the provision of grants-in-aid and fellowships to academic researchers, and the hiring of consultants from academic institutions who would advise firms on matters such as corporate research policy, the recruitment of researchers, and specific research projects.[8] During World War II, these relationships intensified. When the Committee on Medical Research of the Office of Scientific Research and Development contracted with drug companies to develop penicillin, synthetic antimalarial drugs, steroids, and replacement blood products, the companies used their existing connections with academic researchers to meet the wartime demands.[9] These wartime successes confirmed the value of corporate research to drug company executives and by the end of World War II, the leading pharmaceutical companies were expanding their research facilities and staff, increasing the amount spent each year on research, and looking for ways to capitalize on the fundamental biomedical research being carried out in academic laboratories.

The new focus on innovation had a profound effect on the organization and corporate strategy of drug firms after the war. The isolation by drug firms of hundreds of new antibiotic agents (only some of which were clinically useful) led to numerous drugs with very similar therapeutic effects being introduced to the market. Because each of these antibiotics did essentially the same thing, the firms marketing these different drugs could not compete on the basis of therapeutic effects. Instead, to distinguish their products from one another, firms competed for market share through intensive marketing efforts. As a result, those firms that lacked marketing organizations found it incredibly hard to compete with fully integrated firms. This factor led the fine chemical manufacturers, such as Merck and Pfizer, to integrate forward into pharmaceutical marketing in the early 1950s.[10]

At the end of World War II, American drug companies were also dealing with a relatively new regulatory environment. In 1938, Congress had passed the Federal Food, Drug, and Cosmetic Act following the death of 107 people who had taken the sulfa drug Elixir Sulfanilamide. The Massengill Company, which began marketing the new drug in September 1937, failed to test the toxicity of the solvent—diethylene glycol—in which the drug's active ingredient was dissolved. The solvent turned out to be highly toxic. Despite the 107 deaths, the FDA did not have the authority, based on the Pure Food and Drug Act of 1906, to prosecute Massengill for putting a harmful drug on the market. Instead, all the FDA could sue the company for was mislabeling their drug as an elixir—a term used to describe an alcohol solution, which the diethylene glycol solution was not. The failure of the 1906 Act to adequately protect the public's health led Congress to pass the Federal Food, Drug, and Cosmetic Act, which for the first time included a safety provision for drugs. The act mandated that drug manufacturers submit a new drug application, containing documented evidence of their drug's safety, to the FDA. If the agency raised no objection to the application, the drug was considered approved for marketing.[11]

The new regulations had organizational consequences for drug firms. Every new drug—including all its constituent chemicals—produced by the industry's research laboratories now had to be rigorously tested for toxicity. As a result, the medical departments of drug firms became increasingly important; the physicians who staffed and consulted with them were responsible for conducting and analyzing these safety tests. Thus, by the end of World War II, as the innovativeness of research-based drug companies grew, the medical departments of these companies—and their relationships to academic clinical investigators—became all the more critical.[12]

The ability of drug firms to adapt to the changing research, business, and regulatory environments of the 1940s depended in no small part on their ability to call on the advice and experience of researchers and administrators in academia and government. Academic researchers were in the best position to identify and recognize the importance of new research knowledge, while science administrators—especially those with government experience—were skilled at integrating research knowledge with organizational strategy. Merck & Co. was particularly adept at forging relationships with academic researchers and government officials and using those relationships to help create organizational change at the company.

ADMINISTRATIVE KNOWLEDGE NETWORKS AT MERCK & CO.: MANAGING POSTWAR ORGANIZATIONAL CHANGE

By the end of World War II, Merck & Co. was the largest producer of vitamins in the United States, and the second largest worldwide behind the Swiss firm Hoffman–La Roche. Indeed, since the early 1930s, Merck had been at the forefront of research in the identification and synthesis of vitamins, culminating in the company's commercialization of vitamins B_1, B_2, B_6, C, and K by the early 1940s, and vitamin B_{12} in 1949.[13] Merck was also one of the most innovative firms in the antibiotics and steroid fields, introducing streptomycin to the market in 1946, and cortisone in 1948. In the decade after the war, Merck & Co. underwent significant organizational change as it expanded its research programs and developed new marketing capabilities. The company's ability to adapt to the changing business and regulatory environment, and to take advantage of the advances in pharmaceutical-related fields of research, was in large measure due to the knowledge networks it had developed with academic researchers and government officials in the previous decade.

Merck's innovations were the result of the company's growing commitment to research during the 1930s and early 1940s. In 1933, Merck's president, George W. Merck, had established the company's research organization, recruiting to it academic researchers from some of the country's leading chemistry and pharmacology departments.[14] To head the research laboratory, Merck hired the Princeton chemist Randolph T. Major. Major then recruited Karl Folkers from Yale University and Max Tishler from Harvard. Both men—who became research directors at Merck in the early 1940s—brought to Merck links to some of the best chemists in the nation. Folkers, for example, brought the networks he'd developed during his graduate studies in the chemistry department at the University of Wisconsin and his postdoctoral work at Yale University, while Tishler brought his own networks from Harvard.[15]

In addition to building its research networks, Merck & Co. had, since the war, developed an administrative network composed of science administrators. These men (and they were all men) had served in government or military agencies and held appointments at elite universities, in addition to serving either as consultants to drug firms or as company executives.

Because of their diplomatic and bureaucratic skills and through their work with government agencies, science administrators mediated among academia, industry, and government agencies.[16] As they moved among these different institutions, science administrators brought with them research and regulatory knowledge and administrative practices and skills.

The archetypal science administrator was Vannevar Bush.[17] Bush, who served on Merck's board of directors from 1949 to 1962, received his Ph.D. in engineering from the Massachusetts Institute of Technology and Harvard University in 1916. He continued his academic career at MIT, serving as dean of engineering and vice-president of the university from 1932 to 1938. In 1939, Bush assumed the presidency of the Carnegie Institution of Washington, a position he held until 1955. During World War II, he chaired the National Defense Research Committee from 1940 to 1941 and went on to direct, from 1941 to 1947, the Office of Scientific Research and Development (OSRD), which coordinated and sponsored all military research during the war. After the war, the OSRD was dismantled and many of its responsibilities transferred to the newly created Research and Development Board of the Department of Defense, which Bush chaired for one year. In addition to his continuing government service, which included developing the nation's postwar science policy, creating the National Science Foundation, and presiding over the Carnegie Institution, Bush began a career in business, joining the board of American Telephone & Telegraph Co. in 1947, and of Merck & Co. in 1949. From 1957 to 1962, Bush served as chairman of Merck's board of directors.[18]

Indeed, what distinguished Merck & Co. from the other leading pharmaceutical companies at the end of World War II—and which facilitated the creation of its administrative network—was the company's relationship to Vannevar Bush and the OSRD. In part, this sustained relationship grew out of the friendship that developed during the war among Bush, Merck's president, George W. Merck (who served as head of biological warfare in the War Department), and the Merck consultant Dr. Alfred Newton Richards.[19] Like Bush, Richards—a pharmacologist and physiologist—crafted a successful career as a science administrator, moving back and forth among academia, government service, and industry. From 1939 to 1948, Richards was vice-president in charge of medical affairs at the University of Pennsylvania, and from 1947 to 1950 he served as president of the National Academy of Sciences. During the war, Bush appointed Richards to chair the OSRD's Committee on Medical Research (CMR), placing Richards in charge of all military biomedical research. In that position, Richards directed the CMR's projects including the development and mass production of penicillin, steroids, synthetic antimalarial drugs, and synthetic blood substitutes.[20] Richards also served in various capacities within the Merck organization from 1931 through the early 1960s, including serving on the company's board of directors between 1948 and 1960.

A. N. Richards's adept management of the CMR and Merck & Co.'s involvement in the CMR's penicillin, steroid, and antimalarial projects left many researchers involved with the CMR and its projects with a very favorable opinion of the company. So much so that after the war, several individuals who had served in the OSRD found their way to Merck—as executives, directors, and consultants. John T. Connor, for example, who served as the OSRD's general counsel, joined Merck soon after the war. In his position at the OSRD, Connor had responsibility for working out contractual arrangements between the OSRD and its corporate and academic contractors, which included MIT, Harvard, the University of Chicago, Caltech, Westinghouse, and Standard Oil of New Jersey. In negotiating and executing these contracts, Connor became well acquainted with the scientists and business managers working at these institutions.[21] During his tenure, Connor consulted regularly with Richards and worked on several occasions with George W. Merck. Through these interactions and his experience more generally in the OSRD, "it became clear to [Connor] . . . that Merck had the outstanding research organization working on the [penicillin] problem . . . and [he] came to have a great appreciation for the entire company."[22]

George W. Merck recruited Connor in 1947 as the company's general counsel and secretary. As general counsel, Connor was responsible for managing all of Merck's legal issues, which included setting up research contracts and protecting the company's intellectual property, skills he'd acquired during his tenure at the OSRD. As the company's secretary, Connor managed Merck's relationships with state governments and the federal government; a role that also benefited from Connor's experience—and the personal connections he'd made—serving in the wartime federal bureaucracy.[23] Thus, Connor brought to Merck administrative knowledge, experience, and networks from his time serving in the OSRD. Connor was promoted to administrative vice-president in 1951, and served as the company's president and chief executive officer from 1955 to 1965. Returning to government service, Connor served as President Lyndon B. Johnson's secretary of commerce from 1965 to 1967.

Merck & Co.'s involvement in CMR projects, and the close friendship among Richards, Bush, and Merck, led to the establishment, after the war, of an administrative network in which former members of the OSRD moved between Merck, the government, and academia, bringing with them administrative experience and knowledge that, when incorporated into Merck's corporate policy of the early 1950s, proved critical to solving some of the company's most pressing organizational and research concerns.

One such concern for Merck & Co.'s leadership after the war was the state of its research organization. In particular, Merck's leadership feared the stagnation of the company's research pipeline. For help addressing this concern, Merck & Co. turned to Vannevar Bush and A. N. Richards. In 1949, due in part to his long-standing friendship with Merck and Richards, Bush joined the board of directors of Merck & Co.[24] As Richards wrote to Bush in May 1949, Merck & Co.'s board members "are in vital need as I see it of just such counsel as would flow spontaneously from your experience and wisdom."[25] News of Bush's appointment apparently had "an electrifying effect" both within the company and in the broader industrial and research community. As George W. Merck wrote to Bush in November that year, "I have had . . . several messages of congratulations from the outside, each time coupled with the query: How did you do it?" Although Merck believed the answer was "perhaps we deserve it," it is clear that the shared experiences of Bush, Richards, and Merck during the war were in large measure responsible.[26]

Immediately upon becoming a director, Bush, together with Richards, reviewed the company's research and development organization, identifying several major problems with the company's structure and operations. While Bush praised the company for being "refreshingly forward-looking and vigorous" in its research and development, he described "the internal organization of the company" as "atrocious." In particular, Bush found "the lines of authority blurred" and lacking in "clear individual responsibility for each primary phase of the company's functions."[27]

The solution, Bush believed, was for the company to reorganize along more hierarchical—and unmistakably military—lines. In particular, Bush felt the company needed a new chief executive. He outlined to Merck what constituted the "ideal chief executive," and how the company's internal organization should function under that executive.[28] The main elements of Bush's advice were for the chief executive to "delegate effectively and clearly" and to "support decisions of subordinates." As he explained, "When one places in the hands of a subordinate the authority to make a decision . . . that subordinate's judgment must be taken and used even if one thinks it is wrong and that a mistake has been made, and the decision should be reversed only when it is genuinely essential to do so in order to avert catastrophe." The "chief" should also "keep decisions down near the scene of action." In other words, "no decision should ever go above the level at which there is a competent man to settle it. Units should handle their internal affairs, and be responsible only for general results and progress. The chief should not sit in where a subordinate unit is doing business. . . . [C]ompetent men do not like to be watched in detail by their chief as they proceed, for it tends to undermine their own control of their own groups." Finally, Bush maintained, the "chief's office should be simple. It should contain no function that can be placed elsewhere."[29]

In his recommendations, Bush thus sought to institute a clear and authoritative chain of command within the Merck organization—an organizational form with which he had much experience from his tenure as director of the OSRD. Bush's advice was taken seriously; two years later, his suggestions were incorporated into a statement of "Merck Management Fundamentals" that served as a foreword to the company's new organization manual.[30]

Over the next two years, Bush continued to survey and make recommendations to Merck for improving the company's internal organization and, in concert with Richards, for advancing the company's research and development activities. Indeed, in March 1952, Richards noted to Bush that the two of them "have special responsibilities among the Directors to get inside the minds of those in the scientific areas of whom the future success [of the company] depends." Bush agreed with Richards, asserting that if the two of them could identify key trends in the medical field and identify new research areas the company's researchers should look to exploit, "I believe that its influence on Merck thinking could be far-reaching, in fact I think it could snap them out of a groove in which I fear they now are." As Bush continued, "If one knows where the breaks are likely to occur he makes effective contact with those who are at the forefront of the advance, aids them in any way possible, and watches for places where that aid can become independently applied."[31]

Yet as Bush saw it, their foresight alone would not be sufficient to improve the company's research potential. Bush felt that the company needed to improve its use of outside researchers: "We have a good many contacts with outstanding research people in the field I realize, but I am not sure that we have got the critical ones. A more important point, however, is that I am not at all sure that we are in position to make the contacts effective from the standpoint of our own use of them. . . . I do think that unless we have internally some people who have sufficient leisure and interest to think in a highly constructive manner our contacts will be decidedly sterile." What the company needed, Bush surmised, "are some free flowing views ahead, written by men who have vision and also grasp."[32]

Bush also believed that the company's organizational problems revolved around the fact that the company did not engage in long-range planning. As Bush saw it, "the nub of the difficulty appears to lie in the fact that the company has grown up." In previous years, the company's prosperity had depended "upon the occasional adding to its line of products of strikingly new and important items," made possible because of Merck's "early appreciation of changes in medical practice of great moment, a grasp of the significance of valuable products before their full advent and hence an early and advantageous commercial situation." While "it was possible to accomplish this sort of thing by hunch, by playing the matter by ear" when the company was small, this way of operating "no longer applies when the company's business has grown into extraordinary complexity, when there are alert competitors in the field attempting to do the very thing which made Merck grow, and when medical practice is becoming far more scientific and involved."[33]

The solution, Bush proposed, was twofold. First, the company's research and development area had to be reorganized so as to free "some of the individuals at the top" to "have adequate time to think, to consult with specialists in the field, to follow scientific trends, and generally to see where we are going in terms of where we are."[34] Second, Merck needed a central planning group whose function would be to present "complete analyses of the status and probable future possibilities of important products and product lines which might be added to the existing line." Currently, Bush argued, "when a new product looms over the horizon we don't have before us a document that summarizes the nature and extent of the market, the prices that are tolerable, estimated costs of production, the new capital requirements for production facilities . . . and the future outlook for improvements in processes and the like."[35] To rectify this situation, the central planning group would "integrate the thinking," and "tie together the ideas of Research, Development, Production, Sales, Patents, Engineering . . . with adequate contacts with the medical profession and the consumer to an extent sufficient to give a sound foundation to its prognoses."[36] Once more, Bush's advice did not go unheeded. When Bush's former OSRD colleague, John T. Connor, was appointed as Merck's chief executive officer in 1955, one of the first things Connor did was to introduce long-term planning as part of Merck's corporate strategy.[37]

In his first three years as a Merck director, then, Bush played an instrumental role in reorganizing both the company's research and development organization and the company's corporate structure more broadly. In each case, Bush brought to Merck administrative knowledge and practices that he had acquired and developed during his years as a science administrator, first at MIT, then at the Carnegie Institution, and at the OSRD. The most significant of those practices were the hierarchical chain of command and strategic planning.

INNOVATIVE RESEARCH NETWORKS AT MERCK & CO.

To support the company's internal research organization, Merck created and maintained extensive research networks by engaging in collaborative research projects with academic researchers and by recruiting them as company consultants. After World War II, cooperative research with academic researchers grew all the more important at Merck. As the company identified potential new drugs at an increasingly rapid rate, it lacked the in-house biomedical labor to perform all the necessary research itself. Therefore, Merck & Co. supported medical research of two types: specific studies to evaluate or establish a new product and general studies in fields of commercial interest to the company.[38]

Merck benefited from these collaborative relationships by gaining access to and having the potential to commercialize a broader range of research than that being conducted in its own in-house laboratories. For their academic partners, drug company funding was one of the ways academic researchers could support their laboratories and laboratory workers (as I will detail in chapter 2). Furthermore, collaborating with Merck (or any other drug company) represented the only viable way for academic researchers to see their research translated into new therapeutic products and incorporated into medical practice. The expense of drug development and the prevailing attitudes among university administrators and government funding agencies that academic institutions were the site of so-called fundamental research and industrial laboratories the appropriate site for technological development made it infeasible and inappropriate for academic institutions to scale up production and mass-produce new drugs discovered in their laboratories.[39]

The practice of drug firms like Merck providing research grants and research fellowships to academic researchers—on both ad hoc and long-term bases—thus provided academic researchers with an opportunity to translate their knowledge into tangible therapeutic products, while serving

to expand a firm's own research capacities. These relationships also provided academic researchers with access to limited material resources (not
least, new drug products) and research facilities in addition to otherwise
restricted industrial knowledge, all of which helped to advance their own
research interests.

The development and maintenance of Merck's research networks also
depended on the company recruiting academic consultants to its ranks.
These consultants were generally leaders in a specific field who, for an
annual salary or some other form of compensation, kept Merck well
informed about developments in academic institutions and maintained
the company's connections with outside researchers. A key function of
academic consultants—as they moved between Merck's research laboratories and their academic homes—was to facilitate the exchange of biomedical knowledge between academic and industrial laboratories. In addition,
Merck called on its consultants to make recommendations on research
strategies and the recruitment of new scientific staff.[40]

In 1950, for example, the Merck Institute for Therapeutic Research,
a semiautonomous research institute of Merck & Co., retained eight specialist consultants in the fields of nutrition, pharmacology, biochemistry,
veterinary medicine, and pathology. The salaries for these consultants
ranged from a one-hundred-dollar per diem for Dr. H. S. Martland, who
consulted with the institute two or three times a year whenever the institute needed "expert opinion in important and conceivably controversial
matters [such] as histological diagnosis," to Dr. William H. Sebrell, a specialist in nutritional research, who received five thousand dollars a year.
Sebrell's salary reflected the fact that he visited the institute at regular
monthly intervals and the institute's staff frequently consulted with him
by telephone, letter, or personal visits to his laboratory in Washington.
And in addition to advising the company on matters related specifically
to nutritional research, Sebrell also offered guidance in problems outside
of his area of expertise, such as "matters of basic research and personnel
policies."[41]

Some of the institute's consultants functioned more like part-time
employees. For example, Dr. E. P. Pick from Mount Sinai Hospital in New
York City visited the institute's laboratories twice a week, spending an
average of five hours at the institute during each visit. During this time,
he worked in the institute's pharmacology laboratory "on problems suggested to him, but definitely of his own preference." Indeed, by early 1951
Pick had published eight scientific papers from the institute's laboratories
since he joined the institute's roster of consultants in 1939.[42] For Dr. E. G.

Miller from the Department of Biochemistry of the College of Physicians and Surgeons at Columbia University, his role during his first few years as consultant to the Merck Institute was to act "practically as chairman of [the institute's] Biochemistry Department." When Miller joined the institute in 1946, the institute had only a young group of biochemists, who lacked the "experience and scientific stature" to run the department without more senior support.[43]

For Merck & Co.'s corporate managers, academic consultants provided the company with invaluable help beyond their scientific expertise. As R. M. Hayward from Merck's Research and Development Division noted to the company's scientific director and vice-president, Randolph Major, in February 1951, "consultants are valuable for: a. Aiding in the procurement of new personnel; b. Maintaining a high morale of the staff; c. Obtaining a different viewpoint and for preventing the inbreeding of ideas; d. Learning the 'gossip' of the universities and of other industrial organizations."[44] For example, the Merck Institute's consultant Dr. Pick provided the company with more benefits than just his research. As the institute's director, Hans Molitor, explained to Major, Pick's most important contribution was his "influence on the staff, particularly its younger members. He is the prototype of a kindly, wise and thoroughly understanding man and because of his own gratitude to, and high regard for, the Merck Institute, its policies and its management, acts as a morale builder and mediator whenever he senses discontent." And Pick's influence extended beyond the institute's staff. As Molitor noted, "Dr. Pick still maintains close relations with topflight European scientists and thus can serve as a contact with them," on behalf of Merck & Co.[45]

The academic researchers who consulted for Merck & Co. after World War II served as critical nodes in the company's research networks. They provided Merck with connections to other academic researchers—in the United States and abroad—who might be available to collaborate with the company. They kept the company aware of "trends and needs of medicine, human and veterinary, in relation to Merck capacities . . . [and o]pportunities with respect to new products and new or expanded uses of old products." These consultants also provided Merck with their critical perspectives on the company's current research programs.[46] Furthermore, the high status of Merck's consultants and advisors within the academic medical community (Merck's roster of academic consultants and advisors included three Nobel laureates during the 1950s) conferred status and scientific credibility on the firm, making it easier for Merck to recruit other leading researchers.

Merck & Co.'s innovativeness after the war, then, was a product of a concerted effort in the previous decade by Merck's leadership to establish a thriving research organization and to forge extensive relationships with academic researchers—as consultants and collaborators. Reflecting its growing commitment to research, Merck & Co.'s research and development expenditures increased substantially during the 1930s and early 1940s. In 1929, Merck & Co. invested only $36,000 in research and development, by 1940, almost $1 million, and by the war's end, that figure had more than tripled to $3.4 million.[47]

Merck's success building and maintaining its research networks, and the importance of these networks to the company's postwar growth, is seen in the history of one of Merck's most important innovations—vitamin B_{12}. In 1926, the Harvard researchers George Minot and William Murphy had found that feeding liver extract to pernicious anemia patients cured the previously fatal disease in the majority of them.[48] Neither Minot nor Murphy nor any other researchers at the time, however, were able to identify the factor present in liver that was responsible for relieving patients of their symptoms. In the early 1940s, Merck & Co.'s assistant director of research, Karl Folkers, became interested in using chromatographical methods to isolate and identify the antianemia factor. To aid him in this research, Folkers received a sample of fractionated liver from one of Merck's academic consultants, Dr. Henry Dakin, a British chemist. After further concentrating the liver extract on a chromatographic column, Folkers sent the fractions to a hematologist at Columbia's College of Physicians and Surgeons who had agreed to test the fractions in his patients.[49]

To isolate and identify the active substance in the liver fractions, Folkers collaborated with the University of Maryland researcher Mary Shorb. Shorb had developed a bacteriological assay that enabled Folkers to measure the anti–pernicious anemia activity of each fraction. Merck provided Shorb with a fund of about four hundred dollars to test the fractions over the course of several weeks. Thanks to this cooperative research effort, by 1948 Folkers's research group had successfully isolated the so-called anti–pernicious anemia factor, naming it vitamin B_{12}.[50] Although Merck was never able to develop a commercially viable synthesis of vitamin B_{12}, based on Folkers's research the company did develop a process for isolating and mass-producing vitamin B_{12} from the fermentation broth of *Streptomyces griseus*. The company marketed this product as Cobaine.[51]

Subsequently, the company provided Dr. Bacon Chow of the Johns Hopkins School of Public Health with six thousand dollars over the course of the year to study vitamin B_{12} as a growth factor in normal and chronically ill children. The grant money was to pay for "the supervisory help needed to follow the normal children who are in a Catholic home, the need for providing a few special services to assure continued cooperation of the home, and . . . a number of laboratory studies on the etiology of vitamin B_{12} . . . to explain the mechanism of action of this material when given by mouth."[52] Today, of course, such use of experimental drugs on children would be regarded as unethical.

Over the subsequent five years, Hans Molitor, head of the Merck Institute, identified new vitamin research partners for Merck & Co while visiting academic and industry laboratories in Italy, Switzerland, Germany, England, and France.[53] In particular, Molitor pointed to Dr. J. Kuhnau from the Biochemisches Institut der Universität in Hamburg, Germany, who was doing *"by far the most important work* from our point of view,"[54] and Professor F. Verzar, a physiologist from the University of Bale in Switzerland. Verzar's laboratory was engaged in gerontological research, and Molitor suggested to Major that Merck might "buy into this growing establishment" by creating a fellowship in Verzar's laboratory for studying the influence of vitamin B_{12} on aging.[55]

During the 1940s and early 1950s, then, Merck & Co. forged an innovative research network among Folkers's research group and researchers and clinical investigators at various academic institutions in the United States and Europe. People, knowledge, practices, and materials circulated throughout this network: research money in the form of grants and fellowships; biochemical, physiological, and pharmacological knowledge about the vitamins; research materials such as liver extracts, fermentation broth, and the vitamins themselves; and research practices—chromatographic methods and assays the most important among them.

The importance of Merck's research networks, and the innovations they spawned, were reflected in the company's sales growth during the 1930s and 1940s. In 1933—the year the company's research laboratory was established—Merck's annual sales were $10.3 million. By 1939, the company's annual sales had doubled to $20 million. Just two years later, however, those sales had doubled again; by the end of World War II they had reached $55.6 million; and in 1950, following Merck's introduction of streptomycin, cortisone, and vitamin B_{12} to the market, the company's sales reached $139 million.[56]

Despite these achievements, at the end of the 1940s the company's managers were concerned that there were no new products on the horizon. At the same time, Merck & Co. was losing ground in the antibiotics and cortisone markets because of the patent situation of their drugs and the company's inadequate marketing organization.[57] In the case of strepto-mycin, Merck had relinquished its patent rights, assigning them instead to the Rutgers Research Foundation, thus allowing other firms to license that patent and commercialize streptomycin and market it under their own trade names.[58] With cortisone, Merck was not the only company to hold a patent on the synthesis process. Because a number of different people and institutions—including the Swiss drug company Ciba—also held patents on different steps in the synthesis process, a patent pool was established among the various patent holders. As a result, Merck was not the only firm to commercialize cortisone.[59]

Confronted by what some in Merck's management saw as a stagnating research and development program (between 1948 and 1951, the com-pany's annual R & D expenditures had languished around the $4 million mark, finally increasing in 1952 to $5.6 million), and a downturn in the company's competitive position, Merck's leadership turned to its adminis-trative knowledge network for support in resolving the company's declin-ing market position.[60]

ADMINISTRATIVE NETWORKS AT MERCK & CO.: MANAGING THE MEDICAL MERGER

In the early 1950s, Merck & Co. was still primarily a manufacturer of fine chemicals, selling its products to other firms that would then turn those chemicals into finished pharmaceutical products. In the instances when Merck sold finished drug products—as in the case of streptomycin, corti-sone, and vitamin B_{12}—the company struggled to secure a strong market position because it lacked an adequate marketing organization to distribute and sell those drugs. George W. Merck's solution was for the company to integrate forward into the manufacture and marketing of its own finished pharmaceutical products. To market its pharmaceuticals, however, Merck & Co. needed a sales organization and distribution system. Rather than starting from scratch, in May 1953 the company merged with Sharp & Dohme, a pharmaceutical firm with a well-established sales and distribu-tion system.[61]

Until the late 1920s, Sharp & Dohme had an extremely effective dis-tribution network but very little in the way of a research organization. After the company merged with H.K. Mulford & Co. in 1929, Sharp & Dohme acquired a biological laboratory, which it used to research and develop new vaccines and antitoxins. Between 1935 and 1952, Sharp & Dohme's executives worked on developing the company's research and development organization beyond biologicals, and pursued research on sulfonamides and new formulations of penicillin, and on the development of synthetic blood products.[62] Despite the expansion of Sharp & Dohme's research organization during the late 1930s and 1940s and the opening of its new research facilities in West Point, Pennsylvania, in 1952, the company lacked "an in-house level of scientific expertise" high enough to take full advantage of new developments in virology, medicinal chemistry, biochemistry, and pharmaceutical science more generally.[63]

For these reasons, the executives of both firms regarded the merger of Sharp & Dohme and Merck & Co. in May 1953 as mutually beneficial. While Merck acquired expanded marketing capacities, Sharp & Dohme merged with one of the most innovative research organizations in the industry.[64] Although both of the companies recognized the value of—and indeed, need for—the merger, the consolidation of the two companies took several years to complete and was characterized by tense relations between Sharp & Dohme, located in West Point, Pennsylvania, and Merck & Co., located in Rahway, New Jersey.

The integration of the medical divisions of Sharp & Dohme and Merck & Co., and thus consolidation of all medical activities, proved to be particularly challenging. To overcome the challenges, Merck & Co. drew on another of its administrative networks. This network was composed of science administrators—elite academic physicians experienced in medical administration—most notably, Dr. A. N. Richards and Merck's long-time consultants Dr. Dickinson W. Richards (no relation) of the College of Physicians and Surgeons of Columbia University, Chester S. Keefer, and William H. Sebrell.

D. W. Richards was a leader in the field of cardiac and pulmonary physiology. During the 1940s and early 1950s, he and André F. Cournand developed a technique for catheterizing the heart and performed a series of cardiac studies for which they received the Nobel Prize in Physiology or Medicine in 1956.[65] Alongside his academic career, D. W. Richards had administrative experience, serving as medical director of Bellevue Hospital, New York, from 1945 to 1961, chairman of the hospital's executive committee from 1951 to 1953, and deputy chairman of the CMR's physiology division during the war. D. W. Richards had also served during the 1930s and early 1940s as Merck's chief of medical affairs, and continued through the early 1970s as the company's "chief medical adviser."[66] According to A. N. Richards, the "high status of Merck with [the] medical profession is in every important part due to D.W.R.'s [Dickinson Richards's] stature."[67]

Like A. N. and D. W. Richards, Chester S. Keefer and William H. Sebrell had high stature within the medical community and brought to Merck a range of government experience and contacts. Keefer, a professor of medicine at Boston University School of Medicine, had chaired the National Research Council's Committee on Chemotherapeutics and Other Agents and had served as a medical administrative officer of the CMR during World War II. In the former role, Keefer had been in charge of distributing penicillin during the war, earning him the title of "penicillin czar." After the war, Keefer served as special assistant to the nation's first secretary of health, education, and welfare. William H. Sebrell had served as a consultant to Merck & Co. from the late 1940s until his appointment as assistant surgeon general in 1950 and later that year as director of the National Institutes of Health, a position he held until 1955.

The difficulties consolidating Merck & Co.'s and Sharp & Dohme's medical activities, as A. N. Richards noted, was that the "conditions of merger were such as to produce lowering of morale throughout sci[entific] areas of Merck Rahway." In particular, because of its marketing experience, the Sharp & Dohme medical division was given the responsibility of conducting all promotion and sales of Merck compounds, a task previously left to the Merck medical division. The result of this division of labor was to "exal[t] the name Sharp & Dohme in the minds of the medical profession and pharmaceutical trade with corresponding lessening of prestige of Merck." According to Richards, the problem was made worse because "the scientific strength and present scientific leadership of Merck Rahway is much greater and of a different order than those of Sharp & Dohme," which had led in some cases to Merck's researchers treating their West Point colleagues with condescension and little regard for their scientific abilities.[68]

To oversee and give advice on the consolidation process, Merck's scientific director, Randolph Major, established a Medical Coordinating Committee to which he appointed D. W. Richards as chair, along with A. N. Richards and the two medical directors of Sharp & Dohme and Merck & Co.—William Boger and Augustus Gibson, respectively.[69] For D. W. Richards, this meant regular meetings with Boger and Gibson, and frequent visits to both the West Point and Rahway laboratories.[70]

After just a few such meetings, D. W. Richards identified the biggest obstacle to successfully integrating the West Point and Rahway medical divisions as being the matter of who would oversee the company's medical activities: would it be Boger or Gibson, or some third, outside candidate? The problem, as D. W. Richards noted to A. N. Richards in November 1954, was that neither Gibson nor Boger "has gained [status] in the eyes of the Company leaders, but rather that both have lost ground. If we were to bring forward the medical activities of the two companies this is not a good thing."[71]

Furthermore, basic issues that had been impeding the integration of the two divisions since the merger remained unchanged. "The most basic of all," D. W. Richards contended,

> is the difference in attitude or philosophy of the two Companies. The thoughts of Merck & Co. have always been large thoughts; those of S & D are by comparison small, the thoughts essentially of a pharmaceutical sales outfit: "quick profits," "get in with a product fast, clean up and get out again," and "no product lasts longer than three years." . . . How endlessly these are repeated, regardless of what the rest of the argument is. . . . The result is that instead of S & D enlarging the scope of Merck & Co., Merck & Co. is steadily shrinking to the scope of S & D.

For example, D. W. Richards continued, "every time Merck–Medical brings a product to a certain stage, then transfers it to S&D, the thing drops dead, scientifically, clinically, promotionally." As a result, "The Merck–Medical staff's morale is down again about to zero." So much so that "Gus Gibson has come pretty near to serving notice to Major. . . . The other good men in the Division are devoted to Gus and would not stay if he went."[72]

In July 1955, after two years of evaluating and attempting to resolve the problem of medical integration, D. W. Richards outlined to A. N. Richards, Randolph Major, and Max Tishler—the company's research director—his plan for the "Organization of an 'Ideal' Medical Division for Merck & Co., Inc." According to D. W. Richards, the medical division should fulfill the following qualifications: First, "it must be a unified and harmonious group, working together as one team; each separate division well informed of the others' activities and in sympathy with them; the whole group having the same attitude and presenting to the outside medical profession a single point of view." According to Richards, "none of these things prevails at present." Second, Richards asserted, each division of the company needed its own medical department, as currently existed, with each separate medical department working closely with its own chemical and pharmacological research departments to bring forward new products. Third, the medical division should be, as it currently was, a well-integrated collaborative effort with outside clinical investigators. This, Richards believed, "was the key to all practical development of medicinal products." Fourth, the medical division should have an excellent relationship with the medical profession, including the practitioners, the clinical researchers, and organized medicine. And finally, Richards called for the medical department to work closely with the sales and promotion departments.[73]

To effect this change in the organization of the medical division, with each division—West Point, Merck–Chemical in Rahway, and the International Division in Rahway—having its own medical department, D. W. Richards demanded "a single head of all medical divisions." This overall director "would then be responsible to the presidents of all three divisions." In other words, the chief medical director would have a presence in the top level of the company's management. Associate medical directors, who would report to the chief medical director, would then be appointed to head the individual medical divisions of West Point, Rahway, and the International Division.

A final factor that D. W. Richards considered critical to improving Merck's medical division and, more important, the company's market position was to ensure that the medical division was involved in the promotion and sales of Merck's products to a greater extent than was currently the case. Over recent years, Merck had lost some of its market position, especially in the steroids field. For D. W. Richards, the problem was not "solely that MERCK & CO. hasn't had good enough new product; it is also that by skillful and vigorous promotional efforts, competitors like Upjohn and Pfizer have stepped in and taken away Merck's business." D. W. Richards was "convinced that a more likely medical participation in promotion would have helped the Merck cause."[74] The solution, D. W. Richards proposed, was for the chief medical director to "have a controlling and veto power on medical accuracy and ethical acceptability of all promotion to the medical profession."[75] The need for greater accuracy in medical promotion was a pressing concern for drug firms in the mid-1950s, as a small but growing number of prominent physicians had begun criticizing drug advertising as being excessive, misleading, and inaccurate.[76]

D. W. Richards's perspective on the relations between the promotion and sales and medical divisions, highlights the valuable contribution that he, as an outsider advisor, could make to the firm's policies. As an active academic researcher who was very well respected within the medical profession, Richards would have experienced firsthand—and in conversation with his medical colleagues—the detrimental impact that inaccurate and misleading advertising had on Merck's reputation among his medical colleagues. It is likely that, without Richards's perspective, the company's senior management would have had no good avenues for identifying the problems—or potential problems—brought about by the failure of the firm to integrate a medical perspective into its sales and promotional efforts.

In 1955, Randolph Major also recruited Chester Keefer and William Sebrell to help with the company's efforts to consolidate the medical divisions of Sharp & Dohme and Merck & Co. Indeed, A.N. Richards hoped that D.W. Richards, Keefer, and Sebrell would function, in effect, as the company's "Medical Council," providing research and managerial advice to the Sharp & Dohme, Merck, and International medical divisions.[77] During their tenures, Sebrell and Keefer, together with D.W. Richards, consulted twice a year with Randolph Major, the company's scientific director and vice-president, on "the construction and evaluation of programs, and policy matters." They were also available to Max Tishler and L.E. Arnow, the heads of research and development at Merck & Co. and Sharp & Dohme, respectively, "for consultation on any subject." In addition, they met twice yearly with Tishler and Arnow in order to assess the operations of the research and development divisions. They also advised the heads of the three medical divisions—Gibson, Boger, and A.T. Knoppers (of the International medical division)—on their medical programs and personnel, and helped build the status of the medical divisions within both the company and the medical profession. This involved the consultants meeting separately three times a year with the medical divisions at Rahway and at West Point, and once a year with all three medical divisions together. And in keeping with D.W. Richards's push to keep sales and promotion informed by medical opinion, the three corporate consultants were also to be available to review advertising and marketing material when requested.[78]

In late September 1955, D.W. Richard and A.N. Richards reformulated D.W. Richards's memo on his "ideal" medical division into a proposal to George W. Merck for reorganizing the company's medical division. In the end, Merck & Co.'s management incorporated some but not all of the Richardses' recommendations. By 1956, Augustus Gibson had been promoted to the position of executive director for medical research. Yet rather than see the creation of divisional heads of the West Point, Rahway, and International medical divisions, the medical activities of the company were centralized, together with all of the company's research and development, into a single research organization: the Merck Sharp & Dohme Research Laboratories (MSDRL). In 1957, Max Tishler replaced Randolph Major as president of MSDRL, and thus as Gibson's boss. Much to D.W. Richards's disappointment, Gibson was not given a position in corporate management. Instead, his only channel of communication to senior management was through Tishler. In 1959, D. W. Richards expressed his frustration to John Connor, Merck's president, noting "the remarkably high proportion of subjects" discussed by Merck's Management Council over the past few years "in which medicine (active, up-to-date medicine) was immediately relevant," and thus where the council could have benefited from the perspective of the medical director.[79]

That Merck relied so heavily on its medical consultants to develop and administer its medical department highlights two key themes. First, it reflects the critical new linkages forged between drug companies and academic medicine during and after World War II, and the mutually reinforcing nature of those linkages. Second, drug firms' reliance on medical consultants was a product of the regulatory changes that had taken place in the industry over the previous two decades. Prior to the passage of the 1938 Federal Food, Drug, and Cosmetic Act, drug companies had little regard for their medical departments, largely because the work they did— putting together promotional material and literature for the medical profession—was perceived by company managers and researchers to be of little value. Commensurate with this, corporate medical departments were staffed with just a few physicians, often physicians who were no longer practicing. With passage of the 1938 Act and the law's new drug safety provisions, however, rigorous clinical testing of drugs became an integral component of corporate drug development, a responsibility that fell to corporate medical departments. Yet even as firms like Merck came, after the war, to recognize the new and critical role of their medical departments, it did not follow that those departments and the physicians who staffed them were accorded respect. After all, it was not clear to Merck's management that its medical department possessed the requisite skills and stature to do this critical work. As a result, Merck looked to its medical consultants to fill that void and assume leadership of its medical department.[80]

CONCLUSION

Merck & Co.'s merger with Sharp & Dohme and hence its forward integration into pharmaceutical marketing and its building of reciprocal relationships with academic medicine proved to be boons for the company. Although Merck's annual sales stagnated around the $160 million mark in the first two years after the merger, by 1956 they had grown to $173 million, and just two years later they had climbed to $242 million. The company's increasing sales reflected its continuing commitment to research—Merck's research and development investment grew from $7 million in 1953 to $17 million in 1958—and the innovations this commitment spawned.[81] In 1958, nine years after the introduction of its previous "wonder drug," Merck launched Diuril (chlorothiazide), the first drug available for the treatment of hypertension and one that came to transform medical understanding and treatment of high blood pressure. With its fully operational marketing organization, Merck launched a massive and highly effective marketing campaign for Diuril, with sales of the drug reaching $20 million by the end of 1958.[82]

Merck & Co.'s innovativeness and growth in the postwar decade depended on the research and administrative networks it had developed with academic researchers and government officials in the prewar and postwar decades. Academic researchers who consulted and collaborated with Merck provided the company with access to new knowledge being produced in academic laboratories and helped Merck conduct the research necessary to discover, develop, and clinically test new drugs. The science administrators who worked with Merck were equally important, providing the company with critical administrative knowledge, practices, and expertise to help Merck develop its corporate strategy and undergo essential organizational change in the postwar decade.

These same patterns predominated at other core pharmaceutical firms after World War II. Abbott, Upjohn, Eli Lilly, and Parke-Davis & Co., for example, had developed extensive research networks with academic researchers in the interwar years, which they continued to nurture after the war.[83] Like Merck, these other core firms underwent strategic and structural changes in the postwar decade, vertically integrating backward into basic research and forward into marketing. The result was commensurate growth in the American drug industry over the course of the 1940s and 1950s. Between 1947 and 1959, worldwide sales by the American drug industry increased 203 percent from $890 million to $2.7 billion. At the same time, the industry's investments in research expanded from $30 million in 1948 to $170 million in 1958.[84] As a result of its postwar commitment to research and development, the 1940s and 1950s were decades of intense innovation by the American drug industry. Physicians, biomedical researchers, and historians alike consider the period beginning with the introduction of the sulfa drugs in 1935 through the production of penicillin during World War II, the discovery of cortisone in 1949, and the development in the 1950s and 1960s of the first effective antipsychotics and tranquilizers, oral contraceptives, and new vaccines against polio, measles, mumps, and rubella as a therapeutic revolution.[85] It was also the period in which the United States—the principal site of the research, development, and marketing—replaced the German pharmaceutical industry as the leading pharmaceutical innovator in the world.[86] Similar practices and patterns of growth defined the European pharmaceutical industry after World War II. As in the United States, the growth and innovativeness of the leading French and British pharmaceutical firms during the middle decades of the twentieth century depended on the ability of those firms to develop collaborative research networks with academic researchers.[87]

The relationships of drug companies to academic researchers grew all the more important during the 1950s, 1960s, and 1970s. During these decades, drug firms, together with academic researchers and physicians, confronted a series of challenges—in biomedical labor, political pressure, and regulatory change—that threatened to undermine pharmaceutical development and practice. As the following chapters detail, drawing on its research networks with academic researchers and physicians, the American pharmaceutical industry built essential political support for itself in the three decades following World War II by offering to the medical and academic communities solutions to their shared problems. The first of these problems was a perceived crisis in the biomedical workforce in the two decades after World War II.

2 Workforce Relations

The Invention of the Pharmaceutical
Postdoctoral Fellowship

American drug companies and their academic colleagues emerged from World War II with a sense of therapeutic accomplishment. Their prewar and wartime collaborations had produced an armory of new therapeutic innovations that included the sulfa drugs (copied from German firms), synthetic antimalarial drugs, and broad-spectrum antibiotics. For the first time, physicians had the means to eradicate some, if not all, infectious diseases. Yet, in spite of the therapeutic optimism of the period, in the decade after World War II drug companies, research universities, and medical schools were troubled by a perceived crisis in the biomedical workforce.[1] At the same time, drug companies and medical schools were anxious about the federal government's increasing role in medical education as the government became the primary patron of academic biomedical research after the war.[2]

The drug industry sought to tackle the impending shortage of biomedical labor and the threat of increasing government involvement in biomedical research and education after the war by shifting its support toward training the next generation of pharmaceutical workers. Before the war, drug companies had awarded fellowships in pharmaceutical-related fields only on an ad hoc, case-by-case basis to specific university departments with which the firms had standing relationships. After the war, however, firms such as Merck & Co. established annual, competitive, and nationally organized postdoctoral fellowship programs. These fellowships benefited universities by helping them to underwrite the cost of undergraduate and graduate education and by encouraging undergraduate, graduate, and medical students to enter the field of pharmaceutical research. The benefits were no less significant for the industry. First, the fellowships introduced young researchers to the financial and intellectual benefits of working with—and for—industry. And second, these fellowships promoted the exchange of knowledge between academic and industrial research laboratories, as drug company sponsors retained access to the fruits of their fellows' research. By the early 1950s, many firms had established similarly competitive international fellowships sponsoring young foreign scientists to study for up to three years at U.S. universities. And by the close of the decade, the industry's trade association was bankrolling the country's first clinical pharmacology programs at Johns Hopkins University and the University of Pennsylvania in an effort to boost recruitment into the nascent research discipline that was central to the development of new drugs: clinical pharmacology.

MEDICAL SCHOOLS IN NEED OF SUPPORT

World War II had a profound effect on American medical schools. During the war, medical schools had expanded their enrollments in order to meet military and civilian demands for more physicians. At the same time, large numbers of medical faculty had enlisted in the armed services, leaving medical schools with a shortage of faculty with which to teach those medical students. A Survey of Medical Education, conducted by the American Medical Association (AMA) and the Association of American Medical Colleges (AAMC) during the late 1940s, found that the war had "placed tremendous strains on the structure of medical education."[3] Due to these wartime demands, medical school administrators were concerned that the United States had "emerged from the war with a record of accomplishment in the medical sciences, but with a deficit in trained men to carry forward the research upon which new advances depend."[4] As the University of Pennsylvania's president, Thomas Gates, noted to an executive of Sharp & Dohme in March 1944, "The University has many members of its faculty in government service on full or partial leaves." At the same time, Gates explained, "it has turned over its campus and its activities generally toward the training of specialized men in various services. It is using its faculties in training for industry a great number of skilled workers in many production plants." As a result, Gates was "especially concerned with the maintenance of that work in many fields" where "such financial support is lacking." Gates had written to the Sharp & Dohme executive hoping that the pharmaceutical industry would step in to fill such gaps in biomedical research.[5]

After the war, medical schools were faced with increasing costs and medical school administrators worried whether the schools had the financial resources to meet those costs. As the Survey on Medical Education reported, medical school expenditures tripled between 1940 and 1950. In 1940, the total expenditures (exclusive of hospitals and clinics) of fifty-nine of the country's seventy-two medical schools (twenty-two tax-supported or public medical schools, thirty-seven private medical schools) were $27.3 million; by 1950, total expenditures were $85.7 million.[6] The rising costs of medical schools led the federal security administrator Oscar Ewing in 1948 to warn that inadequate financial support of medical schools threatened their ability to produce enough physicians and health personnel to meet the health needs of the nation.[7]

Industry executives were similarly concerned about the financial vitality of the nation's medical schools. As Edward H. Green, a director of Merck & Co., explained to the company's president, George W. Merck, medical schools' and universities' "costs have risen greatly, their income on endowments has gone down, they have already raised tuition fees all that they dare and they have had to call upon alumni and the usual channels of support to make up the deficit from ordinary operations." Without securing new sources of funding, Green warned, medical schools "run the risk of stagnation and perhaps even of losing their men whom they are anxious to hold."[8]

Despite the financial fears expressed by industry executives and school administrators, the income of medical schools, like their expenditures, actually tripled between 1940 and 1950. As the Survey on Medical Education reported, while the percentage of income medical schools received from tuition and endowments had declined since 1940, the percentage of income medical schools received from federal, state, and local taxes had increased over the course of the decade. For public schools, 49.2 percent of their total income derived from tax income in 1940, compared to 70.3 percent in 1950; for private schools, the figures were 2.6 percent in 1940 and 30.5 percent in 1950. The survey also found that income from private sources in the form of gifts and grants had remained fairly stable for both public and private medical schools (public schools: 11.4 percent of total income in 1940 and 12.6 percent in 1950; private schools: 21.1 percent in 1940 and 22.5 percent in 1950).[9]

The economic problem confronting medical schools at the end of the 1940s, then, was not an absolute shortage of income but rather a shift in the way that income was being used from a primary emphasis before the war on instruction to one after the war on research. In 1940, for example, twenty-two public medical schools had spent just 8.9 percent of their budget on research, while thirty-seven private schools spent 13 percent of their budget on research. By 1950, both figures had increased, with public schools spending 24.6 percent of their budget on research and private medical schools spending 37.8 percent. There was a concomitant decline in the percentage of income that schools spent on instruction. Private medical schools, for example, spent almost 60 percent of their budget on instruction in 1940; by 1950, that figure had fallen to 40 percent.[10]

At the same time that medical schools' focus shifted toward research after the war, the source of the income dedicated to research changed as well. In 1941, total medical research expenditures in the United States were $45 million, of which $3 million came from the federal government, $25 million from industry, and $17 million from national and local foundations, health-related associations, and other organizations. In contrast, of the $88 million spent on medical research in 1950, $28 million came from the federal government, $35 million from industry, and $25 million from national and local foundations, health-related associations, and other organizations.[11]

In spite of the federal government's increased support for medical research after the war, medical schools struggled to meet the cost of all other expenses, for which funding remained limited to income derived from student tuition and taxes. Moreover, the research expenses incurred by medical schools also had the effect of raising the school's non-research-specific costs. Sponsored research funding, regardless of source, was restricted to covering only the *direct* costs of research. As a result, medical schools were left to cover the *indirect* costs of research (such as work hours of salaried faculty, and administrative, utility, and facility maintenance costs) out of their general operating funds and funds intended primarily for educational purposes. And when research expenses were high, medical schools found their indirect costs substantial.[12] Yet, while medical schools' research expenditures increased almost 800 percent after the war (from $3.1 million in 1940 to $27.9 million in 1950), they did not see a concomitant increase in their general operating budgets, which rose less than 140 percent, from $24.2 million in 1940 to $57.8 million in 1950. The result, the Survey on Medical Education found, was that the education and service activities of medical schools were less well financed in 1950 than they had been in 1940. This led the administrators of the survey to question whether medical schools with large research budgets could "afford, without weakening their other activities, the amount of research they [were] handling."[13]

Medical school administrators feared the lack of non-research-related funds was having a detrimental effect on America's supply of biomedical labor. As Edwin J. Cohn, the chairman of Harvard's Division of Medical Sciences, outlined in a report to Harvard's president, James Conant, in 1947: "Our changing economic situation is confronting our medical schools with the need to curtail rather than expand their research programs. Curtailment in the training of investigators in the medical sciences at this time cannot but jeopardize the normal, let alone the accelerated, expectation of advances in medicine and the public health. On the other hand, adequate provision for the training of the medical scientist in the very laboratories that are carrying on productive research in the medical sciences is our greatest insurance for advances."[14] Harvard's medical school had dealt with the funding problem by offering the same courses to graduate students in physics, chemistry, and biology, and to medical students. However, as Cohn continued in his report, "no funds have been available . . . for the development of courses and research facilities specially planned to give the most effective training for research." The implication was that Harvard, along with other schools, was being forced to graduate students not fully trained in the specialized research skills of their chosen fields.[15]

Even while the federal government expanded its commitment to medical research through the research programs of the National Institutes of Health, the Office of Naval Research, the Atomic Energy Commission, and, in 1950, the National Science Foundation, there was little direct support available for medical education.[16] Only in the mid-1950s did the federal government, principally through the National Institutes of Health's extramural research programs, begin to emphasize the funding of research *training*. In 1950, for example, the federal government expended $4 million on graduate research training in medical schools; by 1960, that figure had increased tenfold to $41.5 million; five years later, it was $107 million.[17] As a result, in the decade following World War II, medical schools were forced to look elsewhere for support to train the next generation of biomedical researchers. Medical school administrators turned to the drug industry. After all, as Cohn noted, drug firms "depend[ed] for the fulfillment of their avowed aims" on the training of specialized researchers.[18]

Harvard's administrative vice-president (and member of Merck's board of directors), Edward Reynolds, for example, wrote to George W. Merck in May 1948 to suggest ways in which Merck & Co. could help advance biomedical education and research at Harvard. One way was to support specific research "that leads directly towards work [the Company's] own research and development organization can pick up." A second way was for Merck & Co. to support basic research "in a field that is likely to produce new knowledge of interest to Merck & Co." This support, Reynolds believed, should "be annual with some expectancy of renewal for a three to five year period."[19]

Next, Reynolds recommended that Merck & Co. award "an institutional grant to a selected institution, such as Harvard, for work in a broad field of interest to Merck & Co., whether it be research or education of students." Indeed, over the previous two years, Harvard's departments of public health and medicine had solicited Merck & Co. for just such support. Reynolds conceived of such grants as being undirected funds, with the receiving institution free to "decide how to parcel it out among the various participating projects." And in those cases where the company supported education rather than research, Reynolds continued, "it seems to me that it can be justified, even without any commitment that Merck can or will employ any students trained in such fields in the institutions Merck supports, by the probability that we can recruit our fair share of such men by looking over the graduating class as they near the end of their education, in the same way that many large law firms now visit the last-year men in the Harvard, Yale, Columbia, and other Law Schools each year." In this way, Reynolds essentially proposed a recruitment pipeline that would run between Harvard and Merck & Co.[20]

Reynolds's final suggestion was that Merck & Co. contribute to biomedical education "through the foundation mechanism." Merck was already familiar with the concept of supporting education through foundation support. During World War II, the American Foundation for Pharmaceutical Education (AFPE) was established "by various persons in the drug field in view of the need to keep open for young people the avenues of pharmaceutical education."[21] Merck had contributed annually to the AFPE, along with regular contributions to the Nutrition Foundation—similarly established to support nutritional research.[22]

To be sure, the financial concerns expressed by medical school administrators and the funding pleas they made to drug firms included a degree of hyperbole. Nevertheless, throughout the 1950s, the drug industry shared the medical school administrators' concerns about biomedical labor. At the same time, industry executives such as George W. Merck were skeptical of the government's expanded role in peacetime biomedical research and were keen to limit that expansion. As George W. Merck saw it, "we [the Company] have a very real interest in certain wide fundamental fields of research and we are not disposed to leave them to the mercies of a problematical governmental beneficence."[23] The company was particularly opposed to government involvement in the field of biomedicine for fear that such involvement would hasten the country's downhill journey to socialized medicine. As one Merck official noted to his colleagues in 1949, "a critical situation now exists in the financial status of medical schools throughout the country to the extent that a continuation of adequate medical education results in a substantial yearly operating deficit which must be financed in some way. . . . The question appears to be how much of the total medical education should be subsidized by the government. A total subsidy would seem to encourage the trend toward socialized medicine."[24]

Merck was not alone among industry and business leaders in fearing that the government would take over scientific education and training, as *Business Record* reported in 1947. Following a survey of postwar business practices with regard to corporate support of higher education, many executives expressed "fear that government aid may destroy the freedom of thought in privately supported colleges and universities."[25] Indeed, one of the survey's respondents asserted that corporate contributions to universities and colleges served as a "vital part of our free enterprise system," and felt that they "may turn out to be a bulwark against socialized education as a part of complete political and economical regimentation."[26]

To this end, several corporate leaders were seeking ways to help academic institutions meet the cost of providing higher education and limit the need for greater government support. For instance, in 1949 the Standard Oil executive Frank Howard proposed to the president of the National Academy of Science, Frank Jewett, that industry as a group should propose to Congress legislation such as "a special category be established in the income tax law allowing more liberal deductions which would enable corporations and individuals to assist toward relief of education projects."[27] The Ford Motor Company was proposing to turn over annually to a foundation, established by the company, the entire amount (5 percent of earnings) allowed by tax law for deductible corporate contributions and donations.[28] And, as Frank Howard reported to a Merck executive, "This whole situation has led to some private discussion of a plan to organize a nationwide 'Industrial Foundation' to which gifts could be made out of corporate funds by industrial companies, the Foundation to undertake distribution for the best support of privately controlled higher education." As Howard viewed it, the "Industrial Foundation" was an attempt "to apply the 'Community Chest' idea to corporate giving on a national scale and in the field of higher education."[29] That same year, the National Fund for Medical Education (NFME) was established through the cooperative efforts of university presidents, business and labor leaders, and the AAMC and the AMA, with the express goal of developing private-sector support for medical schools.[30]

TO FUND OR NOT TO FUND

Because of their concern over the role of the government in biomedicine, drug industry executives were receptive to the requests of medical schools.[31] Yet, as much as drug firms did "not want to see institutions like Harvard falling back on federal funds, as we see quite enough of the effect of state financing in many of the big Western schools," they had very specific ideas of what shape industry support of medicine should take.[32.] The industry's priorities were laid out in the discussions between executives from Eli Lilly & Co. and Merck & Co. after the dean of Harvard's medical school wrote to both firms in 1947 "seeking to find $27,000 a year for a number of years to permit the addition of personnel, the provision of research expenses, and other matters upon which an adequate expansion of the training of medical scientists depends." Dean Burwell wrote hoping "that three members of the pharmaceutical industry may be found which are willing to contribute $9,000 each per annum to this laudable enterprise." As Burwell explained, the industry should foot the bill because, "first, people with the kind of experience that you yourself have realize the importance of such trainig [sic] to the future of medicine and medical sciences, and, in the second place, the modern development of research laboratories in the pharmaceutical industry means that such organizations have become the large users of the very kind of trained men that this program is designed to provide."[33]

Lilly and Merck, however, were not persuaded by Burwell's proposal. Although, as Hans Molitor, the head of the Merck Institute of Therapeutic Research, noted to his colleagues, "it would be highly desirable to stimulate, if necessary by financial grants, the training of scientists in the pre-clinical sciences," Molitor asked, "Why should Harvard receive such support from industry and not other universities such as for instance, University of Chicago, Pennsylvania Medical School, Columbia University, University of Wisconsin, etc. to name only a few which do outstanding work in training young men in the pre-clinical sciences and which have already given splendid examples of their eagerness to cooperate with industry." Molitor continued that, although he held Harvard Medical School in high regard, he did "not see the justification . . . to single out Harvard for support when so many other first-class universities in various parts of the country, which are just as much in need of support as Harvard, if not more so, are not asking for such support or are not receiving it."[34]

G. H. A. Clowes, the head of the Lilly Research Laboratories, agreed: providing research support was one thing, but funding teaching at individual universities was quite another. For Clowes, "the real crux of the situation is that while corporations like yours and ours can support individual research undertakings in different universities and medical schools, they cannot very well support regular or routine teaching in any form in any one university or medical school without doing the same thing for other similar institutions."[35] There was, of course, a tangible return to be made on investing in the training of young scientists. As Clowes pointed out to Merck, the courses that Burwell was asking them to support were "being particularly arranged so as to provide us in the future with a supply of well trained biological chemists having a really intimate knowledge of the borderline field between chemistry and physics on the one hand and biology, physiology, medicine, and pathology on the other, something which we all sorely need." Indeed, as Dean Burwell had noted in his solicitation, the industry had a vested interest in supporting the development of young biomedical researchers.[36]

The difficulty for industry was in finding a way to support the development of future pharmaceutical workers without arbitrarily favoring individual institutions or creating a relationship of dependency between medical schools and the industry. As George W. Merck warned his colleagues, "a halt has to be called to general dependence on industry to foot the bills."[37] Although the industry had a stake in maintaining the standards of medical education, it was not responsible for funding either the core teaching or the "bricks and mortar" of medical schools and universities. For Merck & Co., if corporate funding would not "benefit the stockholders specifically other than as members of the general public," the company would not fund it.[38] In the end, both Lilly and Merck turned down Harvard Medical School's request for $27,000. As Merck's treasurer John Gage noted, "because of the indirectness of the benefits to corporations," the support of routine teaching as proposed by Dean Burwell "is very difficult to justify."[39]

Drug firms were instead interested in supporting medical schools in projects that were "tangibly connected with the Company's program."[40] This extended to limiting the government's involvement in biomedical research. In 1949, as Congress debated whether a National Science Foundation would be established, Randolph Major, Merck's scientific director, cautioned "that industry should expect and plan to support a greater amount of research in universities than it has in the past, if it does not want to have the support of these activities taken over by the Government to a much greater extent than it has in the past, and that, I think personally, is not desirable." Given the importance of so-called basic research to the discovery and development of new therapeutic compounds, Major continued, "I do not think that industry can be expected to support all the fundamental research which needs support in the universities, but there is much good research in universities which can be supported by industry to its advantage."[41]

But providing grants to support specific research projects would not solve the workforce shortage confronting medical schools and the industry in the early postwar years. Although firms were opposed to footing the bill for medical education, they did not deny that "a very urgent difficulty arises in connection with the supply of well-trained men in medical sciences." As Harvard's Dean Burwell had reminded the executives of Merck and Lilly, together medical schools and the industry faced "a severe shortage . . . in biochemists, bacteriologists, physiologists, anatomists, pharmacologists, and experimental pathologists."[42] In an effort to solve this growing problem and increase the number of young men and women entering biomedical research, drug firms such as Merck & Co. looked to increase a form of support different from that of research and institutional grants.

THE MERCK FELLOWSHIP

In July 1947, Merck & Co. launched the Merck Fellowship, a postdoctoral fellowship program, administered by the National Research Council, to provide advanced training to "young men and women who have demonstrated marked ability in research in the chemical and biological sciences." In particular, the fellowship program was established to promote interdisciplinarity in the biomedical sciences, where applicants could "supplement their mastery of one field by becoming competent in another," the hope being that the fellows would produce "new knowledge, not only regarding the identity and character of cellular processes, but also concerning the action of chemical substances, of whatever origin, upon them."[43] The initial term of the postdoctoral fellowship was one year, but this was extendable to up to three years, with an annual stipend between $2,500 and $5,000, depending on the circumstances of the individual fellow.

The fellowship program was the brainchild of the Merck & Co. president George W. Merck. His experience as the head of biological warfare in the War Department during World War II had exposed him to the new role of the government in biomedical research, and he was eager to shape the postwar political economy of biomedical research in favor of industry interests. By the end of the war, Merck had determined "that the support of advanced training of gifted young persons in fundamental science could properly be regarded as a responsibility of industry as well as of government and private non-commercial institutions."[44]

The Merck Fellowship was to fill, in particular, what George W. Merck and others in the company regarded as a critical gap in advanced scientific training: a lack of postdoctoral fellowships in "the fundamental aspects of the sciences on which our business is founded and in which our research work is focused." Merck referred, in particular, to chemistry, microbiology, pharmacology, and nutrition science.[45] By establishing a prestigious postdoctoral fellowship, Merck & Co. sought to promote interest among young scientists in the fields of research of greatest importance to both the company and the public's health. At the same time, by making the fellowship highly selective and therefore competitive, the company was able to identify those scientists with the greatest potential for research, work to further improve the quality of that research, and attract those young researchers to the Merck corporation.

In these views, George W. Merck was no doubt influenced by his close friend and wartime colleague Vannevar Bush. As director of the Office of Scientific Research and Development, Bush was centrally concerned with ensuring that the United States had sufficient "scientific talent" to carry out the wartime research effort. In the final months of the war, however, Bush published his famous presidential report, *Science, the Endless Frontier*, in which he warned that "with mounting demands for scientists both for training and for research, [the United States] will enter the postwar period with a serious deficit in our trained scientific personnel."[46] To encourage "young men and women . . . to take up science as a career," and reduce the deficit, Bush recommended the establishment of "a reasonable number of (a) undergraduate scholarships and graduate fellowships and (b) fellowships for advanced training and fundamental research."[47] Bush's proposal led eventually, after five years of heated debate among civilian scientists, military leaders, industry executives, and Congress, to the establishment of the National Science Foundation.[48] In the meantime, the U.S. Public Health Service and voluntary health agencies, such as the National Foundation for Infantile Paralysis and the American Cancer Society, launched national postdoctoral fellowship programs. The Merck Fellowship Program was thus part of a national postwar effort to build the scientific and medical workforce through the establishment of postdoctoral fellowship programs. Indeed, between 1939 and 1940, an estimated 47 postdoctoral fellows in the medical sciences were being supported by national agencies. By 1946–47, that number had doubled to 94, and by 1950–51 it was 532.[49]

There was much support among academic researchers for the Merck Fellowship. As George Beadle of the California Institute of Technology wrote, "in supporting these fellowships Merck and Company is doing a great and valuable service to science. It is a service of which your company should be very proud. . . . The influence of the Merck Fellowships on the advances of science in the fields of biophysics, biochemistry, biology and medicine will be increasingly great in directly encouraging the men who will help to make those advances."[50] Within the Merck organization, the postdoctoral fellowship program was viewed as critical to fostering productive and supportive relationships with academic researchers, and thereby extending the company's research networks. As Max Tishler, the company's vice-president and scientific director, reported in 1954, the fellowship program "is enriching science and the company."[51] And as the Scientific Committee of Merck's board of directors noted in 1950, "fellowships . . . create good sources of information and provide good long-range contacts."[52]

In 1950, Merck & Co. awarded one of its postdoctoral fellowships to Dr. Li from the University of California, Berkeley. After two years of support but with little in the way of results that proved of tangible benefit to the company, the question of whether or not to renew Dr. Li's fellowship for another year came up for discussion. Although Li had not managed to achieve his proposed goal (developing a method for purifying and separating peptide-like hormones, such as ACTH, from a mass of peptide impurities), Karl Folkers pointed out the critical networks to which Li gave the company access. First, Folkers noted, "in our past negotiations with Dr. Li, we have been very close to Dr. [Wendell] Stanley," the Nobel laureate, "who has given Li 'paternal' guidance on these matters." If Merck withdrew its support, Folkers feared that the company "will possibly not meet with the understanding of Dr. Stanley." Maintaining good relations with Stanley should be a priority, Folkers asserted, because "Dr. Stanley's new Virus Research and Biochemistry Institute will probably become the outstanding Institute of its kind in the world, and the Company should have an excellent relationship with Dr. Stanley and the Institute."[53]

Second, Folkers reminded his colleagues, Dr. Li had assembled "a very capable group" of investigators "from Europe and America, and he is still collaborating with Professor Tiselius [another Nobel laureate]. It isn't to our advantage for these people [in Europe] . . . to feel that MERCK is withdrawing" its support. And finally, Folkers argued, "Whatever may be the recognition given to Li's research, he is one of the foremost hormone investigators in this country. Since we wish to become stronger in the field of hormones, it is desirable for us to be on good relations with the outstanding people in the field, and Dr. Li and some of his able co-workers are part of this hormone group."[54] In this way, Merck's Fellowship Program was viewed as a critical technique by which the company could build research networks with prodigious academic researchers.

Others in the company lauded the "public relations value to the Company" of the fellowships.[55] The fact that the fellowships "are very widely known among scientists, and naturally have helped to bring good will to the Merck organization"[56] justified the firm's average annual expenditure of $20,000 on the program.[57] Indeed, George Beadle assured George W. Merck, "in terms of good will to Merck and Company it seems to me that the Merck Fellowship program has already had a great influence. I do not know of a single person who is aware of the program who does not have a warmer feeling toward Merck and Company because of it."[58]

Despite the program's success, by 1952 Merck's leadership was concerned that the establishment of the National Science Foundation (NSF) and the creation of national fellowship programs by several other drug firms had diminished the value of the Merck Fellowship. As Paul Weiss of the National Research Council and chairman of the Merck Fellowship Board (the committee responsible for selecting new fellows) observed to A. N. Richards that year, "as a result of the institution of the National Science Foundation fellowships and other changes of economic and educational nature, there has of late occurred a general leveling of postdoctoral fellowships, both in character and stipend." As a major objective of the Merck Fellowship was to distinguish the company from others in the industry by assuring the Merck Fellowship had "higher standards, high stipends, and interdisciplinary training," Weiss feared that "but for minor differences" the fellowships offered by other firms and the NSF "are now essentially all in the same category."[59]

In response, Weiss recommended that "to raise the Merck Fellowships once more into a class of their own" the fellowships should be awarded not to recent graduates but to more experienced candidates "who have already been in the research process long enough to realize from their own experience just what supplemental training they really need." This would mean a successful applicant should have at least three years of postdoctoral experience. In return, the more experienced fellows would receive a higher salary, commensurate with that experience. Weiss suggested that a stipend of at least $6,000 with additional money available for travel and laboratory expenses would be necessary to attract the best candidates.[60]

Despite these concerns, the success of the firm's domestic fellowship program led the company's scientific leadership to extend the program to young foreign scientists. To this end, Merck & Co. launched an international fellowship program in 1952. The fellowships awarded an initial stipend of $6,000 to "suitably trained young research workers" who were seeking to pursue advanced training in the United States in fields such as bacteriology, biochemistry, biophysics, chemistry, microbiology, pathology, pharmacology, physiology, and medicinal chemistry.[61] Like the company's domestic program, the international fellowships were intended to promote good relations and the exchange of knowledge between company and academic researchers, thereby extending Merck's knowledge networks into the international arena.

This general concern over the shortage of biomedical workers must be considered in the context of the efforts made by other scientific leaders at this time to boost recruitment into all scientific fields in the name of national security.[62] Toward the end of the 1950s (as chapter 4 details), the industry espoused the free enterprise system of drug development as a symbol of capitalism and defense against communism and as such saw the strength of the biomedical workforce as central to this.

ATTRACTING ACADEMIC RESEARCHERS TO THE INDUSTRIAL FOLD

Merck & Co.'s workforce problems, however, required more than simply encouraging graduate students and recent graduates to enter fields of pharmaceutical-related research. The company also had to convince those young researchers to leave academia and work for Merck & Co., no small feat as the shortage of skilled biomedical workers meant heightened competition between drug firms for the researchers that were available. A 1958 survey of researchers who had held National Research Council postdoctoral fellowships in the medical sciences (which included the Merck Fellowship) found that only 2.3 percent of past fellows worked in industry, while 66.5 percent held academic appointments, and 5.6 percent worked for the government.[63] The Merck Fellowship was certainly a way of bringing the company prestige, but that alone, the company's leadership feared, would not be enough to secure the continued recruitment of promising young researchers to Merck's research organization. As Hans Molitor reminded his colleagues in 1950, Merck was not only competing with other firms for skilled researchers "but with universities and governmental, state, or municipal agencies." Because salary alone wasn't enough to secure researchers—Molitor noted that these other institutions were paying salaries comparable to industry—Merck had to do more "in order to obtain and keep outstanding men and maintain their excellence after they have joined us."[64]

Molitor proposed establishing a Merck fellowship program that would enable qualified company researchers to spend a year of specialized study in an academic institution in the United States or abroad. Molitor thought such a program "would probably go a long way to make a position in our organization more attractive for a young scientist." It would also carry, he argued, a number of additional advantages:

> (1) it would establish a healthy competition among the members of our research organization to excel in first-class research and to publish their results since obviously the selection of the recipients should be done by a committee of outstanding scientists . . . and should be based solely on scientific accomplishments; (2) a year of study with an outstanding investigator here or abroad would greatly improve the value to our organization of these men after return; (3) by their scientific excellence these men would serve as ambassadors of good-will for the Merck Research Organization and, in turn, their prolonged association with outstanding scientists would greatly widen and deepen our scientific ties.[65]

Molitor suggested, however, that such a program should not be limited to only the company's young researchers. He argued that "one of the greatest dangers against which we must guard at all times is that men who were excellent scientists and full of ideas when they joined the organization grow stale for lack of stimulating contacts with other research men." Although this was a problem shared by universities as well as the industry, Molitor continued, university professors had "two remedies against growing stale which we in industry have not yet fully developed: (1) sabbatical leaves; (2) contact with young men." Molitor urged his colleagues to establish such remedies at Merck. While his proposed internal fellowship could serve as a "sabbatical year" for the qualified and more senior researchers, the firm should also consider establishing fellowships for young academic researchers to spend a year studying within the Merck research organization. This "contact with young people" would provide the "old age cure" for the company's senior researchers at the same time as providing the young academic with an opportunity to experience the benefits of working for Merck.[66]

While these fellowship programs would go some way to resolving the company's concern that the shortage of biomedical labor would make it increasingly difficult for Merck to hire skilled researchers, Molitor added that "such a double fellowship program would [have] considerable . . . public relations value. . . . It would make our facilities and the quality of our research widely known and would not only build loyalty within our own staffs but would also result in a wide dissemination of knowledge concerning MERCK & CO. Inc. 'Merck' could again pioneer a path which probably would be followed, sooner or later, by other members of industry."[67]

Molitor's proposal met with enthusiasm. Merck's study abroad program was up and running by 1952, with the Merck employee receiving a full salary and travel advance of up to $1,250 during their tenure of study abroad.[68] After two years the company considered the program a success. In June 1954, Merck's Science Policy Council agreed that two of the program's primary objectives were being met: "those who had returned from study abroad have gained materially by their experiences" and "scientific contacts abroad have been developed which should be of value to the Company." Moreover, the council found "that those who had had opportunity to be free of routine laboratory administration for an extended period of time have given evidence of increased scientific enthusiasm."[69]

Merck's strategy for attracting skilled academic researchers also included a liberal publication policy. Since 1933, the company's policy was that any findings of scientific interest should be presented to scientific meetings or published in scientific journals.[70] This policy, however, became the subject of debate among Merck's executives in 1949 when officers from the company's sales and commercial departments began pushing for a policy of delaying publications until two to five years after patent applications were submitted. Merck's research personnel were adamant that no such change should be adopted. As Karl Folkers warned, "any change in publication policy requiring the withholding of publications for a long period will bring severe outside criticism, and will lose to Merck & Co. Inc., the position which they now occupy, which is envied by our competitors."[71]

As it was, Merck's liberal publication policy served to distinguish the company from other firms, increasing its attractiveness to academic researchers as both a potential employer and a research collaborator. As one Merck official noted, "By following this policy we receive as well as give. Our scientists have become known throughout the world and learn from contacts with other scientists much that is of value to Merck & Co., Inc. It has also stimulated cooperative research between the universities and Merck which has proved of considerable benefit to us." He cited the development of vitamins B_1 and B_{12}, streptomycin, and cortisone as evidence and warned that any "change in this policy would soon show its effect in the attitude of other scientists towards our men."[72]

Since "the Company's 'liberal' scientific publication policy was an important asset to the Company because of the scientific prestige that it builds and the scientific competence that it fosters," the policy remained unchanged.[73] Indeed, when the company's scientific directors voted on the proposal to prioritize patents over publications, they branded the proposed policy as "incomprehensible, detrimental to the company, and totally unacceptable." To adopt the proposed policy would be to lose the company's best researchers and to make impossible the collaboration with outside scientists.[74]

Merck's scientific leadership hoped that the company's fellowship programs and its policy toward scientific publications together would help the company attract the best and brightest researchers. Yet, as much as the company sought to tackle both the internal and the external labor problems in the biomedical field through the fellowship program, the company hoped also that its fellowship program would help it to build credibility and prestige within the academic scientific community. The fellowship program thus served several key functions for Merck & Co. in the postwar decade. The first was that industry support of advanced scientific training provided an essential alternative to government support of biomedicine. Second, the innovativeness of the company depended on a continuous supply of skilled pharmaceutical knowledge workers—Ph.D. researchers in organic and medicinal chemistry, biochemistry, pharmacology, and other fields related to drug development, in addition to skilled laboratory technicians—and the fellowship program introduced young researchers to the financial and intellectual benefits of working with (and for) industry. Third, these fellowships promoted the exchange of knowledge between academic and industrial research laboratories, as drug company sponsors retained access to the fruits of their fellows' research.

Merck was not the only pharmaceutical company to develop postdoctoral and graduate fellowship programs in the postwar decades. Eli Lilly & Co. and Lederle Laboratories established postdoctoral fellowship programs that were, like Merck's, administered by the National Research Council.[75] Abbott Laboratories and Parke-Davis & Co. also expanded on the ad hoc fellowship programs they had developed during the interwar years, while firms such as Mead Johnson & Co. established new fellowship programs after the war.[76] Elsewhere, the Du Pont Chemical Company began funding

basic chemical research in universities after the war as university administrators increasingly solicited Du Pont and other chemical companies for
financial support. Like Merck, rather than provide universities with unre-
stricted funds for general use, Du Pont's executives established funding
programs that met an institution's specific needs, including the establishment of summer research grants for young faculty, postgraduate teaching assistant awards, and support of undergraduate science instruction in
liberal arts colleges.[77] That a leading chemical company and leading pharmaceutical companies were engaged in developing the next generation of
knowledge workers is suggestive of the broader changes taking place in the
relationships between academic institutions and science-based industries in
the postwar decades.[78] Indeed, by 1956, industry and private philanthropic
foundations were supporting 14.5 percent of the nation's postdoctoral fellowships in the medical sciences, while government agencies such as the
NSF and the National Institutes of Health were funding 57.8 percent, and
voluntary health agencies 27.7 percent.[79]

A FIELD IN DIRE NEED: CLINICAL PHARMACOLOGY

Although the drug industry and medical school and university administrators had shared concern over a general shortage of biomedical workers
since the end of World War II, by the mid-1950s that concern became
increasingly focused on the field of clinical pharmacology. A demand
for specialized researchers skilled in the study of drug actions, metab-
olism, and interactions in humans emerged after passage of the 1938
Federal Food, Drug, and Cosmetic Act, which for the first time required
firms to provide evidence of their drugs' safety prior to receiving
marketing approval from the FDA, and following the explosion of new
drugs after the war.[80] Nowhere was the demand so profound as in drug
firms, which relied on researchers skilled in the clinical study of drugs
to evaluate the safety and effectiveness of all new drugs developed in
their laboratories.

By 1955, medical school administrators were considering ways of fostering the development of clinical pharmacology in order to meet the drug
industry's workforce needs. As the vice-president in charge of medical
affairs at the University of Pennsylvania, Norman Topping, wrote to the
dean of the medical school, John McK. Mitchell, in 1955, through the
school's contacts with the drug industry, it was "quite apparent" that a
teaching and research program in clinical pharmacology "is badly needed.

On the one hand, they have a constant demand for clinical evaluations of new therapeutic agents, and, on the other hand, a dearth of places and people who can accomplish this." At a time when the medical school was struggling for funds, committing to the development of clinical pharmacology served as a way for medical schools to garner the support of drug firms. As Topping noted to Mitchell, the industry trade association, the American Drug Manufacturers Association (ADMA), was considering the possibility of funding a new clinical pharmacology program at the University of Pennsylvania, with the further possibility of endowing a Chair of Clinical Pharmacology.[81]

In 1957, however, the ADMA made its first award to Dr. Louis Lasagna of Johns Hopkins University for the establishment of a fellowship in clinical pharmacology. The initial fellowship amounted to $7,500 each year for a two-year period, but in the second year of the program the ADMA increased the grant to $21,000 for an additional two-year period. Committed to "early and accurate appraisal of the utility and safety of any new drug" but concerned about "the relative lack of specially trained clinical investigators with adequate facilities to carry out and interpret such studies," the ADMA (and its successor, the Pharmaceutical Manufacturers Association) viewed the clinical pharmacology fellowship program at Johns Hopkins University as critical to the industry's continued growth.[82] In particular, the ADMA argued, "the increasing number of potentially valuable new agents now being developed, as well as the demands of teaching assignments and the exigencies of medical practice, makes the current supply [of capable investigators] inadequate for the prompt and efficient completion of all the critical studies which new drugs demand and deserve." Furthermore, the ADMA observed "that at only a very few institutions of medical education is a formal effort being made to train individuals in this critical area of medical research." As such, the ADMA hoped that its clinical pharmacology fellowship program would stimulate such training by allowing individuals with "an adequate research and clinical background to continue their training under a recognized authority in the field," Dr. Louis Lasagna. Although the ADMA had, at that point, raised enough money to support just one fellowship program at a single institution, the ADMA hoped that the Johns Hopkins program "will act as a 'seeding' operation in that individuals so trained may establish similar departments of similar training in other educational institutions, with the result that in this manner the adequate training of appreciable numbers of individuals qualified to conduct clinical investigation will be achieved." Ultimately, the ADMA hoped the program would result in a more adequate supply of suitably trained individuals "available for employment in the medical departments of the pharmaceutical industry, since it follows that the employment of such individuals with sound training and critical judgment will do much to raise the standard of drug evaluation in this country."[83]

In 1959, the Pharmaceutical Manufacturers Association (PMA, successor to the ADMA) established a second clinical pharmacology program at the University of Pennsylvania. Planning for the University of Pennsylvania's clinical pharmacology program had begun in 1955. Norman Topping, the university's vice-president in charge of medical affairs, sought to create an institutional structure that would ensure the program could be responsive to the industry's needs. Indeed, Topping believed the new program should function, essentially, as a service unit for the drug industry. For instance, the individual charged with developing the school's program in clinical pharmacology would hold a joint appointment in the department of pharmacology (where he would be expected to teach) and at the Hospital of the University of Pennsylvania, where his function would be clinical research. However, "he would not be a member of any of the clinical departments in the Hospital, but would be autonomous. This would give him flexibility when approached by Industry to either conduct the clinical investigations himself, or to arrange for members of the appropriate clinical departments to conduct the investigations."[84]

A year later, in 1956, Dr. C. J. Lambertsen from the University of Pennsylvania School of Medicine's Department of Pharmacology began negotiations with the ADMA (which was renamed the PMA in 1958) to secure its support to develop the university's clinical pharmacology program. Three years later, the PMA awarded the medical school an initial grant of $21,000 over a two-year period to support a program in clinical pharmacology.[85] Each year, the grant provided for the partial support of two clinical pharmacology fellows, with the aim of the program being the "training of qualified young physicians in the design and technical performance of drug studies in normal men and patients, and analysis of data obtained in comprehensive studies of new and currently used drugs." The PMA and the University of Pennsylvania hoped that the new fellowship program would "aid in overcoming the present, serious shortage of men broadly trained in Clinical Pharmacology."[86]

Yet, by the end the decade the field was still struggling to recruit. According to Lasagna, the reason was that "all too often the title of clinical pharmacologist raises the specter of the uninspired hack, turning up dreary data on efficacy and toxicity." Lasagna called on industry and medicine "to increase the appeal of clinical pharmacology for talented investigators" by "rais[ing] the prestige value of the field and to make it seem exciting."[87] As such, the ADMA's (and later, PMA's) establishment of the fellowship programs in clinical pharmacology at Johns Hopkins University and the University of Pennsylvania was only a first step toward solving the workforce problem in clinical pharmacology. With the introduction of new drug regulations in 1962 that required drug firms to provide evidence of the safety *and* efficacy of their new drugs through controlled clinical trials, the demand for clinical pharmacologists grew considerably, and with it the struggle of medical schools to secure funding for the development of this all-important field.[88]

CONCLUSION

The establishment of nationally organized, competitive fellowship programs by pharmaceutical companies, and the industry trade association's funding of clinical pharmacology programs, reflected a new strategy adopted by industry leaders to shape the postwar political economy of pharmaceutical research. With the federal government the new principal patron of basic biomedical research, there was less need for drug firms to support the basic research of academic researchers. As drug companies, medical schools, and the scientific leadership came to realize after the war's end, however, the cost of biomedical education and training was increasing without a concomitant increase in support from the federal government. Moreover, these groups worried that greater government support of training and education would represent a move toward socialized education and socialized medicine.

At the same time, industry and biomedical leaders were concerned about an impending workforce shortage in the biomedical sciences in general, and in pharmaceutical-related fields in particular. After all, the innovativeness of the drug industry and the growth of academic fields related to pharmaceutical development were dependent on a continuous supply of skilled pharmaceutical knowledge workers—skilled laboratory technicians and Ph.D. researchers in organic and medicinal chemistry, biochemistry, pharmacology and other fields related to drug development. Drug firms' postdoctoral fellowship programs and the ADMA's and later PMA's clinical pharmacology fellowships represented a major way in which drug firms sought to ensure a pipeline of pharmaceutical workers. The programs also served the interests of drug firms by preserving and indeed intensifying their research networks with the biomedical research community. These workforce concerns formed part of a broader concern among scientific, military, and political leaders regarding the centrality of skilled scientists to national security.[89]

Together with its other network-building strategies—of partnering with academic researchers in the pharmaceutical innovation process and of recruiting science administrators as corporate consultants and directors—the industry's commitment to developing the postwar pharmaceutical workforce constituted an industry-academic-government network that paralleled the emergence of the military-industrial-academic complex. Although the amount of money circulating through this pharmaceutical network was less than that underpinning the military-industrial-academic complex, and the drug industry and medical profession, unlike the military-industrial-academic complex, were skeptical of specific forms of government financing, the scientific—and later political—value of this network was significant. In the postwar decade, the pharmaceutical network produced scores of new therapeutic agents, including the broad-spectrum antibiotics, cortisone, vitamin B_{12}, the minor tranquilizers such as meprobamate, antipsychotics such as chlorpromazine, the Salk and Sabin polio vaccines, and the first antihypertensive drug, chlorothiazide.[90] The pharmaceutical network also supported the development of pharmaceutical-related fields of science and medicine, especially that of clinical pharmacology. And from the mid-1950s on, as the following chapters document, this network played a crucial role in protecting the political interests of the industry and the medical profession, and in establishing the pharmaceutical industry as one of the most powerful interest groups in American politics.

3 Professional Relations

*Crafting the Public Image of
the Health Care Team*

In our zeal to avoid any possible intrusion upon the relationship
of the physician and patient, ethical pharmaceutical manufacturers
have in years past shied away from communication with
the general public. It is human nature to believe gossip and
criticism about a stranger more readily than about someone
whose integrity and good works are well know; therefore,
inadvertently, we have aggravated our present problems of public
understanding.

—EUGENE BEESLEY, chairman, Pharmaceutical Manufacturers
Association, 1962[1]

In the first decade after World War II, the American pharmaceutical industry rode a wave of public and political support. Journalists wrote with awe
about the introduction of new therapeutic innovations such as cortisone
and streptomycin. In the spring of 1949, for example, the *New York Times*
published several articles on the first treatment of patients suffering from
rheumatoid arthritis with cortisone, emphasizing the "dramatic relief . . .
[cortisone] afford[s] in enabling long-time cripples to walk again."[2] Citing
the treating physician, the *New York Times* told of one "woman, unable
to lift herself out of bed or feed herself" who, "within forty-four hours"
of receiving cortisone, "walked and fed herself. After nine days of treatment she literally danced a jig."[3] Similar stories of bedridden, crippled, and
suffering patients saved by the growing cadre of "wonder drugs," such as
the broad-spectrum antibiotics, corticosteroids, and the new psychotropic
drugs, could be found most months in the pages of the *New York Times*,
the *Washington Post, Reader's Digest, Fortune,* and *Newsweek.*

By the mid-1950s, however, the pharmaceutical industry was the
subject of intense government scrutiny as several firms, Merck and Pfizer
among them, were accused of fixing the prices of antibiotics and vaccines,
and of engaging in misleading marketing practices. For all its therapeutic
triumphs and for all its support among academic researchers, the industry
faced a burgeoning problem: public discontent over the cost of prescription

drugs. As it did so, the industry confronted the reality that it operated not just in the realms of commerce and science, but also in the highly politicized—and public—arena of health care. With that realization came the consensus among the industry's leadership that in order to survive *politically,* the industry needed to build not only its scientific networks but also politically meaningful relationships with health care *practitioners,* physicians and pharmacists most critically; so too, the industry needed to develop its relationship with the American public.

THE PRESCRIPTION DRUG MARKET AT MIDCENTURY

In the decade after World War II, the American pharmaceutical industry emerged as a dominant institution in the national and international economy. As chapter 1 detailed, during this decade the industry's core firms underwent strategic and structural changes, vertically integrating backward into basic research and forward into marketing.[4] The result was commensurate growth in the American drug industry over the course of the 1940s and 1950s, with worldwide sales increasing 203 percent, from $890 million in 1947 to $2.7 billion in 1959.[5] The American pharmaceutical industry was a diverse and highly competitive industry in the postwar decades, composed of more than thirteen hundred firms of varying size, degrees of research, marketing, and manufacturing capacity, and extent of vertical integration and product diversification.[6]

The most innovative sector of the U.S. pharmaceutical industry was the large research-based drug firms. These firms (among them, Abbott Laboratories, Eli Lilly & Co., E. R. Squibb, Lederle Laboratories, Merck & Co., Parke-Davis & Co., Pfizer, Schering, G. D. Searle & Co., Smith, Kline & French, Upjohn & Co., and Wyeth Laboratories) developed extensive industrial research laboratories and integrated forward into pharmaceutical marketing. These were the firms that discovered, developed, and marketed the majority of new drugs that constituted the so-called therapeutic revolution, and as such were the most economically important firms of the industry. In 1955, eleven such firms accounted for half of all sales of prescription drugs in the United States; in 1960, twenty firms accounted for 80 percent of all U.S. sales.[7] The majority of pharmaceutical firms, however, did little if any research, conducted minimal promotion, and focused on the packaging and distribution of unpatented or off-patent generic drugs. These firms were typically referred to as generic drug manufacturers.[8]

Generic manufacturers were geographically dispersed and often operated on a state or regional level, while research-based drug firms operated nationally and internationally and were largely concentrated in the Midwest and Mid-Atlantic region. New Jersey, New York, and Pennsylvania, for example, were home to Merck, Smith, Kline & French, Pfizer, Squibb, Bristol-Myers, Lederle, and Wyeth. Abbott Laboratories and G. D. Searle were located in Illinois, Parke-Davis and Upjohn & Co. in Michigan, and Eli Lilly & Co. in Indiana. As will be discussed in chapter 4, the economic development that pharmaceutical firms brought to a region helped the industry secure significant political support in states that were home to the largest firms.

Many of the drugs developed by research-based drug firms were patented and thus marketed under a *brand* name, conferring on the innovator firm a commercial monopoly. In recognition of this, research-based drug firms are often referred to as brand-name manufacturers. In the postwar decades, the awarding of a patent for a new drug conferred exclusive marketing rights of up to seventeen years to the firm that owned the patent.[9] Additionally though, the brand name conferred a significant commercial advantage to that firm. Even after a patent expired and other manufacturers were permitted to develop their own (generic) versions of the drug, the innovator firm could continue marketing (indefinitely) the off-patent drug under its brand name. This had the effect of unofficially extending the innovator firm's commercial advantage in the market for that drug. Despite the "brand name" designator, however, it is important to recognize that the marketing of nonpatented (and thus nonbranded) drugs represented a significant part of brand-name manufacturers' business. Similarly, many so-called generic manufacturers held patents on their work and marketed brand-name drugs.[10]

In addition to being innovative and economically important, the large research-based drug firms were also the most political of the drug industry. Though they were joined by several small and medium-sized research-based firms, the large research-based firms made up the core of the industry's trade associations—the American Drug Manufacturers Association (ADMA) and the American Pharmaceutical Manufacturers Association (APMA), and, later, the Pharmaceutical Manufacturers Association (PMA)—and executives from those companies held many of the leadership positions within the trade associations. It is to these large research-based firms, so-called brand-name manufacturers, and their political activism during the 1950s that we now turn.

MAINTAINING PROFESSIONAL RELATIONS
IN THE EARLY POSTWAR YEARS

Despite the therapeutic optimism of the early postwar years, by 1950, biomedical researchers and physicians were reporting that bacteria were developing resistance to antibiotics and that some of the new wonder drugs were associated with debilitating and sometimes fatal side effects. The press was quick to pick up on these concerns. More worrying for the public and drug companies alike was the news in the spring and summer of 1950 that several people taking Parke-Davis & Co.'s antibiotic Chloromycetin (chloramphenicol) had died from aplastic anemia, a rare blood disorder,. Physicians were also finding that if arthritic patients taking cortisone stopped taking their medicine, their symptoms returned worse than before they started on steroids. By 1953 the press was asking, "Are wonder drugs really wonderful?"[11]

The concern over the safety of new drugs coincided with growing frustration among the general public over the seemingly high prices they had to pay for these wonder drugs. In August 1953, the advertising agency Batten, Barton, Durstine & Osborn reported that 63 percent of people questioned on their attitudes toward the drug trade believed that prescription drug prices were too high.[12]

In spite of the continuing news reports of side effects induced by prolonged use of Chloromycetin and cortisone, and of the mounting incidence of antibiotic-resistant bacteria, drug companies at first appeared little troubled by the negative publicity. As far as industry executives were concerned, the industry's scientific and therapeutic accomplishments meant that "the general public has a more favorable impression of the Pharmaceutical Industry than ever before in its history."[13] The industry felt that it had more to fear from the growing amount of premature or unwarranted publicity on new products and the damage this was doing to the industry's relationship with the medical profession and pharmacy.

In the press's fervor to report on the new drugs being developed by drug firms, journalists were quick to jump on any report, however preliminary, in the scientific and medical press about the discovery of potential new lifesaving drugs. In October 1952, the *New York Times* reported that a "superior" new drug for treating pulmonary tuberculosis was just around the corner after a New Jersey physician published in his hospital's newsletter the findings of a trial of the new combination drug in nine patients.[14] The same month, *Pageant* magazine reported on an "astonishing new drug" against polio, arthritis, and heart trouble, even though the highly experimental drug, Betasyamine, had yet to be studied extensively in patients.[15]

Most physicians regarded advertising by drug companies directly to consumers as an affront to and an unnecessary and indeed dangerous incursion into the doctor-patient relationship. Aware of this and committed to distancing themselves from turn-of-the-century patent-medicine sellers who had advertised—in quite dramatic, overstated, and often misleading ways—their products directly to consumers, prescription drug firms were reluctant to be seen as actively generating publicity.[16] For industry executives, the relationships of primary importance and thus those that required nurturing, were those the companies shared with other members of the health care team, principally pharmacists and physicians. Industry executives held that drug firms should remain largely invisible to the patient, their contact with the patient mediated through their primary contacts with the physician and the pharmacist. As Eugene Beesley, the president of Eli Lilly & Co., explained the industry's reluctance to engage in public relations in the early 1950s, "Our position as an aid to the medical profession led us to feel we had little duty—in fact, little right—to speak directly to the public."[17]

Because physicians perceived premature drug publicity as a way for drug companies to communicate directly with the public, thereby circumventing the physician-patient relationship, this kind of publicity stood to alienate physicians from the industry. Indeed, by the summer of 1952, the American Medical Association (AMA) accused drug firms of using such publicity "to avoid the long but necessary period of evaluation for a new method of treatment."[18] By the end of the year, the AMA had "declared war" on the industry's press activities and accused companies of creating public demand for new and untested drugs.[19] The AMA was particularly troubled by the detrimental effect of these press releases on physician-patient relations, especially the reversal in the balance of power they seemed to inspire. As the AMA's report noted, "following publication of these slanted items, the public is quick to press the profession for employment of newly mentioned drugs or uses and shows little sympathy or understanding for the reluctance and resistance of physicians to accept such publicity as evidence of therapeutic worth."[20]

In the early 1950s, drug firms also faced serious problems in their relationships with pharmacists. In particular, retail pharmacists were increasingly frustrated with the expense of stocking every new drug the industry introduced to the market, especially those drugs that were rarely prescribed. For many pharmacists, the expense of maintaining a full inventory of new drugs was proving too great. In response, as a way of reducing the amount of inventory they needed, pharmacists were engaging in the practice of substituting cheaper generic drugs for brand-name prescription drugs. Although substitution was illegal, the pharmacists practicing substitution hoped to create enough pressure on state and federal legislatures to force the legalization of brand substitution.[21] They were joined in their efforts by small pharmaceutical firms that, lacking research capacities, manufactured generic versions of brand drugs. For these small firms without the capital to develop sufficient marketing capacities, substitution represented a way for them to compete in the pharmaceutical marketplace. In February 1952, for example, a group of small drug manufacturers helped to bring a bill before the Michigan state legislature that would permit the substitution by pharmacists of one drug product for that prescribed by the physician.[22]

Retail pharmacists railed, in particular, against the increasing number of drugs released on the market that were not actually "new products" with unique therapeutic action. Pharmacists complained that the abundance of so-called me-too drugs (drugs that have similar chemical properties and more or less identical therapeutic function) resulted in excessive costs to the pharmacist, who was obligated to stock all varieties of me-too drugs but might sell only a relatively small amount of each. Pharmacists were often left with large inventory that they could not sell. Many individual pharmacists, along with many physicians who were also "confused and troubled" by the increasing number of products introduced to the market that were not major therapeutic advances, were organizing an antiduplication drive. Through this campaign pharmacists, first, sought to restrict the introduction of further me-too drugs and, second, called on physicians to write prescriptions for generic drugs rather than the brand (or trademark) name, thus allowing pharmacists to dispense whichever of the duplicate drugs they stocked.[23]

The pharmacists' substitution and antiduplication campaigns were intrinsically linked reactions to the economic structure of the pharmaceutical industry. Indeed, even as pharmacy leaders condemned substitution, they perceived it to be a symptom of the drug industry's economic practices, specifically pharmaceutical companies' propensity to develop drugs with chemical structures and therapeutic effects nearly identical to those of drugs already on the market. In 1952, for example, the California Pharmaceutical Association's president, John A. Foley, condemned substitution as an "insidious" practice while calling on manufacturers to "desist from the practice of lifting each other's formulas and ideas." Foley believed that in doing so, "the props would be pulled from under" the substituting pharmacists.[24] In turn, brand-name manufacturers accused substituting pharmacists of threatening the economic foundations and the legal system of drug development. As the trade journal *FDC Reports* warned, "by plugging the use of generic names on [prescriptions]," pharmacists were verging on "destroying the value of pharmaceutical trademarks."[25]

For industry executives, the practice of substitution and the antiduplication drive raised far more serious concerns than did the negative headlines in the news media about drug side effects and antibiotic resistance. During the spring of 1952, several firms went on the offensive and instituted antisubstitution campaigns aimed at curbing the practice. These included taking legal action against pharmacists guilty of substitution (on the grounds that substituting pharmacists were engaging in unfair competition) and against the small generic drug manufacturers whose imitation drugs were being substituted for brand-name drugs. Leading the way was Abbott Laboratories, which secured a series of court injunctions against New York City pharmacists guilty of substituting other products for prescriptions written for the company's drugs.[26] As Theodore Klumpp, the president of Winthrop Laboratories (the research arm of Sterling Drug, Inc.), argued before an audience of representatives from brand-name manufacturers, although "it is not good business to sue our customers," because of the "growing conviction that soft words have failed to stop this nefarious practice," it was "time to 'get tough with the chiselers.'"[27] In spite of these efforts, a 1953 mail survey of brand-name manufacturers found that 53 percent of responding firms believed that "substitution of their products is already widespread," with some firms reporting substitution rates for their prescription products as high as 25 percent in some cases.[28]

In getting "tough," brand-name manufacturers sought to reaffirm the economic—and legal—foundation of the pharmaceutical enterprise while reasserting the appropriate professional relationships among physicians, pharmacists, and the prescription. To this end, in December 1953, a group of executives from the leading drug firms determined that in order to improve its relations with physicians and pharmacists, the industry should create an organization to develop an industrywide professional relations program. This new organization, the industry leadership hoped, would promote "the highest professional standards and ethics in the manufacture, distribution, and dispensing of prescription medication."[29] Although the new organization, the National Pharmaceutical Council (NPC), would have other functions, its main objective was to unite drug manufacturers and pharmacists. As the NPC's first president, Theodore Klumpp, described to the Drug, Chemical, and Allied Trades Section of the New York Board of Trade in January 1954, the NPC's member companies recognized "that an industry divided against itself cannot stand. . . . [W]e believe that the interests of all of us [pharmacists and manufacturers] will be best served by strengthening the bonds of common interest that hold us together." Klumpp called on "all those in all branches of our industry who share our common purpose" to work together to "bring our combined influence to bear against those practices that are undermining the ethical principles of fair competition and fair dealing upon which our industry must rest." In particular, Klumpp assured the group, the NPC was committed to squashing the practice of substitution and pharmacists' anti-duplication drive.[30]

The NPC's primary strategy with regard to pharmacists was to develop a public relations program to aid pharmacists in their own public relations troubles. Since the late 1940s, retail pharmacists had faced increasing competition from supermarkets, as supermarkets began dispensing prescription and over-the-counter drugs. The NPC hoped the pharmacy public relations campaign would serve as a "vehicle for a quid-pro-quo arrangement" in which the industry would "undertake to provide the expensive public relations program which leaders in pharmacy have long wanted if pharmacy will cooperate to protect the validity of the trademark system."[31]

The NPC program built on the pharmacy public relations campaigns of Parke-Davis & Co. and E. R. Squibb. After World War II, concerned that the "old-fashioned pharmacist," who compounded his own tablets and operated out of his own store, was being made "almost extinct" by the growth of "the modern drug store" that housed lunch counters and sold a whole range of products, Parke-Davis & Co., organized the first sustained advertising campaign on behalf of pharmacists. The goal of this campaign was to increase the prestige of pharmacists and to emphasize the critical health care services provided by them. One advertisement, for example, told the story of a pharmacist who refused to sell a laxative to a customer after the customer mentioned having severe abdominal pain. The customer, it turned out, had appendicitis and the pharmacist's actions, the advertisement explained, saved the customer's life. Another advertisement described the pharmacist who sent a customer he suspected of suffering from a venereal disease to a physician. Others stressed the precautions the pharmacist took in dispensing poisons (such as arsenic) and narcotics. From 1944 through the early 1950s, these advertisements were published at monthly intervals in the *Saturday Evening Post*.[32]

In addition to conducting a pharmacy public relations program, the NPC also launched a concerted antisubstitution campaign targeted at pharmacists and physicians. Executive officers of the NPC traveled throughout the United States "carrying the 'gospel' of prescription brand names" to state pharmacy boards, state pharmacy associations, and pharmacy students.[33] In his January 1954 speech to the Drug, Chemical, and Allied Trades Section of the New York Board of Trade, Klumpp accused pharmacists who substituted as "cast[ing] a heavy shadow over the entire pharmaceutical family." The substituting pharmacist was guilty of "practicing medicine without a license." After all, "the pharmaceutical industry—all segments of it—is built on certain principles which have stood the test of time. The key principle is that the physician is boss. It is he who prescribes. It is the pharmacist who compounds the prescription. The pharmacist is professionally, morally, and legally bound to fill that prescription precisely as the doctor wrote it." By overstepping these professional, moral, and legal bounds, the substituting pharmacist put not only the "very foundations" of the pharmaceutical industry at risk but, more important, also caused grave danger to the patient. Klumpp warned that the substituting pharmacist's "first victim is the doctor's patient who, at best, got a product of uncertain quality. His other victims are the reputable retail pharmacists in the community who may be accused by the public of overcharging for prescriptions honestly compounded."[34]

The strategy of turning nonsubstituting pharmacists against their substituting colleagues was proving successful by 1956. The new NPC president, Robert Hardt, noted that whereas several years earlier only four or five state pharmacy boards could be counted on to take action against substituting pharmacists, by 1956 the ratio of state boards committed to taking action against pharmacists guilty of substitution had been reversed, with the majority now supporting antisubstitution measures. Furthermore, the rate of substitution had fallen from 14.7 percent in 1953 to 4.3 percent in 1956. Yet for Hardt perhaps the clearest sign of the program's success was the conversion of substitution into a "bad word" in pharmacy circles.[35] A year later, an *American Druggist* survey of brand-name manufacturers found the rate of substitution to have fallen even further, to 3.7 percent.[36] And by 1959, forty-four states had put antisubstitution laws—to be enforced by state pharmacy boards—on the books.[37]

At the same time, the NPC sought to educate physicians on the dangers of substitution in the hope that they would add pressure to state pharmacy boards to prosecute cases of substitution. In 1957, the NPC published and distributed to physicians a twenty-eight-page booklet that highlighted "24

reasons why prescription brand names are important to you." By explain-
ing to physicians that generic drugs were often not therapeutically equivalent to their brand-name counterparts due to differences, for example, in
the drugs' disintegration time, purity, solubility, particle size, quantity
of active ingredient, melting point, surface tension, viscosity, and caloric
values, the booklet sought to educate the physician "to (1) specify brand
names on his prescriptions and (2) insist that the pharmacist supply the
brand ordered."[38]

In addition to the work of the NPC, several firms engaged in their
own professional relations activities. In order to convince physicians that
they wanted to nurture rather than undermine the physician-patient relationship, several pharmaceutical firms engaged in institutional advertising
campaigns that encouraged the public to seek regular and prompt medical
care. In 1952, Parke-Davis & Co. launched a series of advertisements that
appeared in mass circulation publications such as *Reader's Digest, Today's
Health,* the *Saturday Evening Post,* and *Life.* The theme of these advertisements was to encourage the reader to visit their doctor by highlighting how
"YOU [the reader] are medicine's biggest problem." These advertisements
warned of the dangers of ignoring signs of illness and delaying visits to
the doctor. Consider, for example, the 1953 advertisement that berated the
businessman who ignored at his own peril "the danger signals" of heart
disease because he was too busy to visit the doctor "until it may be too
late to take advantage of the help which medical science today is prepared
to give." A second advertisement in the series made very clear the danger
of choosing a friend's advice over that of the physician. Picturing a group
of women playing cards, the advertisements advised, "When you're dealt
a 'sure cure' . . . pass!" Although "Most friendly advice is fairly harmless.
Usually the worst it can lead to is an unbecoming dress, a cake that doesn't
rise, or a plant that doesn't flower," the advertisement admonished that
"when the amateur starts playing the expert in medical counsel—*watch
out!*" The advertisement continued, "Only your doctor's diagnosis can
determine what medicines you need (if, indeed, you need any)." Other
advertisements in the series guided the reader on choosing a family and
community doctor, emphasizing the importance of such a decision to the
health of the reader and his or her family.[39]

By emphasizing the importance of the doctor-patient relationship,
Parke-Davis & Co.'s institutional advertising campaign and that of other
companies through the early 1950s sought to build goodwill with physicians by asserting that the industry knew its proper place in the therapeutic relationship. Together with the NPC's campaigns, the drug industry's

professional relations activities sought to build support for itself among other health care practitioners by promoting the image of the health care team working *together* to protect the public's health. During the second half of the 1950s, this support would prove critical as, facing a rising tide of political criticism, the industry's leadership called on its allies in the health care team to help the pharmaceutical industry educate the public on the industry's lifesaving work.

CONGRESS CATCHES THE "DRUG PRICE BUG"

At mid-decade, the American pharmaceutical industry was an almost $2 billion industry, with worldwide sales in 1955 of $1.82 billion and domestic sales of $1.46 billion.[40] Collectively, the industry was investing $91 million per year in research (5 percent of sales) and operating at a net profit of $191 million per year (10.5 percent of sales).[41] Individually, as table 1 shows, seven of the biggest-selling research-based drug firms had annual sales of between $46 million and $163.8 million, operated at profits (as a percentage of sales) of between 9 percent and 18 percent, and invested between 3.7 percent and 6.6 percent (as a percentage of sales) in research.[42] Those firms responsible for leading the development and marketing of the recent wonder drugs, particularly the tranquilizers, steroids, broad-spectrum antibiotics, and polio vaccine, were showing the greatest gains. Sales at Smith, Kline & French, for example, had increased 40 percent since 1954, due largely to sales of its new tranquilizer, Thorazine (chlorpromazine).[43]

Though the industry was proving economically successful at mid-decade, politically the industry was entering a stormy period. In 1955, a batch of Salk polio vaccine produced by Cutter Laboratories was contaminated with live virus, causing polio in seventy-nine American children.[44] In response, the U.S. surgeon general called for a tightening of vaccine testing procedures. According to press accounts, vaccine producers were unhappy about the plans for more stringent testing of the vaccine. News of these press accounts reached the halls of Congress, raising the ire of Senator Wayne Morse (D-OR). As he addressed the Senate that May, Morse recounted the inadequacies of the government program and emphasized the responsibility of the federal government to see that no further mistakes were made. Morse blamed the government for "simply turn[ing] over to the drug companies" the responsibility for manufacturing, testing, and distributing the vaccine without first having government officials test

TABLE 1. Research Expenditures and Net Profits in Relation to Sales of Selected Pharmaceutical Firms in 1955

Company	Research ($ millions)	Net Sales ($ millions)	Research as % of Sales	Net Profit as % of Sales
Abbott	3.7	91.7	4.0	11
Eli Lilly & Co.	9.3	141.3	6.6	12
Merck	10.3	157.9	6.5	11
Parke-Davis	4.6	123.1	3.7	12
Pfizer	7.0	163.8	4.3	9
Schering	2.7	46.0	5.9	18
Smith, Kline & French	5.0	91.7	5.5	17

SOURCE: Figures cited in *FDC Reports*, April 14, 1958, pp. 4, 5, 10.

each batch. At the same time, he accused the vaccine producers of delaying the start of their polio vaccine programs, arguing that if the drug companies had started their vaccine programs and thus developed their testing procedures sooner, "we would not be in the mess we are in."[45] As Morse saw it, the government had failed to protect the public's health. Worse still, the medical profession and the drug companies were part of a "medical fraternity" that sought to dictate health policy to the federal government. Determined to rein in the "medical fraternity" and return responsibility to the federal government, Morse urged Congress to enact legislation that laid out a framework for public-health policy within which the medical profession and the pharmaceutical industry would be required to operate.[46]

Morse was joined on the floor by Senator Hubert Humphrey (D-MN), who was even more damning of the drug companies efforts to ease the Salk vaccine testing requirements. As far as Humphrey was concerned, "if any drug house or any manufacturer's laboratory had the unmitigated gall or selfishness to tell . . . [the] Surgeon General that any standards or tests he might insist upon were impeding their operations or causing them difficulty, all he would have to do would be to tell a few United States Senators, and we would see who was on the right side." Humphrey continued that it was not a question of whether the manufacturing laboratories were happy or whether they liked the regulations; the government licensed them, and thus it was the surgeon general's duty to impose safety restrictions on the manufacturers. Humphrey admonished, "There is no drug house that dares say to the American people that we must hurry because of their investment."[47] That Morse and Humphrey joined forces to criticize the industry's role in the vaccine program is unsurprising; both were leading members of a liberal coalition within the Democratic party that sought to introduce broad-based legislative reform that included civil rights reform, protecting labor's New Deal gains, and keeping the political power of "big business" in check.[48]

In 1956, the Salk polio vaccine program and the role of drug companies in it came under more intense congressional scrutiny. Troubled by the Public Health Service's mishandling of the polio vaccination program, the House Subcommittee on Intergovernmental Relations, chaired by Representative Lawrence H. Fountain (D-NC), launched an investigation of the program. During the course of its investigation, the subcommittee discovered that several polio vaccine producers had made identical bids to the government for the vaccine contract. Disturbed by what looked like an incidence of collusion, Fountain began an investigation of the pricing practices of vaccine manufacturers. Representative Chet Holifield (D-CA), a member of that subcommittee (and part of the liberal coalition in Congress) recounted to the House in August 1958 that the investigation had disclosed that government agencies throughout the country purchasing polio vaccine had "received literally hundreds of bids which were identical to the fraction of a cent." Even in those few instances where nonidentical bids were found, the investigation had still found evidence of "a price-fixing conspiracy." As a result, polio vaccine prices appeared to be unaffected by conditions of supply and demand, and vaccine manufacturers appeared guilty of violating the antitrust laws.[49]

Following his subcommittee's findings, Fountain pressured the Justice Department to investigate the matter further and in May a federal grand jury in Trenton, New Jersey, concluded that there was sufficient evidence to indict five firms on price-fixing charges. The indicted companies were Eli Lilly & Co., Pitman-Moore (a subsidiary of Allied Laboratories), Wyeth Laboratories (a subsidiary of American Home Products), Merck, Sharp & Dohme, and Parke-Davis & Co.[50] Following the indictment, Fountain's subcommittee unanimously recommended that the Justice Department extend its investigation to determine whether there had been antitrust law violations in the sale of other drugs. For Holifield, illegal price fixing was "far worse when it involves the drugs that are necessary to preserve life and health than when it involves commodities such as cement and gasoline."[51]

The industry's political problems were not limited to vaccine producers. The 1954 Census of Manufacturers identified the antibiotics market as the largest in the pharmaceutical field, with sales of $253 million in the human antibiotics field.[52] The antibiotics field was also one of the most competitive, and conventional economic wisdom led policymakers and the public to assume that competition would drive down prices. Although the price of penicillin had fallen sharply since World War II, the prices of the more recent broad-spectrum antibiotics such as tetracycline had shown no such decline despite the fact that several of the largest firms were producing different version of the drug.[53]

The apparent lack of price competition in the antibiotics market raised concern among legislators.[54] In July 1955, Representative Victor Anfuso (D-NY) proclaimed on the floor of the House that major antibiotic manufacturers were "virtually exercising a monopoly in the field [by] . . . charging the public fantastic prices for antibiotics." Anfuso accused the large antibiotic manufacturers of "fixing prices, and generally pursu[ing] other unfair practices which are . . . driving out competition and pushing out the small firms." Anfuso called on Congress to act either through legislation or by urging "the appropriate authorities to conduct a full-scale investigation of these evil practices."[55]

At the end of 1955, the Federal Trade Commission (FTC) undertook to study the antibiotics industry after Anfuso and other Democrats in Congress threatened to cut the agency's appropriations unless it began an investigation.[56] The FTC was particularly interested in uncovering how much it cost firms to develop and manufacture antibiotics, and determining why the cost of so-called miracle drugs were so high.[57] During its three-year investigation, however, the FTC's focus shifted from an economic study of the antibiotic industry to a police investigation of potential antitrust law violations.[58] By early 1958, the FTC alleged that five pharmaceutical companies were exercising a monopoly in the tetracycline market by maintaining "arbitrary, artificial, non-competitive and rigid" prices.[59]

The congressional and FTC investigations of price-fixing within the drug industry were not isolated instances of government scrutiny of industrial pricing policies. Since the end of World War II, concern about rising inflation and escalating prices for all consumer goods had dominated American politics.[60] In this context, economic New Dealers—schooled in the writings of Gardiner Means—viewed government price controls as a way of curbing inflation, preventing underconsumption, and securing the country's economic prosperity.[61] As part of their effort to rein in excessive

prices, these economic reformers sought to eliminate oligopoly formation, the practice by which a small number of large firms would come to
dominate a market by arranging prices and controlling product supply.
Beginning in 1956 and continuing through 1959, Senator Estes Kefauver
(D-TN), the chair of the Senate Subcommittee on Antitrust and Monopoly,
led an investigation into economic concentration in the automobile, bread,
and steel industries. In each case, Kefauver's investigation focused on the
industry's use of marketing and patents, and its profits and pricing structures. At the end of 1959, prompted by the earlier congressional and FTC
investigations, Kefauver turned his attention to the drug industry (see
chapter 4).[62]

The indictment of the vaccine producers and the FTC's investigation of
the antibiotics industry focused attention on what the trade press referred
to as "the Number One public relations problem in the drug field—the
alleged 'high cost' of medicines."[63] At the same time, it drew attention to
the profitability of the American drug industry. In 1959, the FTC and the
Securities and Exchange Commission (SEC) reported that the drug industry's profits as a percentage of sales averaged 10.3 percent, compared to
average profits of 4.8 percent in all manufacturing industries. When profits
were calculated as a percentage of net worth, the figures were even more
striking, with the drug industry averaging 18.1 percent, compared to 10.5
percent for all manufacturing industries.[64]

The drug industry's profitability served as a powerful rhetorical coun-
terpoint to the apparently high prices consumers were forced to pay for
prescription drugs. As Representative Holifield noted to his congressional colleagues in May 1958, "amounts paid by consumers for drugs
have increased tremendously in recent years. It is estimated that sales
of prescription drugs, which were less than $200 million in the last year
prior to World War II, amounted to $1.7 billion in 1957." Moreover,
citing a *Business Week* survey, Holifield stated that drug manufacturers
"made an average return after taxes of more than 20 percent on their
net assets . . . [and] more than 10 percent of sales. . . . This was double
the average for all industry groups and the highest return of any reporting group."[65]

To be sure, after World War II, the introduction of large numbers of
new prescription drugs had led to rising health care costs. In 1940, for
example, Americans spent approximately $4 billion (4 percent of GNP—
gross national product—or $29.60 per capita) for health and medical care;
in 1955, that figure had more than quadrupled to $17.7 billion (or 4.4
percent of GNP and $105 per capita); and by 1960, health care expenditures

totaled $26.9 billion (5.3 percent of GNP and $146 per capita). Although this increase in Americans' health care expenditures was attributable to several factors, including population growth and changes in the level of use and quality of medical services, critics after the war focused their attention on the rising *cost* of medical care. Those criticisms were not necessarily misplaced; between 1940 and 1950, and between 1950 and 1960, price increases accounted, on average, for 32 percent and 50 percent, respectively, of the total increase in health care expenditures, while population changes accounted for just 11.5 percent and 21.8 percent, respectively, of that total.[66]

Although the average annual price index for hospital, physician, dentist, and other professional fees (so-called medical care services) increased from 49.2 in 1950 to 74.9 in 1960 (which correlated to an average annual percentage change of 4.2 percent between 1950 and 1955, and of 4.4 percent between 1955 and 1960), the cost of prescription drugs remained fairly stable. The consumer price index for prescription drugs over the same period increased from 92.6 in 1950 to 115.3 in 1960, which corresponded to an average annual percentage change for prescription drug prices of 1.9 percent between 1950 and 1955, and 2 percent between 1955 and 1960.[67]

Despite the stability of prescription drug prices relative to other health care and consumer goods, government and public concern about health care costs focused on prescription drugs. In May 1958, for example, the Citizens' Committee for Children of New York City published the findings of its study on the impact of prescription drugs on the family budget. The committee found that patients suffering from arthritis, rheumatism, cancer, heart disease, and tuberculosis "often have great difficulty meeting the cost of medicines essential to survival or alleviation of pain." Citing the cost of brand-name drugs as presenting a "real hardship" to low- and middle-income families, the committee believed that patients would be able to buy drugs "at a fraction of the cost" if physicians used a drug's generic name when writing a prescription.[68] The attention focused on prescription drug prices was in no small part due to the government investigations into allegations of price-fixing among vaccine and antibiotics manufacturers. These investigations underscored to government officials and the public alike just how little they understood about the economics of the pharmaceutical industry.

By the end of 1958, the trade press warned the industry that the "drug price probe virus" was spreading on Capitol Hill.[69] For example, just a few months earlier, in August, Senators Ralph Yarborough (D-TX) and Warren G. Magnuson (D-WA) had argued on the Senate floor that "exorbitant" drug prices justified increasing Social Security payments.[70] As *FDC Reports* noted, "injection of the 'drug price' issue into the Senate floor debate on an entirely different subject indicates the way in which the FTC antibiotic report and complaint will be used in the political arena." The trade journal warned that the recent indictments and FTC complaint pointed to the possibility that drug prices "might be used as the jumping off point for general attacks on the costs of medical care, with every-body—doctors and hospitals as well as pharmaceutical manufacturers and pharmacists—included in the target area."[71]

By aligning the alleged indiscretions of the pharmaceutical industry and high drug costs with the need to secure health care coverage for the poor and for seniors, Democratic health care reformers succeeded in pulling the pharmaceutical industry into the already politicized arena of health care policy. Although the Eisenhower administration made only minimal forays into health policy through the mid-1950s, by the late 1950s health care reformers were pushing Congress to add health coverage to Social Security pensions.[72] By pulling prescription drug prices into the debates over health care coverage, pharmaceutical reformers gave the matter of the industry's pricing policies much greater political traction. Less than a month later, citing the role of high drug costs in contributing to the growing costs of health care, Senator George Smathers (D-FL) was joined by several of his Democratic colleagues when he submitted a Senate reso-lution authorizing the Select Committee on Small Business to conduct an investigation of prescription drug prices. Smathers charged "that the American people, who are fortunate in having the most advanced medi-cines and drugs in the world, share alike the doubtful distinction of paying the world's highest premium for these basic human necessities."[73]

At the same time that the regulatory agencies and Congress were con-cerned with prescription drug pricing, a group of physicians was urging them to investigate the drug industry's advertising practices. Beginning in the mid-1950s, several prominent academic physicians had begun attack-ing drug advertising as excessive, misleading, and often inaccurate.[74] In particular, physicians were frustrated by the large quantity of advertise-ments they received through the mail and the hard-selling detail men that came through their offices. Both practices they deemed were waste-ful and expensive and contributed to the high cost of drugs.[75] Certainly, large research-based drug firms spent significant amounts of their income on the marketing of their products. In 1958, for example, twenty of the largest drug firms reported spending 24 percent of their sales income on marketing compared to between 6.4 percent and 9.5 percent on research.[76]

Leading the charge against "false advertising to the doctor" was Harry Dowling, the chair of the AMA's Section on Experimental Medicine and Therapeutics. In a 1957 *Journal of the American Medical Association* editorial, Dowling called drug advertisements "flamboyant . . . incessant . . . [and] without question confusing." Dowling accused drug firms of diverting energy (and thus money) "from the pathway that leads to the greatest benefit to patients" to the pathway that generated greater profits. Calling on his medical colleagues to "reject misleading information and repudiate those who purvey it," Dowling also charged physicians with "us[ing] every means to make our opinion known" on the matter of pharmaceutical advertising.[77]

At the AMA's annual meeting in June 1957, Representative Oren Harris (D-AR), the chairman of the House Committee on Interstate and Foreign Commerce, noted that physicians' complaints about drug advertising had reached Capitol Hill.[78] By the fall of that year, Representative John A. Blatnik's (D-MN) Legal and Monetary Affairs subcommittee had broadened the scope of its investigation of drug advertising in the proprietary (over-the-counter) field and began investigating the advertising practices of prescription drug firms. Blatnik's subcommittee was concerned, in particular, with the promotional strategies used by drug manufacturers to persuade physicians to prescribe their products.

The 1956 FTC and congressional investigations of the pharmaceutical industry brought home to the industry its mounting public relations problem. In the early 1950s the industry had shied away from directly engaging in public relations, but by mid-decade the industry's leadership realized that its professional relations and scientific network-building activities were not enough to stem the turning political tide. Rather, the industry, in concert with the other members of the health care team, needed a public relations program that would explain to the public the basis for health care costs in general, and prescription drug prices in particular.

CRAFTING A PUBLIC RELATIONS PROGRAM

As early as 1953, the executives of several firms had discussed the need for an industrywide public relations campaign. The trade association, the American Pharmaceutical Manufacturers Association (APMA), published *A Primer of Public Relations for the Pharmaceutical Industry*, which guided individual firms on how to build an effective public relations program.[79] An important element of a successful public relations strategy was, the primer suggested, to avoid the "sensationalism and misleading [press] reports" that the medical profession was railing against. In order to do this, it was necessary for drug firms to become active participants in the making of pharmaceutical publicity by developing professional relationships with science writers and journalists and by handling "publicity in a way that scrupulously respects all the facts, mentioning the limitations as well as advantages of new products."[80]

A year later, in 1954, Theodore Klumpp warned a meeting of drug industry and pharmacy executives that the pharmaceutical industry confronted three problems regarding public perception: "In the first place is that the purchaser can't tell the value and professional content of a pill by looking at it. In the second place the customer doesn't want it and doesn't get any pleasure from it. And, finally, it just isn't human nature to feel deeply grateful for having been spared a perilous illness that he knew wasn't going to happen." Although "in the old days when patients were snatched from death's door after a period of mortal peril and suffering, there was less complaint about the cost of medical care. Let's not forget," Klumpp reminded his audience, "that the drug treatment of an illness seems cheapest when there are no drugs known to treat it."[81] Because of these issues, Klumpp proclaimed, there was a "crying need for the industry to tell its story—which has never been adequately told, and to show the public that the cost of medication is not high."[82]

Despite this earlier recognition that an industrywide public relations approach was needed, the industry's public relations efforts remained uncoordinated and decidedly lackluster. Late in 1955, the trade press explained part of the reason for this, noting that "while almost everybody agreed on the need for an overall PR approach no one pinpointed the specific objectives and targets for such a program."[83] By the spring of 1956, however, it was obvious to the industry's leadership that the most pressing public relations problem was the public and Congress's lack of understanding about the work of the drug industry. The recent congressional scrutiny had made clear to industry leaders the need for educating Congress and the public about the basis for prescription drug prices. In particular, the industry needed to explain that the final price of a prescription drug included not just manufacturing costs but also distribution costs and the dispensing pharmacist's professional service fee. These same events indicated that as the drug industry's points of contact with the public, pharmacists and physicians also had to be taught "how to tell the drug PR story" to customers and patients. According to the trade press, pharmacists would often try to answer customers' complaints about prescription costs by blaming them on the prices charged by manufacturers.[84] Industry leaders also suspected that physicians were shifting the blame for high medical costs to pharmaceutical manufacturers as a way of taking their own fees and practices out of the spotlight.[85]

In response, the industry's two trade associations—the APMA and the ADMA—created an industry public relations organization in the spring of 1956. The priority of the Health News Institute (HNI) was to educate the public on the role of all members of the health care team in distributing to the consumer the drugs developed by the pharmaceutical companies. After a year in operation, HNI's director (and former editor of *Newsweek*), Chet Shaw, asserted that in order to successfully tell the industry's story, the industry needed to be more forthcoming about the facts of the business. In particular, the public needed to be educated on the industry's "continuous and relentless struggle against obsolescence" and about how much money the industry spent annually on research. Although, Shaw noted, "We've done a lot of talking about an estimated $100 million . . . we'd be hard put to document it. What if someone questioned it—someone whose voice we couldn't afford to ignore?"[86]

Shaw cited the industry's use of the oft-quoted study of the comparative cost of pneumonia before and after the advent of sulfa drugs. Here, Shaw referred to a study made by a Philadelphia physician who calculated that a case of pneumonia in a Philadelphia hospital in 1927 cost an average of $358 with a hospitalization period of five weeks. Accounting for the loss of earnings incurred during the hospitalization and convalescent period, the total cost of the illness was approximately $1,000. In 1953, however, the average duration of a case of pneumonia was two weeks, with no period of convalescence required. With most cases treated at home with antibiotics that ranged in price from $15.12 to $29.68, depending on the antibiotic used, and considerably less lost earnings, the example of pneumonia was used by the industry to show the great economic savings made by drugs.[87] In addition, Shaw continued, the industry had "told and retold how the price of penicillin has declined 99 percent." What the industry now needed "is the same idea with a new look—for instance, some examples of price reductions that you have made voluntarily, without the goad of competition, and while you still retained the patent on the compound."[88]

To aid with the industry's fact gathering and dissemination, the HNI commissioned Bertrand Fox, the director of research for the Harvard Business School, to conduct an independent economic study of the pharmaceutical industry. When Merck's president, John T. Connor, announced plans for the study at an APMA meeting in December 1957, he argued that the industry would not be able to do an effective job of informing the public about its activities unless it had specific facts on hand to substantiate its claims. Connor was concerned that with the FTC's ongoing investigation of the antibiotics industry, the government agency had "at its command many more facts about the industry than we ourselves possess." Believing that the FTC investigation would not be the last governmental or congressional inquiry into the industry, Connor asserted that the ability "to communicate to the public the facts about the industry and its accomplishments . . . is likely to be the price of survival of the pharmaceutical industry as we know it."[89]

To disseminate information about the industry and its work, the HNI's public relations program included organizing symposiums for newspaper editors and science writers in which the "facts of the drug industry" could be relayed and discussed; publication of a booklet titled *Facts about Pharmacy and Pharmaceuticals*, distributed to the press, schools, and community organizations; and speaker's kits containing industry facts, statistics, and "quotable quotes" for ready reference for any industry representative preparing speeches on the drug industry.[90] In each case, the HNI promoted telling of "the drug story," which explained the high level of risk and research expense involved in drug development, the health care savings made possible by new drug developments, and the therapeutic gains already achieved by the American public thanks to the innovations of the American drug industry.

The industry-funded Health Information Foundation (HIF) served as another informational resource for the drug industry.[91] The HIF was established in 1950 as a nonprofit educational organization by several leading pharmaceutical, drug, and allied companies including Merck, Eli Lilly, Johnson & Johnson, Sharp & Dohme, G. D. Searle, and American Home Products. With an annual budget of a half million dollars, its mandate was to conduct research on the social and economic aspects of health care, to publicize the results of that research, and to increase public understanding of the health care system. Although the HIF's board of directors was composed of the presidents of major pharmaceutical and chemical companies, nonindustry people staffed the foundation. For the first four years, the foundation was led by Admiral W. H. P. Blandy, with Kenneth Williamson, a former administrator with the American Hospital Association, as its executive secretary. Following Blandy's death in 1954, George Bugbee, the executive director of the American Hospital Association and a respected health policymaker, assumed the presidency of the HIF. In 1952, Blandy had hired the medical sociologist and leading health services researcher Odin Anderson to serve as the foundation's director of research. Under Anderson, the HIF conducted extensive research throughout the 1950s on the status of health services in the United States and abroad.[92]

Although the HIF was explicitly *not* a public relations vehicle for the drug industry, the research produced by the foundation benefited the industry's public relations activities by helping the industry identify the targets for those activities. In 1955, for example, the results of an interview survey of the public's attitudes toward health care problems conducted for the HIF by the University of Chicago's National Opinion Research Center revealed that the public still knew very little about the work and accomplishments of the drug industry. The survey also revealed that while the industry's research story was getting across to the public, the public did not understand the story of drug distribution and its costs.[93]

The following year, taking heed of the survey's findings and hoping to counter the public's lack of understanding about prescription drug prices, Parke-Davis & Co. launched a series of advertisements that defended the costs of prescription drugs and of medical care more generally. These advertisements appeared in *Reader's Digest, Newsweek, Life,* the *Saturday Evening Post,* and other major newspapers and magazines. By emphasizing the increase in life expectancy and the reduction in mortality and morbidity associated with infectious and other diseases, and by highlighting the reductions in hospital costs made possible by prompt treatment with drugs such as antibiotics, the campaign asserted, "more than ever before, prompt and proper medical care may well be one of the biggest bargains of your life!" A 1957 advertisement in the same campaign suggested that the next time you are sick and you question the price of the drug prescribed by your physician, just "think what the prescription may do for you . . . get you well, get you back on the job sooner and possibly even save your life." For this reason, the Parke-Davis advertisement continued, "when you consider what today's more effective medical care can do for you and your family—in saving lives, speeding recoveries, preventing complications, easing worries—you appreciate what good value you're getting."[94]

Adopting a different public relations strategy, Pfizer began publishing its annual report to stockholders in the *New York Times* in 1956. In its first year, Pfizer's annual report reached more than 3.5 million readers, appearing as a sixteen-page supplement in the March 23 issue of the Sunday *Times,* followed two weeks later by publication in the Sunday *Chicago Tribune* and the *Los Angeles Times.* The company hoped that by showing how Pfizer turned "its scientific knowledge and business resources to the task of creating the raw materials of human betterment," the widely circulated annual report would "convey an intimate picture" of the company and of a modern American business enterprise more generally.[95]

While individual firms and the HNI focused on telling "the drug story" to the general public, the NPC committed to educating pharmacists and physicians. In an effort to persuade physicians to stop shifting the blame for medical costs, the drug industry launched a professional relations campaign targeted at educating physicians—through advertisements and the work of detail men—about drug costs. The goal of this campaign was twofold: first, it explained that drug costs had increased proportionately less than any other segment of health care costs, and that by reducing patients' hospital stays drugs actually reduced the overall cost of health care. Second, the industry's campaign emphasized that physicians shared the same interest as the industry when it came to criticisms of health care costs.[96] Any attack on health care costs, the industry warned, was an attack on the capitalist system of medical care. Thus by attacking drug costs, physicians were effectively threatening the stability of the health care system—the very system that allowed them to treat patients autonomously. By situating the critique of drug costs in this way, the industry made a persuasive argument, as physicians were embroiled in an ongoing battle to preserve their autonomy and defeat health care reformers seeking to nationalize health care in the United States. In this way, the industry was able to draw on the medical profession's long-standing concern about the expanding role of the federal government in medicine.[97]

TOO LITTLE, TOO LATE

Despite mobilization of an industrywide public and professional relations campaign, the industry's efforts were neither extensive enough nor early enough to quell the burgeoning public and congressional critique. At the December 1957 APMA meeting, the *Saturday Evening Post*'s executive editor, Robert Fuoss, warned that things were likely going to get worse for the industry. Fuoss warned that because the public was fascinated by articles about medicine, there would continue to be extensive press coverage of the pharmaceutical industry. "The very fact that millions of people can identify their personal interest with a flu shot, a polio vaccine, a tranquilizer, a possible chemical solution to the cancer problem," Fuoss noted, "means only that, henceforth, there is an entirely new dimension to your corporate enterprises," that of public relations.

According to Fuoss, this heightened public interest was already manifesting signs of danger for the industry. Recounting the kind of letters he had been receiving over the past several months, Fuoss summed up the public's critique of the industry:

> A lot of people are complaining about the high cost of new drug products. My mail also shows that druggists are griping about the vast proliferation of drug products that they are forced to stock; that some doctors and some science writers feel you are exerting too much pressure to win too rapid recognition for products in which your investment is great; that some ordinary folks are pushing for a tougher food and drug law. And . . . at least three letters this past fall . . . flatly accused your industry of collusion to create a flu scare in order to sell unnecessary flu vaccine.

The lesson to be learned from his inbox, Fuoss concluded, is "that as your industry moves closer to the public interest, so, too, do you become ever more vulnerable to the slings and arrows of outrageous fortune."[98]

In a speech to the same industry audience, the Washington antitrust litigator H. Thomas Austern predicted an acceleration in government and congressional investigations into the industry's activities. Like Fuoss, Austern regarded the industry as a victim of its own success, citing as the reasons for the increased political attention "the personalized, constantly growing public interest in drugs—derived in no small measure from your own achievements. The expenditure of large sums of public money for drugs needed for the armed services and other agencies. The acclaim, as well as the claims, for each new discovery." Austern also credited the political climate, where anyone "interested in posing as a guardian of the public health and pocketbook" could "make charges . . . pursue investigations, and . . . instigate attacks."[99] Just a few months later, the president of both Schering Corp. and the APMA, Francis C. Brown, repeated the warning at the APMA's annual meeting. He blamed the increasing government attention to the drug industry on "the fact that health is politically popular. Our industry has necessarily grown and prospered as it has brought out of its laboratories to the world important new pharmaceutical products." This interest, he continued, "is a symptom of our maturity."[100]

If the political attention on the industry was a symptom of its maturity, the merger of the industry's two trade associations—the APMA and ADMA—and the creation of the Pharmaceutical Manufacturers Association (PMA) in the spring of 1958 signaled the beginning of the pharmaceutical industry's transformation from a disparate collection of manufacturers with overlapping political and economic interests into a unified and activist trade association. Although prior to the merger the two groups had overlapping membership, the activities and priorities of the two groups often differed. In particular, the APMA included a greater number of smaller manufacturers, whose political and economic interests sometimes diverged from those of the larger manufacturers, which dominated the ADMA's membership.

During the spring of 1956, at the height of the government's investigations into vaccine and antibiotic manufacturers, the APMA and ADMA initiated informal discussions of a merger. Given the heightened attention on the industry, the leadership of the two groups were particularly concerned that having "two legislative or legal groups speaking for our industry," which often failed to present a united front, was having a detrimental impact on the industry.[101] Although it took two more years before the merger was formalized, the establishment of the PMA in July 1958 created "a single voice for the pharmaceutical industry," which would act as a united front for the industry "in its relations with the medical profession, pharmacy, and related professions, with other scientific organizations, with government agencies, and with the public." The unification also brought consolidation of the industry's finances, with the new trade association owning about $400,000 of assets and with potential annual income of more than $350,000.[102]

With the establishment of the PMA, however, a clear distinction was drawn between those firms that engaged in innovative research and marketed patented and thus, brand-name prescription drugs (eligible for membership), and those firms that lacked any commitment to original research (excluded from membership) and marketed only unpatented drugs or generic versions of off-patent brand-name drugs. Because small firms usually lacked the capital necessary to engage in innovative research, the PMA consisted mostly of medium- and large-sized firms. In 1960, for example, of the more than 1,300 firms that made up the U.S. drug industry, just 140 of them belonged to the PMA. The PMA's member firms, however, produced approximately 95 percent of all the prescription drug sales in the United States, with twenty of those member firms accounting for 80 percent of those sales.[103]

During its first year of operation, the PMA was led by George F. Smith of Johnson & Johnson, who worked in the position unpaid, and a board of directors staffed by executives of the leading drug firms. The PMA's board soon realized, however, that the task of leading the trade association should be a full-time paid position, and that the new president should serve as "a spokesman for the industry." Reflecting—and institutionalizing—

the industry's commitment to building supportive relationships with the medical profession, the PMA board elected an AMA old-timer as its first full-time paid president. Austin Smith had joined the AMA staff after completing his residency in the mid-1940s, serving as editor of the *Journal of the American Medical Association* from 1949 to 1959.

Despite the unification of the industry, government and congressional scrutiny of the pharmaceutical industry escalated through the end of the decade. The limited success of the industry's public relations campaign hit home when, in October and November 1958, *Consumer Reports* published two articles on the high cost of prescription drugs, which criticized the drug industry and called for the federal government to launch a comprehensive investigation of the industry.[104] In November, Senator Estes Kefauver (D-TN), the chair of the Senate Subcommittee on Antitrust and Monopoly, promised Congress that his subcommittee would begin an investigation of the pricing structure and policies of the pharmaceutical industry in the next session of Congress. Ten months later, Senator Smathers, frustrated by "the extremely high cost of antibiotics and other medicines and drugs which must be borne by every American family," and committed to discovering "the extent to which pharmaceutical houses are ballooning drugs costs," echoed the call for Congress to "undertake to discover whether the naked law of supply and demand has forced upon the needy group of Americans who are ill . . . an unreasonable financial strain for an inseparable human need." Smathers congratulated Kefauver on his plan to investigate the high cost of drugs and promised that if Kefauver's committee were too busy to go forward with its investigation, then the Small Business Committee (of which Smathers was the chair) would readily undertake the investigation.[105] Smathers's offer was unnecessary, however. Four months later, on December 7, 1959—"the pharmaceutical industry's own 'Pearl Harbor Day' "—Kefauver's investigation of administered prices in the drug industry began.[106]

CONCLUSION

While industry executives believed the public and political attention focused on the pharmaceutical industry at the end of the 1950s was due, essentially, to a lack of understanding on the part of the public, Congress, and government about all that the pharmaceutical industry did and how much it cost the industry to achieve it, the reason for the industry's burgeoning crisis is, unsurprisingly, more complex. To be sure, the drug industry was not entirely innocent of all the charges arrayed against it in the late 1950s. As George F. Smith, then president of the PMA, admitted to an industry audience in 1958, "it is nevertheless true that a few in our own group have been guilty of questionable promotional practices."[107] Yet four factors in particular help account for the timing and intensity of the critiques against the pharmaceutical industry at the end of the 1950s.

First, by the end of the 1950s Americans were spending more on prescription drugs than they had in any previous decade. Despite the fact that the therapeutic arsenal available to physicians and patients before the 1950s was significantly smaller—and less effective—than that available to them in the 1950s, Americans did not expect to have to pay more for increasingly efficacious drugs. Theirs was a consumer culture in which a new innovation begat competitor products, which in turn begat a reduction in the prices paid for those innovations. Seeing little difference between the pharmaceutical economy and the consumer goods economy, the American consumer expected the typical laws of the marketplace to apply also to drugs, so that every time a new drug was joined by a succession of similar (me-too) drugs, they expected a marked reduction in the drug cost.[108]

Second, health care costs were already a subject of intense political attention by the time health care reformers pulled drug industry pricing policies into the center of their reform efforts. This meant that there was a ready-made, organized, and highly motivated lobby in place to attack prescription drug prices.

Third, the government's newfound interest in the pharmaceutical industry in the 1950s occurred in the midst of the government's postwar commitment to Keynesian economics. In a measure to boost American consumption and ensure the country's continued economic growth, the government sought to stamp out the uncompetitive practices of business more generally. The FTC and the Fountain subcommittee investigations of charges of price-fixing among pharmaceutical firms were thus part of this broader critique of and effort to wipe out monopolistic practices in the American marketplace.

Finally, the pharmaceutical industry's failure, in the mid-1950s, to grasp the extent of its escalating public and political relations problems helps explain why the public and congressional scrutiny of the industry exploded as it did at the end of the decade. For despite the early warning signs that Congress and the public were growing increasingly disgruntled, the industry was in general slow to respond to the emerging political trouble. Rather than engaging in specific strategies to defend itself and undercut the congressional and regulatory challenges facing it, the pharmaceutical industry preferred instead to let its past therapeutic achievements stand as its defense and focus its efforts on curtailing the medical profession's critique.

By the end of the decade, however, the politicization of prescription drugs had made starkly clear to the industry's leadership that it operated not just in the realms of science and commerce but also in the public realm of health care politics and practice. While its scientific networks might ensure the continued innovation and economic growth of the industry, without an equal commitment to bolstering its public image and developing productive alliances with health care practitioners, the industry recognized that it would suffer politically. This fact, and the political significance of the relationships the industry had developed with academic researchers and physicians during the 1940s and 1950s, were nowhere clearer than during Senator Kefauver's investigation of the pricing and business practices of the American drug industry.

PART II

Allied against Reform

4 Cold War Alliances

Kefauver's Bid for Pharmaceutical Reform

> Now that we are forced to take stock, we find that our
> industry has grown into a significant national asset, these daily
> contributions to the war against disease are well known . . .
> but whose potential contributions to the world struggle against
> communism are only beginning to become apparent.
> —JOHN T. CONNOR, president, Merck & Co., 1959[1]

By the time Senator Estes Kefauver launched his Senate Subcommittee on Antitrust and Monopoly investigation into the alleged administered pricing in the drug industry in December 1959, the American drug industry was finally taking its political troubles seriously. As Kefauver indicated in his opening remarks, the aim of the hearings were to determine whether the antitrust laws as applied to the drug industry were adequate "and, if not, to devise specific remedial legislation."[2] At the center of Kefauver's concern was the purportedly high price of prescription drugs and what seemed to him to be an absence of price competition in the industry. Kefauver was concerned that, rather than drug prices being determined by the market (and thus by fluctuations in supply and demand), instead they were being set by the companies that held patents—and thus, a monopoly—on specific drugs.

Through his investigation of the drug industry, Kefauver focused his investigation on the pricing policies and marketing strategies employed by firms in the research, development, and distribution of four types of drugs: antibiotics, corticosteroids, tranquilizers, and oral antidiabetic drugs. Kefauver's research into the pharmaceutical industry—and the bill he subsequently introduced in Congress—was the first attempt to regulate the price of prescription drugs, earlier drug legislation having focused on regulating the accuracy of the industry's advertising and product labeling claims and on the safety of its products.[3] Moreover, the Kefauver hearings marked the beginning of what would become two decades' worth of congressional investigation into the business and pricing practices of the

American drug industry, the focal point of a pharmaceutical reform movement, led by Democratic congressional reformers and with the support of labor leaders, consumer groups, and patient advocates, to rein in the perceived excesses of the drug industry and force a reduction in prescription drug prices.

In reaction to Kefauver's investigation, the drug industry mobilized the scientific networks and medical alliances it had developed during the previous decades. As Austin Smith, the president of the Pharmaceutical Manufacturers Association (PMA), announced to an industry audience in 1959, a successful defense against pharmaceutical reform depended on the "industry using all its talents and the help of its friends, present and acquired, to pursue objectives in which there is a mutuality of interest." Industry's "friends in medicine"—and specifically their shared concern over the increasing role of government in medicine—were particularly critical to this task.[4]

At the same time, Smith called on the industry to tell its story to the American public. Smith believed that educating the public on the "technics, facts, and actions" of the industry and helping the public to "develop a healthy respect for the free enterprise system" would be the industry's best defense against its critics.[5] A year later, Smith's words were echoed by William Graham, the chairman of the PMA's board of trustees: "I am convinced that the continued success, in fact even the very existence of our industry in its present form, depends upon our demonstrating, even more effectively than we have to date, the benefits of the competitive system in our industry. We must bring the public to understand that this competitive system of drug research, manufacture, and distribution, works more to the benefit of society than could any other system." In particular, the industry's leadership sought during the Kefauver hearings (and afterward) to promote the industry as a critical national asset in the global war against communism. As Graham asserted in his chairman's address to the PMA in 1960, "Probably through no other industry can the superiority of our American competitive system be demonstrated so impressively."[6] Thus, in the midst of the Cold War, the pharmaceutical industry hailed itself as a model of American free enterprise and sought, through the development of more and more products and through donations of drugs and other pharmaceutical supplies to aid missions in the Third World, to disseminate its message to those developing nations deemed susceptible to communism.

The industry argued that any challenge to the system of free enterprise not only threatened the country's international fight against communism but, potentially worse, invited socialism into the domestic political economy. Indeed, the industry's primary defense strategy was to assert that the government's relentless encroachment on private enterprise, particularly in the health care field, signaled America's ready sprint toward socialized medicine—a situation, the pharmaceutical industry and the medical profession warned, that every American should fear.

By packaging the system of drug development and regulation as the marker of free enterprise, the drug industry sought to win the support both of organized medicine and of the public and to derail Kefauver's efforts to increase the government's control over the drug industry. The drug industry's Cold War strategy was neither novel nor unique. The industry drew from and reinforced the pervasive anticommunist political culture of the 1950s and early 1960s, which, as one historian of Cold War science describes, "took perpetual U.S.-Soviet conflict for granted and invoked anticommunism as a shorthand to simplify and avoid the consideration of complex political issues."[7] In every political arena, "conservatives used anticommunism not only to dismiss the prospect of reform but to impugn the motives and loyalties of reformers."[8] The drug industry's Cold War political strategy was part and parcel of this political and cultural milieu.

FREE ENTERPRISE UNDER ATTACK: THE KEFAUVER HEARINGS

Kefauver came to drug prices having already conducted lengthy investigations into administered pricing in the auto, steel, and bread industries. Since 1957, Kefauver had chaired the Subcommittee on Antitrust and Monopoly of the Senate Committee of the Judiciary, where he was aided by thirty-eight subcommittee staffers, the most influential of whom were John Blair, a Federal Trade Commission (FTC) economist who served as Kefauver's chief economist; Dr. Blair's former FTC colleague and fellow economist Irene Till; and Paul Rand Dixon, an FTC lawyer who served as Kefauver's staff director and chief counsel. Having both been involved in the FTC's investigation of the antibiotics industry earlier in the decade, Till and Blair convinced Kefauver in the fall of 1958 that the subcommittee should next investigate the drug industry's pricing structures.[9]

Through their investigation of the American drug industry, Kefauver and his staffers sought to determine whether or not prescription drug prices were reasonable and thus whether price competition existed in the drug market. To establish this, during the hearings Kefauver sought answers to three fundamental questions. The first was how drug companies determined the price they would charge for a drug. Using data provided by the companies themselves, together with the testimony of those responsible for purchasing drugs for the military or for hospital pharmacies, Kefauver and his staff accused firms of marking up drugs as much as 7,000 percent from their production costs. The second question was why many drugs could be purchased more cheaply abroad than they could in the United States. Was it, as Kefauver believed, because other countries did not grant product patents on drugs, only a much weaker form of protection—process patents—thus avoiding the creation of a monopoly by individual patent holders? The third question posed by Kefauver was why the drug industry was able to make such high profits—up to 20 percent of sales—significantly higher, he charged, than any other U.S. industry.[10] To Kefauver, these profits were evidence that firms holding drug patents exercised excessive control of the market. Kefauver believed these firms were able to set the price of drugs as high as they liked because of their monopoly, making drugs prohibitively expensive to patients throughout the country.

After two years of investigative hearings, Kefauver and his staffers decided the evidence proved that drug companies were able to retain a monopoly in the pharmaceutical market and secure their high profits through three major mechanisms. The first was the government's granting of product patents with seventeen years of market exclusivity to the developers of new drugs. The second was the expense and intensity of firms' advertising and sales efforts to physicians. Kefauver singled out the work of "detail men" as particularly troubling. These were the pharmaceutical sales representatives who regularly visited physicians' offices presenting physicians with prescribing information about their company's drugs.[11] Kefauver argued that not only was detailing costly, but drug companies attempted to pass the activity off as educational rather than the advertising he believed it clearly was.[12] Kefauver also saw the fact that advertisements failed to include details about side effects and contraindications, and that they emphasized the brand name rather than the generic name, as contributing to the drug companies' "duping" of the busy physician. The third mechanism, Kefauver claimed, was the ability of companies—through their marketing activities—to persuade physicians to prescribe using brand names rather than generic drugs. It was the physicians' dependence on brand names that helped enforce a drug company's monopoly, Kefauver charged.

Thus, for Kefauver the key to reducing the price of prescription drugs and improving the nation's health was to limit the power of drug patents and trademarks. To this end, after the conclusion of his investigative hearings, Kefauver and his staffers prepared a bill that sought to curtail what Kefauver perceived to be the more "malignant" practices of the drug industry. In particular, the bill, S. 1552 (and its companion bill in the House, H.R. 6245), sought to eliminate the industry's "excessive" promotional practices and its use of patents and cross-licensing agreements between drug firms to create monopolies that brought the firms high profits while denying patients lifesaving drugs.

Four of the major provisions of S. 1552 called for a revision of the patent law such that companies granted a patent would have only three years of market exclusivity as opposed to the standard seventeen; patent-holders would be forced to cross-license their patents to other qualified manufacturers after three years for a fixed royalty fee of 8 percent; only one trademark or brand name (granted the original patent-holder) would be permitted per drug product; and, in a measure to limit the number of "me-too" drugs on the market, Kefauver called for patents to be awarded only to those drugs that had a significantly different molecular structure and that had significantly greater therapeutic effect than other drugs already on the market.

The remaining provisions of S. 1552, though less contentious than the patent provisions, sought to increase the safety of prescription drugs and to increase competition in the drug field by extending the government's authority over drug development, distribution, and practice. To improve the safety of drugs, S. 1552 required all drug manufacturers to be licensed by the FDA.[13] In order to retain their licenses, manufacturers were to meet strict standards of quality control, to be determined by FDA inspectors who would periodically visit manufacturing plants. The bill also granted the FDA authority to withdraw any new drug application at any time if it believed a drug showed signs of toxicity. For drugs already on the market, S. 1552 required the secretary of the Department of Health, Education, and Welfare (HEW) annually to publish a list of harmful prescription drugs, and called for all antibiotics to be certified by the FDA for quality, strength, and purity before being released on the market. The bill also required that before the FDA could approve a new drug for marketing, it must be proven to be effective as well as safe; as the current Food, Drug, and Cosmetic Act stood, a firm had only to show that its drug was safe before it could be approved. The final safety provision of Kefauver's bill mandated that all drug advertisements contain information about a drug's side effects and contraindications.[14]

To increase competition and make it easier for small firms to enter the pharmaceutical market, Kefauver sought to encourage physicians to prescribe by generic name rather than brand (or trade) name. Seeing the complexity of generic names—especially when compared to the simplicity of brand names—as a significant deterrent to physicians prescribing by generic name, Kefauver's bill gave the secretary of HEW the authority to review and revise all current generic names and establish new ones on the basis of usefulness and simplicity. At the same time, however, the bill called for a drug's generic name to be featured in equal prominence to the drug's brand name on all drug labels, advertisements, and promotional material.[15]

Although the patent provisions of S. 1552 were the most radical, taken together, the provisions of Kefauver's bill promised to reform the system of drug development, distribution, and practice, reduce the drug industry's profits, and give the federal government greater authority over the practices of both the industry and the medical profession. Kefauver introduced S. 1552 to the Subcommittee on Antitrust and Monopoly on April 12, 1961, and on March 4, 1962, a slightly revised version of Kefauver's bill reached the Senate.

During both the investigative and legislative hearings, the major strategy adopted by the pharmaceutical industry to defend itself against Kefauver's charges was three-pronged and built on the scientific networks, medical alliance building, and public relations efforts of the previous decade. First, the industry attempted to sell Congress on the centrality of the drug industry to America's ongoing battle with communism. For each class of drug, the industry emphasized the effectiveness of the free enterprise system in motivating American drug firms to repeatedly innovate new drugs, to promote competition within the industry, and to foster both American health and economic growth. Second, the industry hoped to tie the industry's strategy of defending the system of free enterprise with the medical profession's war against socialized medicine, thus making a political ally of an already well-organized and strong medical lobby. And third, the industry launched a massive public relations campaign that sought to tell the drug industry's story—and sell free enterprise—to the American public.

"HEALTH FOR PEACE": PHARMACEUTICALS AS FOREIGN POLICY

Throughout the hearings, the drug industry and its supporters drew on the rhetoric of the Cold War to promote its cause. This approach took advantage of rhetoric already in use by legislators who for several years had argued that prescription drugs were necessary weapons for winning over the people of underdeveloped and undecided nations in capitalism's fight against communism. Before turning to the drug industry's defense during the Kefauver hearings, let us first consider some of these earlier Cold War arguments in support of the U.S. drug industry.

After the Soviet Union's surprise launching of Sputnik in October 1957, American policymakers feared the Soviets were going to surpass Americans in all things technological and economic. For pharmaceutical industry executives and policymakers, the concern was not that the Soviet Union would jump ahead of the United States in a pharmaceutical arms race, or that there would even be a drug race—after all, noted an analyst of Soviet medical research in November 1957, "Russia has no medical sputnik up its sleeve"—but rather that the Soviets would use their medical personnel, know-how, technologies, and drugs to capture the support of people in underdeveloped countries.[16]

Beginning as early as 1957, legislators argued in Congress and before industry audiences that drugs—and by extension the drug industry—were going to be critical weapons in the ongoing war against communism. On June 3, 1957, Senator Hubert Humphrey proclaimed to a meeting of pharmaceutical advertising executives the value of using pharmaceuticals to free people in underdeveloped countries from both disease *and* the communist threat. As he noted, "No amount of diplomacy or armament can bring peace where the bodies and minds of men are sick." Humphrey recounted how, on a recent fact-finding mission of the Senate Foreign Relations Committee to the Middle East and Far East, he had seen "poverty and misery provide the fertile ground for the very dissatisfactions that so often made communism acceptable." As the Soviets were moving into the Middle East and Far East, "areas where the greatest doubt and misunderstandings as to our way of life exist," Humphrey advised, "we are now, more than ever, challenged to help the starving and disease-ridden people of the world to raise themselves out of their misery." After all, Humphrey continued, "People can start thinking of freedom and the rights of the individual when they are freed from the day-to-day concern of trying to eke out a bare survival and are in good enough health to turn their attention to matters other than sheer subsistence. In helping others to help themselves, we are achieving in a practical way a means for these people to live fuller lives." By committing to fight disease in these countries and sharing technical assistance and scientific know-how, the United States would "demonstrate in unmistakable terms our genuine concern for the rank and file of humanity, and our willingness to build them a better life."[17]

As such, the American pharmaceutical industry had a crucial role to play in this battle for control of underdeveloped nations. Only through the industry's work of developing and distributing drugs could America "hel[p] suffering people rid themselves of disease" and "place those people on a firm foundation." To this end, Humphrey called on American drug firms to become leaders in promoting international health, first, by providing drugs such as antibiotics and vaccines to undeveloped countries and, second, by promoting the development of pharmaceutical research in these countries by establishing "agreements between a needy country's government and American pharmaceutical firms" to develop pharmaceutical and medical institutions that followed the American model. In other words, Humphrey saw the work of American drug firms as a critical vehicle in which the American system of free enterprise could be delivered to those undeveloped and undecided nations in Asia, Africa, South America, and the Middle East. To achieve this, Humphrey suggested that American firms send out teams of research chemists, pharmacologists, and clinical investigators to help other countries set up professional schools, and establish fellowships to encourage students in these countries to enter these fields and thus alleviate the shortage of pharmaceutical workers.[18]

Humphrey's comments in 1957 strike a tone distinctly different from the criticisms he lodged against vaccine and pharmaceutical manufacturers earlier in the decade. Yet as much as Humphrey abhorred the power wielded by large corporations, he was a dedicated cold warrior committed to fostering stability and security among potential American allies in South America, Africa, Asia, and the Middle East. Ultimately, Humphrey's efforts to secure international cooperation on medical research played a crucial role in advancing his presidential aspirations. In 1958, during a visit to Moscow to explore how the United States might achieve such cooperation, Humphrey was called into a surprise meeting with the Soviet premier, Nikita Khrushchev. The meeting, which lasted eight hours and centered on the issue of disarmament, propelled Humphrey into the spotlight of national—and international—politics.[19]

Aware of the threat posed by creeping communism, several pharmaceutical firms had been engaged in efforts to reach out to the research talent in Europe and in underdeveloped nations since the mid-1950s. As chapter 2 described, Merck & Co., for example, had, since 1952, organized an international postdoctoral fellowship program. Although the majority of the program's fellows came from industrialized European countries, in 1956, the director of scientific personnel at the National Research Council, M. H. Trytten, approached Merck & Co. about the possibility of the company establishing programs in less developed and more politically sensitive countries, such as India. Trytten's suggestion came from the perceived efforts of the Soviet Union to secure technological development in these uncommitted, nonaligned countries.[20]

By the time Humphrey made his 1957 speech to industry's advertising executives, then, the industry was sufficiently concerned that the Soviet's biomedical workforce would be wielded against America in the Cold War theaters of Asia, Africa, and South America. In fact, the year after Humphrey's address, Smith, Kline & French Laboratories had sent a delegation of its researchers and executives to the Soviet Union for a month in an effort to evaluate the extent of the Soviet Union's pharmaceutical development capabilities. There the delegation visited medical and pharmaceutical research facilities in Moscow, Leningrad, and Kharkov. In exchange, the Soviet Union sent five representatives of Soviet medical and pharmaceutical research to U.S. laboratories. Although it was clear to the industry that the Russians did not possess superior drugs to those in the United States, the Russians did, however, have a much larger pool of biomedical labor, and it was this labor that posed the real threat in America's battle to win over to the side of capitalism the undeveloped and undecided nations of Asia, Africa, and South America. As Merck's president, John T. Connor observed in June 1958, the Soviet Union had more physicians per 100,000 population than the United States (164.2 versus 130). Connor worried that the "Soviets plan to 'export' their medical talent to underdeveloped countries in their effort to 'sell Communism.'" Repeating Senator Humphrey's proposal of the previous year, Connor called on U.S. drug firms and medical schools to train more physicians and "embark on a foreign medical aid program in a 'longevity race' with the Russians, raising the life span throughout the world."[21]

The work of historians of the Soviet pharmaceutical industry makes clear that the fears of U.S. policymakers and drug industry executives were overstated.[22] The Soviet Union certainly did have a significantly larger pool of biomedical labor than the United States and Western Europe did.[23] But as Mary Schaeffer Conroy has documented, after World War II the Soviet pharmaceutical industry "lagged behind the West and Japan in producing breakthrough medicines of good quality and in sufficient quantities," developing most of its pharmaceuticals by cloning and licensing foreign methods rather than by the innovative research of its own scientists.[24] Despite the inadequacies of the Soviet pharmaceutical industry, there is evidence that the Soviet Union did export pharmaceuticals to developing countries (in addition to other communist states) throughout the Cold

War.[25] The extent and specific destination of these exports is currently unknown, however. Thus, as was often the case in Cold War America, the rhetoric of the Cold War—and the anxieties that rhetoric fostered—tended to exaggerate reality.

Nevertheless, Americans believed that the threat of Soviet superiority was real, and this threat ultimately led to legislation such as the 1960 Health for Peace bill. In President Dwight D. Eisenhower's 1958 State of the Union address he characterized the Soviet Union as "waging a total cold war" against the United States. Eisenhower called on "all peoples, especially those of the Soviet Union" to engage in "Works of Peace" rather than continue down "the present plunge toward more and more destructive weapons of war." As an example of such Works of Peace, Eisenhower proposed establishing an exchange of medical research information between the United States and the Soviets as part of a joint international effort, along with several other nations, to eradicate malaria within five years.[26] Eisenhower proposed that Russians and Americans should collaborate to discover new drugs to rid the world of epidemic diseases rather than competing in the development of nuclear weapons. Over the course of the following year, Eisenhower's Works for Peace agenda was translated by a bipartisan group in Congress into a "Health for Peace" bill, which proposed the establishment of a National Institute of International Medical Research (as part of the National Institutes of Health), which would be responsible for coordinating the medical research being done around the world and providing research funding and facilities for the field. The bill was signed into law, with the support of the American drug industry, in July 1960.[27]

The industry's potential role in foreign policy coincided with the political foment over high drug prices and excessive pharmaceutical advertising that was heating up elsewhere in Congress. Indeed, when Kefauver began congressional hearings on the drug industry on December 7, 1959, he did so in the midst of congressional efforts to get the Health for Peace bill passed. Because of this timing, and because Kefauver sought to criticize the system of pharmaceutical development and distribution, the rhetoric of the Cold War framed the debate over the political economy of drugs. In fact, after Kefauver delivered his introductory remarks at the hearings, he yielded the floor to the Democratic senator from Florida, George Smathers. In his support of Kefauver's investigation, Smathers recounted the experience of his friend, Governor Leroy Collins, who had recently visited the Soviet Union. While there, the governor had been taken ill with a sickness that had struck him previously in Florida. Smathers explained that the governor had managed to find in the Soviet Union the same medicine he had taken in the United States. However, "in our United States the prescription cost him in the neighborhood of something like $18, compared to the cost in the Soviet Union of something less than $2."[28] That on the opening morning of the Kefauver hearings, Senator Smathers compared the cost of prescription drugs in the United States to the cost of drugs in the Soviet Union was no coincidence. In doing so, Senator Smathers plugged into the fear that had gripped American policymakers since Sputnik's launch.

THE COLD WAR OFFENSE

Capitalizing on the growing Cold War concerns of Congress and the public more generally, representatives of the drug industry infused their testimony before the Kefauver subcommittee with the rhetoric of the Cold War. Merck's president, John T. Connor, for example, described his firm's role in fighting the spread of communist ideology as evidenced by Merck's efforts to establish corticosteroid manufacturing plants in Third World countries. Connor noted, in particular, how Merck had won "an initial skirmish with the Soviet Union in India last year," as Merck and the Soviet government fought for the right to establish a manufacturing plant in India. The result of this win was that Merck was now "building pharmaceutical plants in that country, though the Russians are still very much in the picture there as well as in many other underdeveloped countries." Although Connor emphasized that the Soviet pharmaceutical industry was inferior to that in the United States (noting that "Soviet drug research is still in the horse-and-buggy stage"), he warned that Americans should be worried about the Soviets' ability (and indeed history of) duplicating the discoveries made in American laboratories and distributing them to Third World countries.[29] By drawing on the same language that legislators and industry executives alike had used during the late 1950s, Connor reminded the subcommittee that the drugs manufactured by American firms served as both important symbols of American capitalism and necessary vehicles of foreign policy.

To emphasize the drug industry's commitment to fighting the spread of communism and disease in underdeveloped countries, the PMA's president, Austin Smith, invited Dr. William B. Walsh, a clinical professor of internal medicine at Georgetown University School of Medicine, to testify on the industry's behalf. In addition to his academic role, Walsh was founder and president of the People to People Health Foundation, a nonprofit organization committed "to improving the health opportunities for less fortunate persons both at home and abroad" through the work of medical missionaries and volunteer health professionals.[30] As part of its mission, the People to People Health Foundation had in 1958 established Project HOPE (the acronym standing for Health Opportunities for People Everywhere). Using money donated by the pharmaceutical industry, Project HOPE transformed a U.S. Navy ship donated by the Eisenhower administration into "a floating hospital, medical center, and school."[31] The ship, S.S. *Hope*, was fully equipped and staffed to "carry American medical knowledge and health care to isolated areas of the world which need it most," most notably in Asia, the Middle East, and South America.[32]

Project HOPE, then, was a manifestation of legislators' and the drug industry's earlier plans to use pharmaceuticals as foreign policy. As Walsh testified to Kefauver's subcommittee, the purpose of the project was "not only to heal the sick" in those countries "but also to improve, by means of teaching and training, the abilities of the people of newly independent nations to help themselves." In addition to providing Walsh with the necessary startup funds, American drug firms had also committed a million dollars worth of drugs each year to Project HOPE. As Walsh noted to the subcommittee, "I have never asked for an iota of support in funds or drugs, on the basis of potential profit or future market. My only plea to the numerous executives with whom I have spoken has been based upon the appeal of help to the needy and the obligatnion [*sic*] of good citizens to improve the understanding of the people of the United States by others throughout the world. I have never been refused." The industry's generosity, Walsh continued, should be recognized as its "compassion for the needy and a deep sense of the duties of American citizenship," none of which would be possible if the present free enterprise system were compromised.[33]

Project HOPE was one of several Third World aid missions to which the pharmaceutical industry contributed during the years of the Kefauver hearings. The chairman of the PMA's board, William B. Graham, reminded his industry colleagues in 1960 to emphasize in their congressional and press dealings the important donations the industry had made during the previous year. For example, following the 1960 earthquake in Agadir, Morocco, American drug firms responded immediately by contributing medical supplies "and substantial gifts of drugs." The industry had also "given almost half a million dollars worth of drugs" in a period of six months to the American Medical Missionary, whose executive director noted the "invaluable aid" given by the American drug industry to the Missionary's "fight against communism." Another project "of importance to our Western freedom," Graham added, was the Polish medical aid program in which the industry, under agreement with the Gomulka regime in Poland, was "allowed to ship American drugs direct to Polish hospitals. These drugs—donated by some 20 companies from our competitive American pharmaceutical manufacturing industry—are either in short supply or non-existent behind the Iron Curtain." Through these donations, Graham asserted, "probably through no other industry can the superiority of our American competitive system be demonstrated so impressively," something that the industry's representatives should try to remind the subcommittee of in their testimony.[34]

The Republicans on the Senate subcommittee, who overwhelmingly sided with the drug industry, were also quick to mobilize the language of the Cold War to defend the pharmaceutical industry. Senator Alexander Wiley (R-WI), for example, argued in the published report of the hearings that "it is part of a free enterprise system to permit differences in income and profit, to allow free use of advertising and promotion, and to leave business management to those responsible for it." To challenge that system, as Kefauver was doing, was to challenge "the core of democracy" and destine Americans "to follow the example of totalitarian governments."[35] Wiley warned that although "it is easy . . . to accuse the drug industry of unconscionable profits and to demand Government controls . . . it must be remembered that the Soviet Union, in which the profit motive does not exist and in which the drug industry is completely regulated, produced no single new drug since the Communist revolution."[36] There was no incongruity for Wiley or the industry representatives to argue that a nation that had not produced a single innovative drug should be feared: in the logic of Cold War America, one should never underestimate the Soviets' capacity to make technological advances or communism's ability to infiltrate American society. Although the drug industry and its allies may have exaggerated the Soviet threat, the threat still felt real to Cold War Americans.

For the drug industry, however, to effectively mobilize the rhetoric of the Cold War as a defense against Kefauver's criticism required more than simply comparing the achievements and capacities of the American industry with those of the Soviet industry. As part of their defense, the industry and its supporters argued that with the introduction of S. 1552 Kefauver sought to undermine the very system that distinguished America from the Soviet Union and that made all of America's pharmaceutical achievements possible. As Senator Wiley charged, "the cures that have been suggested for dealing with the drug evils—real or illusory—are sufficiently drastic to kill . . . the whole concept of free enterprise."[37]

The patent provisions of S. 1552, in particular, raised very pragmatic—indeed, technological—questions for academic physicians who were involved in developing new drugs. A parade of academic physicians, many of whom had collaborated with drug firms during the previous decade and thus were part of the industry's research networks, testified in opposition to the provision of S. 1552 that called for granting patents only to new drugs with therapeutic effects or molecular structures significantly different from those of existing drugs. As Dr. Edward W. Boland, professor of medicine at the University of Southern California School of Medicine and consultant to the AMA's Council on Drugs, wrote to the Kefauver subcommittee, "during the last 8 years much knowledge has been gained regarding the effects of chemical alterations on the physiologic properties of steroids." It was exactly these kinds of molecular modifications that would enable chemists "to create anti-inflammatory steroidal agents which are more efficient and safer than those that are now available." To pass legislation that would deny the granting of patents to new drugs generated through such research, Boland continued, "would indeed be a severe blow to the progress of medical research" by "discourag[ing] continued efforts to modify the molecular structures of steroids and . . . imped[ing] the introduction of new drugs that may result from such efforts."[38]

Dr. Philip S. Hench, a Nobel laureate and collaborator of Merck & Co. in the development of cortisone, concurred, asserting that he found the proposed patent reforms "astonishing" when the "supreme lesson, which the current history of corticosteroid pharmacology has taught us is . . . that marked, indeed profound, physiological and therapeutic changes can be, and have been, obtained from making what had appeared to be minor molecular changes."[39] Hench also reminded the committee of the importance of industry-academic collaborations made possible by the free enterprise system to the successful development of new drugs like cortisone. Arguing that only the drug industry had the financial resources to "compulsively sustain the pursuit of almost hopeless investigations" that would lead to the discovery of new drugs, Hench questioned the rationale behind the "sharp limitation of patent rights and other restraints in this bill which tend to reduce incentive and impose psychological handicaps" on the industry's continued investment in drug research. Moreover, Hench expressed his confusion as to why "at this time when we are in a most serious scientific race with Russia," Congress would "endanger by legislation the scientific, professional, and industrial teamwork that has been responsible for putting us far ahead of the Russians in at least this one regard."[40]

Other physicians testified to the importance of molecular modifications in fields other than steroids. Lowell Coggeshall, a vice-president of the University of Chicago, reported on his own work in the development of antimalarial compounds, noting that the drug primaquine, discovered during the National Research Council's antimalarial research program, had turned out to be almost identical chemically to the already known pamaquine.[41] Coggeshall recalled that despite the fact that "every element of predictability suggested that this compound was unworthy of detailed further investigation" because of its similarity to an already available drug, the program's researchers "recognized the value of pursuing the close chemical relatives. As a result, thousands of returning Korean War veterans were spared the discomfort and, indeed, the danger of vivax malaria." This experience made clear the "vital importance of having laws that do not discourage the testing, development, and marketing of drugs simply because they are similar to some other drugs."[42] Coggeshall further warned that S. 1552 threatened the country's position in the Cold War, noting that the United States' "excellence in the treatment of disease may very well be decisive in the ultimate outcome" in the war against communism. So far, the United States was leading in this area, in large measure due to the industry's continued development of new drugs. "Surely," Coggeshall continued, "our efforts should be directed to maintaining and increasing our leadership. This is no time for legislative changes that even create a possibility of retarding our continued progress. S. 1552 not only entails such a possibility but, in my judgment, would almost certainly do precisely this."[43]

For other industry supporters, the danger lay not only in compromising the U.S. industry's capacity to keep ahead of the Soviet industry in a putative therapeutic arms race but, more important, in seriously endangering the public's health while the nation was engaged in a cold war that could turn hot at any moment. When Vannevar Bush, former head of the Office of Scientific Research and Development (OSRD) during World War II and recently retired director of Merck & Co. testified against S. 1552, he was quick to remind Kefauver's subcommittee "that we live in hazardous times, and that a great war might be started, perhaps by accident or irresponsibility. If it came," Bush continued, "it would be far more terrible than any war in history. This time, in addition to hydrogen bombs, with their burns and radiation, we might also meet a still more appalling weapon in the hands of men with no conscience: biological warfare." Because of the severe health threats posed by nuclear and biological warfare, Bush exclaimed, "This is no time to weaken our medical system, or the pharmaceutical industry which supports it." In particular, Bush singled out the American patent system as being fundamental to the preservation of the American medical system. As such, Bush argued, "It needs to be strengthened for its intended purpose," not weakened. With S. 1552, Bush told the subcommittee, "you gentlemen have a blunt instrument in your hands. If you use it you will do great harm."[44]

During Bush's testimony, Kefauver pushed Bush to consider the OSRD's wartime penicillin program as an example of Kefauver's patent reforms in action. As part of that program, Bush had required participating firms to license their penicillin-related patents at a fixed royalty rate of 5 percent to all other participating firms.[45] Kefauver argued the success of the penicillin program was evidence that mandatory compulsory licensing was an effective mechanism for ensuring the production of lower-priced drugs. Bush disagreed, pointing out that the program's licensing arrangements and the "complete interchange of technical information" made possible by them actually constituted a violation of the antitrust laws and thus were viable only during wartime. Instead, Bush insisted, to guarantee the development of new and reasonably priced drugs Congress should "support the present pharmaceutical industry, which is doing a magnificent job of doing just that."[46]

Neither Kefauver nor his staffers attempted to discredit the testimony of the academics with ties to industry. It is likely that Kefauver realized that their status as leaders in their fields (for example, Bush as former OSRD director, Hench as a Nobel laureate, Coggeshall as former special assistant to the secretary of HEW) made any attack on their credibility a fruitless and potentially risky endeavor. Instead, Kefauver held up the Swiss, German, and Italian pharmaceutical industries as examples of firms innovating in climates of lesser patent protection (in each case, these countries allowed only process patents on drugs) and as justification for his patent reforms. The academics who testified against S. 1552 remained unconvinced of the bill's merits. Rather, they countered that the U.S. industry's post–World War II rise to leadership in the global pharmaceutical marketplace was predicated on the superior patent protection afforded by the U.S. patent system.

While Kefauver's patent reforms faced substantial opposition from the industry and its allies, Kefauver found significantly more support for his efforts to reform the industry's marketing practices. A group of prominent academic physicians, which included Louis Lasagna of Johns Hopkins University, Maxwell Finland of Harvard Medical School, Walter Modell of Cornell Medical School, and Harry Dowling of the University of Illinois, criticized the industry for each year introducing a "plethora of poor compounds," with little to no therapeutic advantage over existing drugs and yet marketing them as if they were groundbreaking therapeutic innovations. Most troubling for these physicians was the industry's recent practice of combining two or more old drugs and marketing—and patenting—the resulting drug as a new drug without any evidence that the combination drug had any therapeutic advantage over its constituent drugs. These same physicians further warned that drug companies were usurping the role of "medical educators" in providing physicians with up-to-date information about new drugs and advances in the field of therapeutics. Because the "average" practicing physician had neither the time nor knowledge to keep up with the barrage of new drug products introduced each year, and because neither medical schools nor medical societies were inclined to or able to meet the challenge of continuing medical education, pharmaceutical firms—and their teams of detail men—had stepped in to fill the role. As a result, physicians were confronted daily with advertisements and promotional materials put out by drug manufacturers that were often hyperbolic, inaccurate, and misleading.[47]

Kefauver's reforms also found support as the subcommittee heard testimony from consumer and seniors groups, representatives of hospital formularies, and representatives of the military's procurement agency, who reported being able to purchase generically named drugs at significantly lower prices than those listed for brand-name drugs. These witnesses argued that the pricing policies of generic firms were evidence that brand-name manufacturers were overcharging consumers. Representatives from the brand-name manufacturers, however, argued that generic manufacturers could sell their drugs more cheaply because they engaged in neither innovative research nor the extensive educational programs of the brand-name firms. They also questioned the quality and therefore safety of drugs produced by small generic manufacturers, arguing that unlike the large, research-based drug firms, generic manufacturers did not institute adequate quality controls and were often guilty of producing substandard, even harmful drugs. The repeated claims of hospital officials, physicians, and members of seniors groups, who regularly used generic drugs without harm, however, gave credence to Kefauver's reform efforts.[48]

In spite of such evidence, the industry's strategy of mobilizing the rhetoric of cold war and emphasizing the necessity of the free enterprise system in the field of pharmaceuticals to win that war served as an effective defense for the industry. Equally critical to the industry's efforts to defeat Kefauver's bill, however, was the support the industry secured from the medical profession by linking the fate of the industry and the system of free enterprise with the fate of private medical practice.[49]

WINNING THE SUPPORT OF PHYSICIANS

At the 1960 annual meeting of the PMA, Austin Smith warned the audience that the drug industry and the medical profession had "between 1960 and 1964 to make up your minds whether you want socialized medicine in this country or whether you want a so-called free enterprise system."[50] In case the consequences of socialized medicine were not clear to the audience, Smith yielded the floor to William Apple, the president of the American Pharmaceutical Association. Offering a glimpse of the bleak future promised by Kefauver's reforms, Apple painted a dystopian picture of illness two decades in the future:

> Today—April 5, 1980—the citizen desiring medical attention merely dials the nearest government health center which arranges for his transportation to the nearest government diagnostic center. Physicians have long ago been relieved of such professional decisions as where, when, or how to practice. The physician's diagnosis today consists of performing government-prescribed tests, and completing "United States" mark sense data cards. The patient is no longer subject to the anxiety of listening to the physician describe his diagnosis and prescribed treatment. This information will be communicated by an agent from the government health center. The patient knows that if he requires medication it will be supplied without effort or cost on his part and without choice on the part of the physician. The diagnostic data card is sent to a "United States" decoding center. The electronic brains, which have been government programmed, will prescribe the "correct" drug. There is no problem of competing brands to be concerned with because everything today is the "United States" brand, which, in the field of pharmaceuticals, is readily identified by the letter "K." There is no problem of competition or concentration since each pharmaceutical manufacturer is assigned the products it can produce, the quality specifications it must not exceed, the price it must charge. There is no problem of distribution through wholesalers and retail pharmacies; they have been eliminated. The distribution of drugs is accomplished through government depots

which distribute directly to the government hospitals and to the general public.[51]

According to Apple's description, this "hyper-rational," state-controlled system of health care would eliminate physicians' autonomy and the industry's profit margins by subjugating all health care decisions to the state.

While the bleak picture painted by Apple might have seemed a little fantastic, Apple warned the industry audience, "We need only look around us now in 1960. . . . We are currently experiencing the seeding required for generic prescribing, for establishing the ethical drug industry as a public utility, for eliminating the incentive of the patent process, for substituting mail-order prescription depots for community pharmaceutical service."[52] Because of the shared threat faced by the drug industry and medical profession, the PMA leadership called on the industry to join forces with physicians and unite against Kefauver.

The AMA was known as a powerful lobby by the end of the 1940s when it defeated the Truman administration's efforts to pass a national health insurance plan.[53] For the AMA leadership, Kefauver's efforts to increase the authority of the FDA over therapeutic practice marked a dangerous trend in health care policy at a time when reformers were pushing for nationalized health insurance for the elderly. As the AMA's president, Leonard Larson, told an industry audience early in 1962: "One of our mutual problems is that we suffer from the *dubious benefits of too much supervision*. . . . [T]oo many people still turn around and insist they are competent to tell the physician *how to practice medicine*. Labor leaders, the Secretary of H.E.W. [Health, Education and Welfare] . . . the FDA, the Senator from Tennessee . . . —all of these and others are eager to dominate the practice of medicine and the behavior of the physician."[54] For Larson and the industry's leadership, the legislative efforts of Kefauver were part of a larger struggle confronting the health care team. The attempts by pharmaceutical and health care reformers "to wreck the patent system in the pharmaceutical industry, to have the government purchase medical care for the aged, to put the FDA in charge of the clinical evaluation of drugs, and to censor drug advertising are all phases of a single effort." For Larson, these efforts signaled that the medical profession and the drug industry were "involved in a large scale war. . . . [W]e should recognize that there are many facets involved in what must be viewed as a broad-scale attempt to make health care a government responsibility."[55]

Against this backdrop, leaders in the medical community worried about what Kefauver's bill would mean for the practice of medicine. As Hugh Hussey, the chairman of the AMA's board of trustees, argued during the legislative hearings, it was not the FDA's responsibility to determine the efficacy of a drug but rather the physician's because only he "has the knowledge, ability, and the responsibility to make that decision [about efficacy] in regard to that particular patient." The physician, he continued, "should not be deprived of the use of drugs that he believes are medically indicated for his patient by a governmental ruling or decision."[56] The AMA, however, did not speak for all of the medical profession. Leaders in academic medicine, including members of the AMA's own Council on Drugs, supported the efficacy requirement, contending that the practitioner did not have sufficient expertise in clinical research or pharmacology to make judgments about a new drug's efficacy. As the renowned pharmacologist Louis S. Goodman testified, "the average practicing physician—and I have helped to train hundreds of them—does not have the time, the facilities, the skill, nor the training to be an expert in determination of drug efficacy."[57] The PMA also diverged from the AMA on the efficacy provision. As far as the PMA was concerned, the FDA was already evaluating drugs on the basis of efficacy.[58] Rather than see the efficacy requirement as a threat, the PMA instead saw it as an opportunity to reduce competition. By raising the standards for drug approvals and thus barriers of entry into the marketplace, the efficacy requirement would, the PMA believed, eliminate many of the small, so-called fly-by-night manufacturers from the marketplace.[59]

The potential for political alliance between the medical profession and the drug industry was laid out in an editorial in *Science* in July 1961. Assessing the AMA's testimony before the Senate subcommittee on Kefauver's bill—in which the AMA opposed every aspect of it—the editorial noted how "the AMA naturally finds itself sharing the views of the conservatives [on the subcommittee], not only because the leaders of organized medicine are themselves conservative, but because their greatest political interest is in opposing the development of socialized medicine, and they cannot help feeling, probably correctly, that any increase in the federal role in medicine weakens the resistance to a national health service."[60]

But the AMA's interest in the drug bill was not simply political, the editorial continued. As the AMA had discovered in the 1950s—when its membership rolls were down and it was low on funds and had turned to drug advertising to restore its revenues—it was sorely dependent on the drug industry for financial support of its operations.[61] The editorial suggested that the drug industry spent "some $4 million annually on advertising in AMA journals, for over half its annual budget." For economic reasons then, reasoned the *Science* article, the AMA would present even greater opposition to Kefauver's drug bill because "the professed aim of the bill is to alter the circumstances that make the industry's heavy investment in promotion profitable." The Kefauver bill "would make the drug business less profitable, thereby reducing the economic power of a principle political ally of the AMA. It would, if it serves its purposes, sharply reduce the amount of promotion, and this would reduce the AMA's own resources, since the AMA, in fighting the increasingly expensive battle against government-financed health service, has come to rely heavily on the money its journals earn from advertising."[62] For the AMA and the drug industry, then, there were very clear political and economic benefits to be gained by mobilizing a political alliance against Kefauver.[63]

The drug industry and medical profession had shared the threat of increasing government oversight—and marshaled the specter of socialized medicine to defend against that threat—for several decades.[64] Yet the political alliance forged between the drug industry and medical profession during the Kefauver hearings differed from these earlier alliances in important ways. For the first time Kefauver's investigative and legislative hearings put the spotlight on the research and marketing practices of the drug industry, and questioned the physician's ability to make the best choices for their patients given those practices. The hearings also revealed the degree of financial interdependency between drug firms and physicians, and Kefauver's bill—by proposing economic reform of the industry— threatened to limit the financial relationship between the industry and medical profession. For the AMA, this meant a potential reduction in the funds available to it with which to wage its ongoing battle against national health insurance. Thus, both the drug industry and the medical profession had political and economic stakes in defeating Kefauver's reforms and maintaining the regulatory status quo.

The mobilization of anticommunist rhetoric by the industry and medical profession during the Kefauver hearings also differed somewhat from its previous incarnations. Although the industry's strategy of framing Kefauver's proposed reforms as the first step to socialized medicine was a familiar one (the industry had made similar arguments regarding the FDA's proposed labeling regulations in the late 1940s), the industry's assertion that opposition to Kefauver's reforms would guarantee the industry's ability to contain communism abroad—thereby extending their anticommunist ideology into the international arena—was a new element in the fight against socialized medicine.

SELLING FREE ENTERPRISE TO THE AMERICAN PUBLIC

The drug industry's strategy to defeat Kefauver extended beyond securing the support of physicians and beyond the power corridors of Washington, D.C. Due to the masterful use of publicity by Kefauver and his staffers, newspaper and television coverage of the Kefauver hearings was extensive and tended to emphasize Kefauver's most negative assertions against the industry. As Richard Harris has documented, Kefauver was "a genius for publicity creation," making "it a point to bring out his biggest guns half an hour or so before the reporters" covering the hearings "had to leave to file their stories."[65] In the first three months of the hearings, for example, the *New York Times*'s headlines included: "Senate Panel Cites Mark-ups on Drugs Ranging to 7,079%"; "Big Profit Found in Tranquilizers: One 6 Times Costlier Than in Paris"; and "Inquiry Finds Drug Production Controlled by a Few Companies."[66]

To counter the negative publicity, the third component of the industry's defense strategy was to extend its public relations efforts of the late 1950s and tell "the story of the American enterprise system" to the American public. As the president of the public relations firm hired by the PMA proclaimed to an industry audience in 1960, by proving to the public that *"our American competitive system is more productive and efficient, applied to industry in general,"* the pharmaceutical industry would convince the public that *"the job of producing drugs in particular . . . must continue to be entrusted to such a system."*[67] A year later, as the Kefauver bill reached Congress, the chairman of the PMA and president of Parke-Davis & Co., Harry Loynd, reiterated the necessary approach, calling on his industry colleagues to "preach the principle that made our country great. Tell the free enterprise story. Stand up and say, 'It is no crime to make money providing you make it honestly and distribute it properly.'"[68]

To this end, the PMA launched a public relations program that told "the drug industry story" through a series of institutional advertisements, the public speaking activities of industry representatives, letters to news and medical editors and congressional members, and individual in-house corporate publications. In telling the drug story as the story of the free enterprise system, the drug industry was engaged, along with other American corporations at that time, in "selling free enterprise." America's business leaders had feared since the second New Deal the gains being made by organized labor in both the workplace and policymaking.[69] In the immediate postwar period, the business community, led by the National Association of Manufacturers, launched a far-reaching public relations campaign that sought to "reorient workers away from their loyalties to organized labor and government" and to "undercut . . . the ideological hold" of labor and the state on the American people by "selling free enterprise" to the American public.[70]

The drug industry's public relations efforts in the name of free enterprise were part of this larger business project. Because drugs affected all Americans, the industry's mobilization of "the drug story" extended the "business assault" of the postwar period beyond the political machinations of business and organized labor, connecting the interests of business with those of the medical profession, biomedical researchers, and patients everywhere The result was to bring home to all Americans—irrespective of their stance toward business and labor—the seemingly very real dangers of letting socialism get a grip on the American political economy.

Adopting an approach similar to its congressional defense, the drug industry centered its overall public relations strategy on a message combining the fear-augmenting rhetoric of the Cold War with the triumphant rhetoric of the therapeutic revolution. In particular, the American pharmaceutical industry presented its role in the therapeutic revolution as powerful evidence of the superiority of a capitalist mode of pharmaceutical production (especially compared to the lackluster performance of the Soviet pharmaceutical industry). And it argued that any effort to undermine *corporate* drug development by inviting, as the industry's challengers in Congress proposed, greater government involvement in drug development promised to threaten the public's health and the technological superiority of the United States, and lead the country down the perilous path of socialized medicine. Casting corporate innovation as the key to winning "the human race" against the Soviet Union proved critical to the industry's efforts to build political support for itself in this period.

The key elements of this drug story focused on the therapeutic achievements made possible by the drug industry's investment of millions of dollars in research, oftentimes in research that dead-ended without a product ever reaching the market. Through that investment, as Theodore G. Klumpp, the president of Winthrop Laboratories, relayed in his commencement address at the University of Chattanooga in June 1960, Americans' life expectancy had increased "from 49 years in 1900 to 70 in 1959." Furthermore, "among infants the revolution is even more marked.

At the turn of the century, of every 1,000 babies that survived birth, 162 died within the first year, whereas today only 26 succumb. And of the 20 million babies born in the last 5 years, 80,000 are destined to live to a hundred." Other evidence of the drug industry's contributions was "the almost complete elimination of such killers as cholera, yellow fever, smallpox and the plague." At the same time, Klumpp continued, "the deadly sting has been drawn from diphtheria, scarlet fever, typhoid fever, typhus and an array of other diseases too numerous to mention." These victories were also accompanied by substantial reductions in morbidity and mortality rates from tuberculosis and pneumonia due, the industry claimed, to the development of antibiotics. Klumpp, for example, assured his audience that "in half a century the greatest reaper of them all—pneumonia—has been all but defeated as witnessed by the fact that the death rate has declined from 152 per 100,000 to 12."[71]

Lest the public believe the drug industry's work was almost complete, a second element of "the drug story" was to emphasize the work that still remained to be done. As Klumpp reminded his Chattanooga audience, "There are still bacteria that haven't been mastered. . . . [T]here is still a whole host of virus diseases that are as yet untouched. Cancer is still a murder mystery to which there is still not a single basic clue. . . . A whole host of endocrine, mental and neurological disturbances still defy the best research brains. Arteriosclerosis, the greatest killer of them all and the ultimate limiting factor in our life span, is still beyond our grasp."[72] Because of the numerous medical challenges still confronting Americans, the industry asked that the incentives needed to continue their research not be taken away. The brand name, which Kefauver sought to all but abolish, was one such incentive, Klumpp explained. "Our entire system of free enterprise is, in fact, based on brand names," because, Klumpp continued, "brand names enable the consumer to reward the product which is proved good . . . through repurchases of the product. If a product proves unsatisfactory, the consumer has the means of punishing it—by refusing to buy it again." Because "brand names facilitate reward or punishment" they are "a prime factor in stimulating reputable manufacturers to produce the best product." In the drug industry story, the brand name was associated with the quality of drug and the reputation of the manufacturer producing that drug. As Klumpp explained, when the doctor prescribes by a brand name he can be sure he's purchasing a quality product. However, "if his only way of identifying a drug is by generic name, rather than by brand name," as Kefauver would have it, "he will have no way of knowing the true quality of the drug which he prescribed." Not only would the abolishing of brand names lead to a decline in drug safety, Klumpp continued, but the substitution of generic for brand name would mean that "little incentive would remain for a pharmaceutical manufacturer to engage in research when, if it is successful, the resulting product cannot be identified by the manufacturer's own trademark or brand name."[73]

The most significant part of the drug story, however, was to challenge the public's "deeply ingrained impression that medical care and the drugs that are a part of it, cost too much." In this instance, industry executives like Klumpp gave examples of the great savings made possible by the development of drugs "costing perhaps several dollars" that cure "what used to be a perilous illness with long disability, loss of earnings, hospital and nursing expense and a convalescence that sometimes lasted for months." For instance, they compared the cost of lobar pneumonia in 1927 (approximately $1,000) with the cost of treating the disease with antibiotics in 1953 (no more than $29.68). Moreover, they were quick to emphasize that drug prices had actually risen "far less than that of most other commodities during the past 15 years of inflationary pressures"; an element of the drug story supported by contemporary economic data documenting the cost of prescription drugs relative to other health care services. According to Klumpp, "In 1958, the per capita consumption of drug preparations and sundries was $19," compared to the $53 spent on alcoholic beverages, $37 on tobacco products, $24 on "auto repair, greasing, washing, parking, storage, and rental," and $10 on "admissions to specified spectator amusements." Yet, as Klumpp pointed out, these figures "say nothing of the savings in health and in hard dollars which the American people have made by virtue of the contributions of scientific research." Thus, when compared to the amount spent on these other nonessential commodities, was not "health and what it cost . . . the biggest bargain available to the American people[?]"[74]

Not incidentally, since the early 1950s the AMA had employed the same strategy of likening medicine to other consumer products.[75] Throughout the decade the AMA tracked "medical spending on alcohol, tobacco, recreation, and jewelry in order to point out both relative inflation and consumer 'choices.'"[76] In 1960, for example, as part of its efforts to defend against the Forand bill, the AMA compared the rise, between 1939 and 1959, in medical care costs (107 percent) with the rise in the consumer price index (109.8 percent), men's haircuts (218.3 percent), and "commodities" (126 percent) to show that "the real cost of medical care has not been rising; indeed, it has been falling over the inflationary period."[77] By comparing medical care costs with the costs of other commodities, both the industry and the AMA sought to show the public that when considered in perspective, neither medical costs nor drug costs were as high as critics claimed and thus both government-subsidized health care and greater regulation of the drug industry were unnecessary measures. Moreover, they implied that it was not the health care system that needed fixing but rather the choices consumers made about how and where to spend their money.

In addition to the elements addressed by Klumpp, the drug story also included an explanation of the high risks taken on by drug firms that were involved in the research and development of new drugs. An article in *Business Week* in 1960, for example, emphasized these risks as it took the reader through the stages of researching, developing, and manufacturing a new drug. The article noted that all the research being conducted by drug firms was extremely costly, citing that in 1959 "the pharmaceutical industry spent an estimated $200 million on research—as much as $40 million of it on basic activities." The reason drug research was growing increasingly expensive was that "researchers have apparently come just about to the end of their string in reaping great rewards from chance discoveries. . . . And now the research emphasis has turned toward finding drugs that will halt the progress" of more complex diseases such as cancer and atherosclerosis. As "chance discoveries here are even more problematical," the article continued, the cost of research increases as "researchers are now convinced that the only way heart diseases and cancer will be brought under control will be by uncovering something basic about their causes."[78]

Juxtaposed against the increasing cost of drug research, Parke-Davis's president, Harry Loynd, pointed out in the *Business Week* article that because of the high levels of research and development, many new drugs were being made therapeutically redundant after just a few years as even newer and more efficacious drugs reached the market. The result was that "the sales life of a new product can hardly be estimated for more than five years." Because of this high rate of product obsolescence, firms had even less time to recoup their investment costs from the sales of new drugs, which in part explained why new drugs cost as much as they did.[79] The high rate of product obsolescence and the high risk of failure associated with researching and developing drugs also explained why the drug industry operated at such seemingly high profit levels—a source of much criticism in Congress. As Loynd stated, "because of the risks in this business . . . we have to operate on a wide margin of profit." Loynd, for example, recounted how he had committed Parke-Davis "to purchase $1.5 million worth of material for a new ulcer product" (when the firm's sales were $40 million a year), "gambling on favorable test results. The product," however, "proved to be a failure when clinical investigations were made," resulting in a considerable loss of investment for the company. This, Loynd explained, characterized the nature of the drug development business. Indeed, industry executives were often wont to quote that for every success in drug development there were almost three thousand failures.[80]

The "drug story" did not go unchallenged. Kefauver and his staffers, along with several physicians, made sure to qualify what they regarded as the industry's more grandiose claims. Harry Dowling, for example, reminded a group of Canadian physicians that while "the pharmaceutical industry deserves a share—perhaps a lion's share—of the credit" for the postwar reductions in mortality and morbidity from infectious diseases, "surely, improvements in sanitation, better public health organization, research by universities and government, increased diagnostic and therapeutic skills of practicing physicians and more intelligent co-operation on the part of the public have also contributed to better health."[81] During the hearings themselves, Kefauver's staffers pointed out to the industry's representatives that many of the drugs credited with significant reductions in mortality and morbidity—such as the sulfa drugs, penicillin, and tranquilizers—were first discovered in Europe and not in the United States, as the "drug story" implied. Kefauver and his staffers also contended that of the drugs discovered and developed in the United States, the majority of the research that led to these discoveries had actually taken place in government-funded academic laboratories, rather than in the laboratories of American drug companies.[82]

Critics of the industry also challenged the drug story's contention that high research costs justified the prices American consumers paid for their prescription drugs. In particular, critics accused the industry of spending more on marketing than they did on research. The Senate Subcommittee on Antitrust and Monopoly's final report, for example, charged that while the industry spent, on average, 6.3 percent of its sales on research, eleven of the largest firms "spent 5 to 11 times as much in advertising, promotional and selling expenses."[83] Several physicians, including some who had previously worked for drug companies, criticized firms for directing too much of their research to minor molecular modifications of existing drugs rather than to finding completely novel drugs.[84] Dowling, for example, perceived that it was the very competitiveness of the industry that pushed firms to invest in less productive forms of research and to overmarket their products. As he explained in an editorial in the *New England Journal of*

Medicine, "to obtain enough profits to provide capital to go on with its work, a successful pharmaceutical company apparently has to divert its research facilities to make minor modifications in the original product to compete with other companies that had promptly started making minor modifications of the first company's discovery. Furthermore, each company has to step up its advertising campaign to compete with the others."[85] It was "the predominance of this kind of imitative research," argued Frederick Meyers, a pharmacologist at the University of California, San Francisco, "and not the rate of medical progress that accounts for the rapid obsolescence that manufacturers complain of."[86]

Despite these qualifications, the industry's representatives continued to proclaim "the drug story" at every opportunity. To this end, the main elements of "the drug story" were captured and delivered to the public in the Pharmaceutical Industry Advertising Program, launched by the PMA in May 1962. The goal of the program, which included a series of advertisements published in national magazines such as *Reader's Digest,* the *Saturday Evening Post,* and *Look,* was "to win widespread understanding for the industry by presenting to the public its record of achievement in protecting health, prolonging life and lowering the costs of illness."[87] Several advertisements told of the diseases already made curable and the lives saved by the industry's developments. Others emphasized the earnings and health care costs saved because of the reductions in duration of illness, hospitalization, and convalescence made possible by prescription drugs. Three of the advertisements described the nature of drug research: the high risk of failure, the length of time invested in finding a cure, and the cost of developing a new drug.[88]

One advertisement in particular that captured the essence of the industry's defense was the advertisement that asked, "Who's winning the human race?" As an answer the advertisement recounted the "75 new drugs important to modern medicine" that American drug companies had developed between 1939 and 1962. Compare that, the advertisement stated, to the fact that in the "forty-six years of Communist rule Russia has not developed a single new drug of consequence." Lest the reader miss the implication, the advertisement explained, "The pharmaceutical industry in Russia is owned by the state," whereas the new drugs developed by American firms "were made possible by a competitive American drug industry and medical center research. And by a patent system that encourages new inventions and discoveries." Protecting the system of free enterprise and keeping the government's hands off the American drug industry meant that Americans could count on American drug companies to continue "spending hundreds of millions of dollars in research every year to find still better drugs against a host of ills." To let Kefauver have his way would guarantee Americans no such protection.[89]

The PMA also disseminated "the drug story" through *Medicine at Work*, the PMA's monthly magazine that circulated among "14,000 opinion leaders," which showcased the industry's work with other members of the health care team to "solve community health problems on a voluntary cooperative basis without government interference."[90] The PMA published pamphlets, distributed to physicians' offices, pharmacists, and hospitals, aimed at educating readers on specific issues of concern to pharmaceutical consumers.[91] And the PMA and several of its member companies organized speakers bureaus, which supplied industry representatives to tell the "drug industry story" to community groups like the Kiwanis and Rotary Clubs. In 1961, the PMA reported that "well over 500 field representatives" had "reached more than 2,500 groups—more than 100,000 community leaders."[92]

The industry's public relations campaign also disseminated the drug story to drug firm employees in the hope of motivating them to spread the story to their friends and to ask their representatives in Congress to oppose Kefauver's bill. Parke-Davis, for instance, dedicated the entire July 1961 issue of its in-house publication, *Parke-Davis Review*, to the matter of Kefauver's bill. Capitalizing on the rhetoric of war, the editors of the *Review* introduced the edition by announcing that "at this very moment a lethal weapon is being pointed at you and at me. It [Kefauver's drug bill] hovers threateningly over the entire drug industry. . . . If passed, [the bill] could undermine the very roots of our free enterprise system." Because of the dangers posed by the bill, Parke-Davis wanted its employees and stockholders to fully understand those dangers and know the facts about the industry, not what it saw as the distorted impressions and false conclusions conveyed by Kefauver.[93] Parke-Davis hoped that by setting the facts straight in the *Parke-Davis Review*, its employees and stockholders who read the issue would then discuss those facts with their family, friends, and neighbors. And, if they shared "the grave apprehensions already felt by many others, in and out of the industry," the company hoped they would "*do* something about it by expressing [their] views to [their] congressmen and senators."[94] The strategy seems to have had the desired effect: during the spring of 1962, as the Senate debated Kefauver's bill, Senator Philip Hart (D-MI) received "scores of letters from constituents in Detroit [the home of Parke-Davis]—most of them identical"—opposing the Kefauver bill.[95]

CONCLUSION

Despite the fact that the patent provisions of Kefauver's bill would have significantly altered the pricing and profit structure in the industry and potentially contributed to a reduction in drug prices—the goal that Kefauver was trying to achieve when he began his investigation of the drug industry—the patent provisions were the first things to be written out of the bill. In the end, Congress would not vote against securing greater reductions in morbidity and mortality or freedom from the forces of socialism and communism.

Without the support of President John F. Kennedy's administration, which, having barely squeaked through the 1960 election, had no interest in pursuing such controversial legislation, Kefauver's bill was dead until the summer of 1962, when news broke of the thalidomide tragedy. Reports that thousands of babies had been born in Europe with severely shortened limbs because their mothers had taken the drug thalidomide during pregnancy brought home to Americans the dangers of taking potent pharmaceutical agents and the potential limits of the regulatory system in the United States. Although the FDA had denied marketing approval to the manufacturers of thalidomide, some twenty-thousand Americans (including 624 pregnant women) had taken the experimental drug, leading to the birth of seventeen thalidomide babies in the United States (compared to the approximately ten thousand born elsewhere). The tragedy renewed support for pharmaceutical reform in Congress and a significantly revised version of Kefauver's bill passed unanimously on both floors of Congress in October 1962.[96]

The final bill, however, was remarkably different from Kefauver's original bill: gone were the provisions to limit the period of exclusivity for firms holding patents on drugs from seventeen years to a mere three years; gone also were the compulsory licensing provision and the provision that called for the abolition of trademarks in pharmaceuticals and mandatory generic prescribing. Kefauver's fingerprints were barely visible on the final bill. Frustrated by Kefauver's obsession with reforming the patent system and finding his bill altogether too radical, the Department of Health, Education, and Welfare had put together its own version and submitted it to Congress under the sponsorship of Representative Oren Harris (D-AR). It was essentially the administration's bill that was ultimately signed into law that fall (Kefauver's reform efforts were, however, reflected in the naming of the new drug regulations as the Kefauver-Harris Act).[97] In the end, the bill that finally passed did very little to challenge the practices of the industry that Kefauver thought were responsible for the high price of drugs and the large profits of the industry. In the final bill, the emphasis was on ensuring the safety of drugs—a consequence of the thalidomide tragedy—rather than on reducing the price of drugs. The amendments to the Food, Drug, and Cosmetic Act, thus, reflected a broader transformation in the American political economy from a politics of production to a politics of consumption.[98]

Although the drug amendments improved the safety of prescription drugs, they also strengthened the economic position of PMA member companies—brand name manufacturers. They tightened restrictions on pharmaceutical advertising by—among other measures—mandating that all advertisements contain information about a drug's side effects and by transferring regulatory authority over drug advertising from the FTC to the FDA. But as Merck's president and chief executive officer, John T. Connor, noted, the advertising provisions could prove beneficial to companies like Merck. The hearings, after all, had made "clear that there is a large amount of dissatisfaction with the advertising and promotion practice of some of the companies." As industry leaders saw it, it was no longer "practical to think in terms of continuing the status quo because there's been attracted to the pharmaceutical industry many fringe operators." Rather, Connor continued, "from the point of view of protecting the honest firms and the firms that have some scientific practices and try to do a good job on the commercial side I think it's absolutely necessary that we have stronger Government regulations and this view is now rather generally accepted in the industry."[99]

The drug amendments also required that drug manufacturers submit to the FDA evidence not only of the safety but also of the "substantial efficacy" of their drugs before the FDA would grant marketing approval. The efficacy requirement, however, merely codified what the FDA had been doing for the previous decade and, together with the increased factory inspections mandated by the new regulations, raised the barrier of entry into the pharmaceutical marketplace. The result was to reduce competition from the smaller companies unable to afford the costs entailed by these new requirements.[100] In many ways, then, the pharmaceutical industry gained more than it lost from passage of the drug amendments. Three months after the drug amendments were signed into law, Merck's Connor announced to a group of Texas physicians, "the new law—on the whole—is sound." Connor recalled that of the provisions included in the final bill, "many grew out of proposals that had either been advanced or advocated by the drug industry itself."[101]

The industry's strategy to mobilize the rhetoric of the Cold War in its defense against Kefauver's reforms helped it secure the support of key congressional members (particularly fiscal conservatives who were eager to protect the free enterprise system from the incursions of an overreaching government) and organized medicine. Although the Cold War context may not have been the most important consideration for physicians during the early 1960s, what made the industry's efforts to garner the support of physicians successful was the industry's ability to tie the fate of the system of drug development to the privatized system of health care. In arguing that socialized medicine was the inevitable next step in the government's effort to increase its control of drug development, the industry made the threat more palpable to the public and to physicians. Citing evidence that the Soviet Union's efforts to disseminate communist ideology, as it related to health care, to nonaligned countries were proving effective, the industry argued that it would be possible for the Soviets and their domestic allies to introduce socialism in the United States.

5 Expert Alliances

The Creation of the Drug Research Board

> The pharmaceutical industry and the medical profession have
> stood shoulder to shoulder in the past and will continue to do
> so in the future, wherever the health of the public is at stake.
> We are both dedicated to pursue our chosen fields in the public
> interest. We both seek the same goal—better health for the
> American people.
>
> —LEONARD LARSON, president, American Medical Association, 1960[1]

Passage of the 1962 amendments to the Food, Drug, and Cosmetic Act
marked a victory for pharmaceutical reformers. Although the drug industry had derailed much of Senator Kefauver's reform agenda, the amendments did grant the Food and Drug Administration (FDA) significantly
greater authority over the clinical testing, marketing, and distribution of
drugs. Recognizing the limits of that victory, however, pharmaceutical
reformers continued throughout the 1960s and 1970s to agitate for even
tighter government control over the drug industry.

At the center of the battle over pharmaceutical reform in the 1960s were
questions about expertise, authority, and physician autonomy. Congressional reformers, FDA officials, industry leaders, the American Medical
Association (AMA), and leading academic physicians debated who were
the appropriate purveyors of pharmaceutical information and education,
who had the expertise to make pharmaceutical policy, and what should
be the limits of the FDA's authority to regulate pharmaceutical practice.
Increasingly, the drug industry and the leadership of the medical profession viewed the FDA as having overstepped its authority. Both groups,
for example, balked as the FDA began institutionalizing the regulatory
power granted to it by the drug amendments in new rules governing the
conduct of clinical trials.

In response, the American pharmaceutical industry drew on the medical
profession's concern about expanding government oversight over therapeutic practice and called on academic physicians to join forces with the

121

industry to establish an expert advisory body, the Drug Research Board, to guide government officials on pharmaceutical policy. By positioning themselves as experts, this alliance gave industry a seat at the policy table and enabled it to challenge the efforts of pharmaceutical reformers to further increase the government's role in drug development. This chapter details the development of this political alliance between the drug industry and the medical profession, and shows the ways in which this industry-medicine alliance worked to circumvent the FDA's increasing authority over pharmaceutical practice in the post-Kefauver years.

THE SHARED THREAT OF GOVERNMENT OVERSIGHT

As the previous chapters have documented, since the 1950s the drug indus-try had drawn on the medical profession's long-standing concern about the expanding role of the federal government in medicine to help stultify the efforts of reformers to increase the government's control over the drug industry.[2] Part of this concern related specifically to the authority of the FDA over pharmaceutical practice. Indeed, since passage of the 1938 Food, Drug, and Cosmetic Act, the FDA had been pushing to increase its authority over prescription drug labeling. Its efforts provoked a decade-long response from the drug industry as it worked to curtail the agency's authority. This effort included warning physicians of the impending social-ization of medicine if the FDA were allowed to have its way and dictate to physicians which drugs they could and could not prescribe.[3]

The drug industry's and the medical profession's unease over the FDA's burgeoning authority was exacerbated throughout the 1950s by their con-cerns about the intellectual and material weakness of the FDA. A citizens advisory committee evaluating the agency in 1955 emphasized the FDA's inadequate budget and lack of scientific prowess and called for a three- to four-fold increase in the agency's budget and the addition of a thousand new field inspectors.[4] Although industry and the medical profession dis-cussed their worries that the agency did not have the resources to ade-quately protect the public's health, they did little to tackle the problem. In 1959, the Johns Hopkins University clinical pharmacologist Louis Lasagna suggested to the Pharmaceutical Manufacturers Association (PMA) that one way of solving the FDA's workforce and intellectual crisis was for "universities and the pharmaceutical industry . . . [to] join forces in pro-viding reasonable advice to government." Such a solution, Lasagna sug-gested, would strengthen the FDA *and* "preven[t] unwise participation of the government in drug development."[5] Although the PMA agreed that an industry-academic advisory body was desirable, it did not act on Lasagna's recommendation.

Concern about the FDA's inadequate resources and calls for creating an advisory body of pharmaceutical experts to aid the FDA in its mission were voiced repeatedly by the leading academic physicians who testified during the Kefauver hearings. Harry F. Dowling of the University of Illinois School of Medicine, for example, urged the FDA to appoint "a council of leading scientists, who would advise it regarding overall policies," a measure that was strongly supported by Harvard Medical School's Maxwell Finland and the University of Utah's Louis Goodman.[6]

When Kefauver's investigation of the pharmaceutical industry culminated in October 1962 with passage of the drug amendments to the Federal Food, Drug, and Cosmetic Act, the drug amendments significantly altered the political economy of drug development in the United States, making more urgent the industry's and academic physicians' concerns about the FDA. Two provisions of the amendments were particularly important for drug developers and their academic colleagues. First, the amendment granted responsibility for approving the clinical testing of drugs to the FDA. Before enactment of the amendments, a firm had been able to undertake clinical testing of a new drug at any time without any prior notification of the FDA. Thus it was the responsibility of the firm and its team of clinical investigators to determine whether or not it was safe to proceed from in vitro and preclinical studies in animals to testing in humans. The new law, however, transferred that responsibility to the FDA, requiring that firms receive approval from the FDA for their testing procedures *before* proceeding with clinical studies of an investigational new drug.

Second, the amendments now required that a drug firm provide proof of safety *and efficacy* to the FDA (before the new law, the FDA required only evidence of safety to grant a firm marketing approval for a new drug). The efficacy requirement, which mandated that all new drugs—including those *already* on the market—have "substantial evidence" of efficacy, threatened to deprive physicians of drugs they had long held to be effective and charged the FDA with greater authority over the prescription practices of physicians. Together with the clinical testing provisions of the new law, this meant that clinical investigators were expected to provide a lot more documentation about the drugs they were studying. This new level of oversight raised the ire of drug firms and academic researchers alike, as both parties feared that the new levels of bureaucracy would deter researchers from engaging in clinical studies, hindering the development of new drugs and thereby jeopardizing the public's health.

In July 1963, less than a year after the drug amendments were passed, the medical director of Eli Lilly & Co., Dr. Raymond Rice, reported to an AMA audience "that qualified investigators are indeed giving up clinical research rather than bother with all the paperwork" necessitated by the new regulations. The number of investigators registered with his company had dropped by half in the previous two years.[7] Earlier that year, the director of medical research at Lederle Laboratories had reported similar problems confronting his firm, noting that the time and cost of adapting to the new regulations had forced Lederle to "close out a lot of projects." The Lederle executive warned that the "increased research, testing, and development costs" incurred by the new regulations would force "industry [to] take long searching looks at all research programs before they are instituted. There will be less inclination to take the long gamble."[8]

Industry leaders also feared the added strain the drug amendments placed on the FDA's already limited resources. As Lilly's Rice asked an AMA audience in 1963, "how critical can be the evaluator of a new drug application within the FDA[?] I recently saw the data for one such application," he continued, "which consisted of a stack of paper six feet tall—how can one man cope with dozens of these and how can Dr. Kelsey [the director of the Division of New Drugs] supervise the evaluation of hundreds of them?" Rice further warned that just as drug companies were struggling "to enlist the cooperation of qualified investigators," so too would the FDA "find it difficult to recruit men of the caliber needed."[9]

The FDA's recruitment difficulties were made worse by the agency's persistently inadequate funding, as Merck's John T. Connor noted to a group of Texas physicians: although "at the height of the thalidomide furor President Kennedy had announced a 25% increase in the FDA staff . . . a few months later, came Congressional action eliminating the necessary supplemental appropriation." How, Connor asked, "can an understaffed, overworked and underpaid FDA be expected to cope with this onslaught of data" produced by the new regulations? This concern extended beyond the industry. In 1962, a second citizens advisory committee of the FDA (on which Connor served) had warned of the continuing material and intellectual weakness of the FDA, and called for the agency's personnel to be upgraded and its scientific orientation and leadership improved.[10]

Academic researchers were equally concerned about what the new regulations meant for clinical research, as William M. M. Kirby, a professor of medicine at the University of Washington and the chairman of the Committee on the Study of New Drugs of the Association of American Medical Colleges, reported in October 1963. Based on the results of a questionnaire circulated among the deans of the country's medical schools (which included 650 replies from seventy-five medical schools), Kirby's committee found "that the new regulations have not been received enthusiastically by medical school investigators. Far from participating more actively in studies involving new drugs, thereby improving scientific merit as well as increasing drug safety, clinical investigators in academic institutions are likely to undertake less and less of this type of research."[11]

While their academic colleagues were concerned about the implications for biomedical research, leaders in the nonacademic medical community worried about what the new drug amendments meant for the practice of medicine. As we saw in chapter 4, Hugh Hussey, the chairman of the AMA's board of trustees, had argued during the hearings on the drug amendments that only the physician had the knowledge and authority to make determinations about a drug's efficacy. To place such decisions in the hands of the FDA was to undermine the physician's expertise, subvert his or her autonomy, and endanger the public's health.[12]

The challenges posed by the new regulations represented a mutuality of interest between the drug industry and the medical profession. In addition, the industry and the medical profession shared a second problem after 1962. At the same time that they were confronted with an increasingly powerful government agency that lacked the resources to meet its responsibilities, both groups faced a growing labor shortage in clinical pharmacology.

A SHORTAGE OF SKILLED PHARMACEUTICAL LABOR

Testimony during the Kefauver hearings and the failure of European and American physicians to adequately test the safety of thalidomide had shed light on the paucity of standards among clinical investigators charged with testing the safety of new drugs. As Harry Dowling wrote to Maxwell Finland in September 1962, "many drugs are sent out to *hundreds* of doctors for clinical trial." This was one reason, Dowling believed, that following the findings that thalidomide was unsafe the FDA had difficulty securing both the clinical trial records and the drug itself from the hundreds of clinical investigators engaged in testing the drug. As Dowling noted, "many of the doctors had kept no records and did not know where his supply of the drug was." Dowling also feared the lack of qualifications among many of those charged with testing the safety of new drugs, with "many so-called clinical investigators . . . unable to determine whether animal experiments are safe." What was needed, Dowling asserted, was for poorly qualified clinical investigators to be "prevented from operating" and for drug companies to take "a more active part in the training and the *long-term support* of clinical investigators" so as to upgrade the standards of clinical investigation and increase the pool of well-trained clinical investigators available to both drug firms and the FDA.[13]

Clinical pharmacologists—physicians specialized in the clinical study of drugs—were those best suited to the task of drug evaluation and became increasingly important to industry and the FDA following passage of the 1962 drug amendments and enactment of the FDA's investigational new drug (IND) regulations in 1963. The IND regulations classified the testing of drugs into three phases of preclinical and clinical studies and required extensive safety and efficacy data for each phase. The industry, after all, needed clinical pharmacologists to perform the clinical studies necessary to determine the safety and efficacy of drugs, and the FDA needed them to enforce the new regulations.[14] Yet prior to passage of the drug amendments and IND regulations, academic physicians had made little effort to formally define the requisite qualifications of physicians who investigated drugs in humans. By the early 1960s, only a handful of institutions—most notably the medical schools at Johns Hopkins University and the University of Pennsylvania—offered training programs in clinical pharmacology. Even where such programs existed, young physicians were often reluctant to enter the field of clinical pharmacology, believing it to be a field with little prestige and with limited research funding, offering only routine and mundane research opportunities.[15]

BUILDING ALLIANCES

The shortage of clinical pharmacologists and the growing authority and attendant weakness of the FDA were two problems shared by the drug industry and academic medicine in the 1960s. They represented the "mutuality of interest" that the PMA's president, Austin Smith, had referred to in 1959.[16] Yet, the medical profession was itself divided in its position toward the drug industry. Even as academic leaders like Harry Dowling and Maxwell Finland called on the pharmaceutical industry to increase its support of clinical pharmacology, they criticized the industry for its heavy-handed marketing tactics. As Daniel L. Shaw, a physician with

Wyeth Laboratories, explained to an industry audience in November 1964, "We must divide physicians into at least two groups: 1.The practicing physician . . . a friendly neutral who, if made better informed, could become one of our most prized assets." And "2. The investigator," of whom there were three kinds: "1st: Friends, 2nd: The Indifferent, and 3rd: The Academic Prigs."[17]

The industry's investigator-friends (friends "because they have a common goal in therapeutics with us") were the industry's "best offense if through them we can practice 'third-person sell' . . . [to] the FDA and [to] the medical community at large." The "indifferent investigators" (those who "are content to participate in clinical pharmacology and clinical trials without becoming involved in the scientific or political problems that surround their activities") "could become a compelling force . . . if properly molded" by the industry. The academic prigs, however, posed the biggest problem for the industry. These, Shaw asserted, "are the therapeutic nihilists, the smallest group, but the loudest in their denouncements. They usually hold high academic appointments. Their administrative duties and their approach to life have taken them out of contact with day-to-day common programs. Yet they no longer do research, they only talk about it. They rarely see patients, yet they consider themselves, and are looked upon by others, as experts. They have status. These are our most severe critics . . . and must not be ignored." As experts, these were physicians who possessed a significant degree of political capital and, as such, were the physicians whose support the industry was most keen to secure.[18]

Throughout the 1960s, relations between academic and nonacademic physicians had grown increasingly antagonistic. Nowhere was this antagonism more pronounced than over the question of who had the authority to evaluate the safety and efficacy of drugs. Many academicians believed that practitioners did not have sufficient expertise in clinical research or pharmacology. As William Coon, a professor of surgery at the University of Michigan Medical School, explained, "I feel that the practicing physician has neither the inclination, breadth of experience or background of research experience necessary for objective evaluation" of the safety and efficacy of new drugs.[19] Nonacademic physicians, for their part, believed that academic physicians lacked the clinical expertise to make pronouncements on drug efficacy. As Sidney Merlis, the director of psychiatric research at Central Islip State Hospital in New York, argued, both the industry and government suffered from "excessive acceptance and dependence on the academician"; he called on drug firms to reevaluate the role of the academician. In particular, Merlis warned that "the influence of the academician must not be permitted to extend beyond the limits of their knowledge. Their 'ivory tower' position and their prestige often permit their statements to have much greater weight than experience or practical clinical data would support. The industry must make some effort to place the academic viewpoint in proper perspective." That proper perspective would be achieved, Merlis continued, if the industry—and government committees—would balance the academic perspective with that of the practicing physician.[20]

If the industry wished to win the political support of all physicians, it would have to take note of these differences and build alliances where possible. Because of their political capital, the drug industry was especially keen to secure the support of the so-called academic prigs. To do so, Shaw urged his industry colleagues to "recogniz[e] these people for what they are and . . . [be] willing to take the time to penetrate their hard shell." One way of doing this was to establish cooperative committees with academic researchers, such as the Greater Philadelphia Committee for Medical-Pharmaceutical Sciences (GPCMPS).[21]

Established in the spring of 1963, the GPCMPS was composed of the deans of Philadelphia's five medical schools, the deans of its two pharmacy schools, and representatives from the region's major drug firms, and operated under the aegis of the College of Physicians of Philadelphia.[22] The committee met regularly to discuss and develop strategies for solving the problems facing clinical researchers in the wake of the drug amendments. According to Shaw, the early meetings of the GPCMPS "were quite strained and restrained. Those of us from the industry were sure we had B.O. [body odor] and quite probably a police record." But "with time—lots of time—and patience . . . barriers were gradually broken." Eighteen months later, Shaw could confidently report that while not "all of Philadelphia's academic prigs are . . . on 'our side' . . . at least we can talk with them, we can make them aware of our problems. They in turn have learned that we can be helpful to them."[23]

The experiences of industry and academic physicians on the GPCMPS reminded both groups that underneath their differences they shared certain key interests: neither group wanted the federal government to wrest further authority away from physicians or to circumscribe what the physician could prescribe. Similarly, academic physicians and the industry both regarded the scientific weakness of the FDA as a very real threat to the integrity of pharmaceutical innovation and to clinical research, and thus to the public's health.

The need for alliance building between industry and medicine grew all the more pressing during the mid-1960s as health care reformers continued to advocate for national health insurance, and pharmaceutical reformers continued to push for legislation that would reduce the cost of prescription drugs. In 1964, for example, as the AMA fought in Congress against the Kerr-Mills legislation, Senator Philip A. Hart (D-MI) chaired a Senate subcommittee hearing into charges that U.S. drug firms were fixing the price of the antibiotic tetracycline. These hearings resulted in antitrust charges being filed against Pfizer, Bristol, and American Cyanamid.[24] That same year, during Senate and House subcommittee investigations into FDA procedures, the safety of pharmaceutical agents was again called into question as Senator Hubert Humphrey (D-MN) and Representative Lawrence Fountain (D-NC) highlighted several instances of serious adverse reactions induced by FDA-approved prescription drugs.[25] The most publicized of these adverse reactions were those associated with the use of oral contraceptives. Although it took the FDA until late 1968 to confirm that the long-term use of oral contraceptives increased women's risk of blood clots and until the 1970s to confirm that oral contraceptives increased women's risk of cervical cancer, the safety of the birth control pill had been hotly contested in the national and medical media since 1961.[26]

Congressional and public debate over the cost of prescription drugs also continued through the 1960s. In May 1967, Senator Gaylord Nelson (D-WI) began what would become a decade-long investigation of the American drug industry. As chair of the Senate Subcommittee on Antitrust and Monopoly, Nelson was concerned, as his predecessor, Senator Kefauver, had been, "with the important matter of the health and pocketbook of American citizens." In particular, Nelson's hearings examined "such matters as restraint of trade, drug pricing, scientific and technological progress in the industry, the comparative cost and effectiveness of generic and trade-name drugs, the welfare of the consumer and of small business."[27] As a way of reducing prescription drug prices and thus putting a break on escalating health care costs, Nelson, like Kefauver before him, pushed for legislation that would require physicians to prescribe by generic name rather than by brand name. As chapter 6 describes, the drug industry and medical profession were vociferous in their opposition to mandatory generic prescribing.

The drug industry, of course, fought back against these challenges, its political mobilization during the Kefauver hearings merely a warm up for the battles that ensued. As described in chapter 4, during the Kefauver hearings the PMA had hired the public relations firm Hill & Knowlton and launched a massive public relations program that told "the drug industry story" to the American public. This public relations effort expanded after 1962. Through the public speeches of its executives, a series of advertisements that were published through the late 1960s in national magazines such as *Reader's Digest*, the *Saturday Evening Post*, and *Look*, the writing of letters to news and medical editors and congressional members, and individual in-house corporate publications, the industry presented "to the public its record of achievement in protecting health, prolonging life and lowering the costs of illness."[28]

The industry also worked to establish a stronger political presence in Washington, D.C. In addition to hiring a cadre of lobbyists to promote the industry's interests in the halls of Congress, firms established programs that worked to get "business-oriented, free-enterprise philosophy individuals" elected in congressional district elections instead of those congressional members who pushed for "Fabian-socialist type of government controls."[29] To help with this, firms sought to make connections with as many elected officials as possible, passing along information to these officials and in return receiving information from them. The industry also sought to insinuate itself into state and local politics. Eli Lilly & Co., for example, encouraged its employees to run for elective office in the Indianapolis community, seeking "such spots as precinct committee man, ward chairman, state representative, city council members, members of town boards and trustees, board of education members." The firm established a company policy that granted leave to employees who worked on political matters.[30]

More than anything, however, the industry's ability to draw on the "mutualities of interest" it shared with the academic medical community proved critical to its political efforts. Although the drug industry and academic medicine had shared the threat of increasing government oversight since the end of World War II, passage of the 1962 drug amendments—by expanding the FDA's authority over drug development and therapeutic practice—transformed that threat into reality. In response, the pharmaceutical industry joined forces with academic physicians to circumvent the FDA's new authority and shift the balance of power back toward industry and academic medicine.

NETWORKED SOLUTIONS: THE COMMISSION ON DRUG SAFETY

During the summer of 1962, in response to the thalidomide disaster, the PMA created the Commission on Drug Safety, a body of pharmaceutical experts from industry and academic medicine. The commission was charged with guiding industry and the FDA on the issues raised by thalidomide and other problems relating to drug safety. Composed of medical scientists and physicians that were roughly half from industry and half from academia, the makeup of the commission highlighted the "revolving door" that characterized pharmaceutical industry–medicine–government relations throughout the twentieth century.[31] Included on the commission were the Nobel laureate Philip S. Hench (who had shared the 1950 Nobel Prize in Physiology or Medicine for his work on the corticosteroids); the former special assistant to the secretary of the Department of Health, Education, and Welfare Chester Keefer (then a professor of medicine at Boston University School of Medicine); the former director of the Drug Division at the FDA Theodore Klumpp (then the president and a director of the drug firm Winthrop Laboratories); the former surgeon general Leonard Scheele (then a senior vice-president at Warner Lambert Pharmaceutical Company); the former editor of the *Journal of the American Medical Association* and the current president of the PMA Austin Smith; and two additional industry executives and eight academic researchers, several of whom had ties to drug companies.[32] In this way, the commission also embodied the pharmaceutical networks that characterized drug industry–academic-government relations in the postwar decades. For example, Hench had collaborated with Merck & Co. on the development of the corticosteroids and Keefer had served as a longtime consultant to Merck.

The aim of the Commission on Drug Safety was to guide industry and government on improving the policies and methods by which new compounds were tested for safety and efficacy.[33] To this end, the commission formed seventeen subcommittees (composed of nearly two hundred scientists), which evaluated each of "the critical phases of the complex problems of drug safety."[34] These included the study of prenatal malformations, the principles of clinical trials, and the respective responsibilities of industry, universities, and the state and federal governments regarding drug safety. The PMA's chairman, Eugene Beesley, also hoped the commission would help to undermine the image—portrayed by the industry's critics in Congress and the press—of the industry as greed-driven and quick to exploit the sick patient with costly and dangerous drugs, by making "it more clear to all people that the prescription drug industry is truly going their way, seeking what they seek—the conquest of disease."[35]

The ad hoc commission was in operation for eighteen months, funded entirely by the PMA. At the end of its tenure, the commission published a final report detailing 116 recommendations based on the evaluations of its seventeen subcommittees. Of those recommendations, three in particular were aimed at shifting the balance of power within the regulatory environment back toward academic medicine and industry. The first called on academic medicine to "take an aggressive role in training programs for those disciplines directly concerned with drug investigation, particularly clinical pharmacology." The expectation was that with better investigators on hand to predict and interpret drug actions, there would be less cause for FDA intervention.[36] The key to expanding training in clinical pharmacology, however, was increased financial support for the field. Although the PMA had been tackling the workforce problem since the late 1950s, establishing fellowship programs in clinical pharmacology at Johns Hopkins University and at the University of Pennsylvania, the commission made clear that this was only a beginning, calling on "both government and private granting agencies [to] consider immediate increase of support for the universities that now offer these educational programs or that wish to institute them."[37]

The commission's second recommendation sought to tackle the intellectual weakness of the FDA. Concerned that the FDA remain fully engaged with advances in pharmaceutical knowledge but aware of its stretched-thin resources, the commission recommended that the agency engage in "wide consultation" with leaders in pharmaceutical research. By outsourcing its scientific expertise, the FDA could "take full advantage of the knowledge" of pharmaceutical experts in academia and "close the gaps in [the FDA's] knowledge." In particular, the commission suggested that the FDA use ad hoc advisory panels to help guide the agency in making decisions about the safety and efficacy of drugs. In this way, the commission sought to make pharmaceutical experts outside of government the designators of regulatory requirements.[38]

The third and most significant of the commission's recommendations went a step further and aimed to secure for academic medicine and industry a role in making pharmaceutical policies. As the commission's chairman, Lowell Coggeshall, testified before the 1964 Senate Subcommittee on Drug Safety, the commission recommended the establishment of a permanent advisory body similar to the Commission on Drug Safety, "composed of men whose scientific ability and integrity is not questioned—if you will, a supreme court that might serve as a reference body to all the problems that currently exist or will exist in the future."[39] Such a body was needed, Coggeshall explained, because as new and increasingly potent drugs were developed, the processes of drug development and testing were certain to grow more complex. And if a major problem or crisis was to arise, the government "should not and could not await a regrouping of ad hoc committees to consider each" problem.[40] Rather, the commission urged the government to retain an elite group of pharmaceutical experts with whom it could consult on everyday issues and should a crisis emerge.[41] These experts would also guarantee that industry and academic medicine had a permanent presence in the policy arena, thus ensuring that their interests would be protected even as federal reformers sought to further expand the government's authority over pharmaceutical practice.

ESTABLISHING A "SUPREME COURT" ON DRUG POLICY: THE DRUG RESEARCH BOARD

The Commission on Drug Safety recognized that, as an industry-funded entity, it could not function effectively as a permanent advisory body because its motives and the objectivity of its advice would be questioned. Such a body needed instead to be independent of both business and government influence. As both a nongovernment and nonbusiness scientific organization with "the stature, the tradition, and the capabilities of effectively assuming an advisory function," the commission regarded the National Academy of Sciences–National Research Council (NAS-NRC) as the ideal home for the "supreme court" of pharmaceutical experts.[42] In the spring of 1963, Lowell Coggeshall approached the NAS-NRC to see about transferring the commission's operations to the Academy and setting up a permanent advisory body.

The NAS-NRC accepted the commission's proposal, having already determined that the FDA's "woefully inadequate resources" jeopardized the public's health. Like the drug industry and academic medicine, the NAS-NRC was keen to balance the FDA's new authority with that of academic researchers. At the end of 1963, under a three-year contract with the National Institutes of Health (at up to $75,000 a year), the Drug Research Board (DRB) was established. The primary objectives of the DRB were to evaluate "the policies, principles, and practices" of pharmaceutical research, to provide a forum for academic medicine, industry, and government to discuss "the problems, responsibilities and opportunities" of drug research and practice, and to make policy recommendations to government.[43]

Like its predecessor, the DRB relied on a system of subcommittees— composed of non-Academy scientists considered experts in their field—to evaluate and make recommendations on key issues in drug policy and practice. And like the commission, the membership of the DRB consisted of high-ranking industry and academic physicians, and many of the latter had affiliations with industry and thus were part of the pharmaceutical network.[44] Although Congress had raised some questions about the role of industry in any such advisory body, the DRB sidestepped the specter of "conflict of interest" charges. The DRB's members insisted that their industrial affiliations actually gave them the expertise to deliberate on issues of national drug policy rather than undermining their authority to speak on such matters.[45] In a statement made to the FDA in 1963, the DRB asserted, "almost inevitably, those individuals with the greatest experience in the study of the action of drugs will be found to have developed working relationships with the pharmaceutical industry."[46] The Academy was confident that it "has sought out the best men for the job as it sees it, confident in the belief that one has less to fear from asking the counsel of the best men than one has to fear from rejecting their counsel because of suspected possibilities of conscious or unconscious bias."[47] The FDA agreed; its commissioner assured the DRB that when seeking its advice the agency would not question conflict of interest in any individual selected by the board.[48]

The DRB operated for twelve years (from 1964 through 1975), during which time it was at the center of the industry's and academic medicine's efforts to reshape the regulatory environment to better serve their interests in the years after passage of the 1962 drug amendments. In particular, as pharmaceutical reformers in Congress pushed to further increase the government's authority over pharmaceutical practice, the DRB's work proved critical in circumscribing these efforts. Nonetheless, the DRB was not a straightforward proxy for the industry. During the DRB's tenure, there was often disagreement among its members over how best to resolve the problems confronting the pharmaceutical field. The discussions and work of the DRB, however, show that in its efforts to reshape the regulatory environment for prescription drugs, the shared interests of the industry and academic physicians were far more important than their differences.

Four issues, in particular, dominated the work of the DRB during its tenure: the shortage of clinical pharmacologists, the production and dissemination of drug information, the FDA's informed consent regulations, and the therapeutic equivalence of generic drugs. Each case served as an issue around which the drug industry and academic medicine forged a political alliance, and each reveals the extent to which both groups perceived the FDA to have significantly overstepped its authority in the wake of the 1962 drug amendments and sought—through the work of the DRB—to rein in that authority. The remainder of this chapter will describe the work of the DRB as it relates to the first three issues; chapter 6 considers the work of the DRB as it relates to the therapeutic equivalence of generic drugs, a subject of significant controversy and government, academic, and industry debate from the late 1960s through the 1970s.

DEVELOPING THE FIELD OF CLINICAL PHARMACOLOGY

Building on the recommendation of the Commission on Drug Safety, the problems of recruitment, training, and funding in clinical pharmacology became an early—and major—priority of the Drug Research Board. Before discussing the DRB's efforts to tackle these challenges, let us first review the status of clinical pharmacology in 1964. As Dale Friend of Harvard Medical School and Peter Bent Brigham Hospital had explained to the AMA's Section on Experimental Medicine and Therapeutics in June 1963, very few highly trained individuals were entering clinical pharmacology because the field "does not yet command the prestige that leads to rapid academic advancement." The reasons, Friend explained, were that the field was new, having emerged only in the previous two decades with the explosion of pharmaceutical innovation in the 1940s. As such, the field "is not well understood even by experienced colleagues." In addition, Friend continued, the "clinical pharmacologist is not an essential member of the modern hospital team, but crosses many disciplines and he, therefore, does not fit easily into the usual clinical categories." Finally, Friend argued, "it is more remunerative to be a surgeon, internist, or other clinical specialist."[49] In a fee-for-service medical economy (in which physicians were paid for every service or procedure performed rather than a fixed salary), a physician's remuneration depended on the number of patients seen and the number of procedures performed on those patients. Without their own patients, clinical pharmacologists were not able to command the levels of pay of their patient- and procedure-oriented colleagues.[50]

The political economy of biomedical research and of academic career building further impeded efforts to recruit young and talented physicians to clinical pharmacology. Clinical pharmacologists looked to the National Institutes of Health (NIH), the primary patron of biomedical research after World War II, to support their research. Yet the NIH's mandate was to support basic research and, although clinical pharmacologists argued that their work was fundamental in nature, the NIH and its advisory committees, which were responsible for selecting projects for funding support, perceived the evaluation of drugs to be too applied—and too mundane—to fund. In reality, clinical pharmacology stood at the intersection of basic and so-called applied research, bridging basic and clinical science. In today's parlance, clinical pharmacologists were engaged in translational medicine, moving new therapeutic agents from the laboratory bench to the patient's bedside. But because the work of clinical pharmacologists occurred at the intersection of clinical research and practice, they more often than not found their funding requests rejected by the NIH.[51]

The interdisciplinary status of clinical pharmacology further relegated clinical pharmacologists to the lower rungs of the medical hierarchy. As clinical pharmacologists often held dual appointments in departments of pharmacology and one of the clinical departments (usually medicine), there was uncertainty as to which department would evaluate the clinical pharmacologist for promotion, and what those standards for promotion should be. In 1963, for example, of the twenty-seven formal programs of clinical pharmacology within American medical schools, eighteen were located jointly in departments of pharmacology and medicine.[52] Even within their own pharmacology departments, clinical pharmacologists garnered less respect than their "basic" pharmacology colleagues. With their own institutional pressures to perform under the academic standards of the day, academic departments placed their intellectual emphasis on the fields that garnered the most federal funds. In the case of pharmacology, this meant research oriented toward the biochemical mechanisms of drug action rather than on the clinical study of drugs.[53]

By 1963, it was clear to academic physicians that clinical pharmacology needed to professionalize beyond what had already been achieved for the field. In practice, this meant formalizing the degree and types of training required for clinical pharmacologists, increasing the number of training programs, and establishing the clinical pharmacologist as a critical member of a medical school faculty and hospital staff. In doing so, leading academic physicians hoped to raise the prestige of the field, which would in turn, they hoped, encourage young physicians to enter it.

Prior to passage of the 1962 drug amendments, the nature of training required for a clinical pharmacologist was undefined. Academic leaders such as Harry Dowling and Dale Friend contended that the clinical pharmacologist should have training in both medicine and the basic sciences, including biochemistry, pharmacology, physiology, and statistics. However, they were undecided as to whether that basic science training should come before or after internship and residency.[54]

Exacerbating the problem of establishing training standards, there was but a handful of medical schools with programs in clinical pharmacology and experienced clinical pharmacologists on faculty that could train new generations of clinical pharmacologists. Of eighty-one pharmacology department chairs surveyed by the American Society for Pharmacology and Experimental Therapeutics (ASPET) in 1963, only twenty-seven reported having some formal teaching and research program in clinical pharmacology.[55] Among those programs, very few had more than one clinical pharmacologist on staff, and the functional activities of those programs varied greatly from institution to institution. In some medical schools, for example, the work of the clinical pharmacologist was limited to giving a series of lectures on therapeutics during the medical school's second-year pharmacology course and serving on university committees concerned with clinical trials. In others, the clinical pharmacologist's principal function was to perform controlled drug trials.[56]

In June 1963, ASPET (the main professional association for clinically oriented pharmacologists) considered the possibility of establishing qualifying boards in clinical pharmacology. The board certification of clinical pharmacologists served as a two-pronged effort to raise the status of clinical pharmacology. On the one hand, board certification would designate the minimum qualifications for entry into the field, thus providing a guarantee that all clinical pharmacologists would be adequately trained before they were certified to practice. On the other hand, board certification would make clinical pharmacology more comparable to that of the other medical specialties and thus, the proponents of board certification hoped, more attractive to medical students picking their specialties. Ultimately, though, ASPET rejected the 1963 proposal to establish a qualifying board in clinical pharmacology, arguing that there was no precedent for certifying *scientists* for *research*, and that the medical specialty boards related only to medical *practice*. Specialty boards did not designate a physician qualified for *research* in that medical specialty. Moreover, ASPET was concerned that certification of clinical pharmacologists would impede drug evaluations by restricting the clinical investigation of new drugs only to "qualified" clinical pharmacologists, thereby eliminating many good clinical *investigators* who could not qualify for board certification—not an insignificant consideration, given the shortage of clinical pharmacologists.[57]

The rationale behind ASPET's rejection of calls to establish qualifying boards in clinical pharmacology reflects the tension inherent in the debate over the pharmaceutical workforce: academic physicians, the

FDA, Congress, and patients were demanding that physicians charged with evaluating the safety of drugs should be better trained in order to avoid another thalidomide disaster, but many physicians were reluctant to relinquish their role in the clinical investigation of drugs and to cede authority to a new specialty group—clinical pharmacology—that in many physicians' eyes lacked the status of their colleagues engaged in full-time clinical practice.

Despite a degree of uncertainty over the appropriate training and qualifications of those charged with the clinical study of drugs, there was a clear expectation that all those trained as clinical pharmacologists should serve as teachers and should be responsible not only for training the next generation of clinical pharmacologists but also for educating their clinician colleagues in the fundamentals of drug evaluation and research. In other words, clinical pharmacologists would be responsible for training *clinical investigators* with respect to clinical pharmacology, thus further increasing the pool of skilled researchers available to study drugs in humans.[58] A further area of consensus was that programs in clinical pharmacology, and the clinical pharmacologists on staff at teaching hospitals, would provide a service function to hospitals. As Dale Friend described it, the clinical pharmacologist should "serve as a consultant for all drug evaluation programs" and should "teach and set forth patterns of excellence in drug therapy. Furthermore, he can head the therapeutic and adverse drug reaction committees and assist the hospital pharmacy by serving as an effective liaison between the pharmacist and the staff."[59] In Friend's vision, the clinical pharmacologist would become an invaluable member of the hospital team. In providing a service function, clinical pharmacologists—and their home programs—while giving up some institutional autonomy, would in return secure a degree of institutional stability and financial security. Indeed, for every consultant service performed for the hospital, clinical pharmacologists would be paid a fee. As other medical specialties that lacked their own patients, most notably, pathology and radiology, had done earlier, clinical pharmacologists constructed a functional niche within the hospital that designated their unique expertise as critical to the safe and efficient operation of the clinical team.[60]

By 1964, then, the field of clinical pharmacology lacked organizational, financial, and institutional stability. At its first meeting in January 1964, the DRB highlighted the major challenges confronting the field: the lack of a standardized training program for clinical pharmacologists, the absence of a consistent organizational form for existing programs or "units" of clinical pharmacology, and insufficient levels of government and industry funding for research, teaching, and training in the field.[61]

Recognizing that it was not the only organization interested in tackling these issues, in October 1964 the DRB invited representatives from the NIH and the Association of American Medical Colleges (AAMC) to discuss those organizations' efforts to increase the number of clinical pharmacologists. Reflecting the ongoing debate about how best to train those preparing for careers in clinical pharmacology, those in attendance at the fall meeting debated the necessary qualifications of a clinical pharmacologist. The DRB asked: Could "a physician trained solely in a medical specialty" be considered a clinical pharmacologist or was that physician more accurately termed a *clinical investigator?* Should a clinical pharmacologist be defined only as an individual who had training equivalent to a "doctorate in both medicine and pharmacology"?[62]

Attention at the conference also focused on assessing current and future funding sources for the field and discussions of how best to increase the funding available for the education and training of clinical pharmacologists. George J. Cosmides of the NIH's Research Training Grant Branch, for example, reported on the recent efforts of the National Institute of General Medical Sciences (NIGMS) to support training programs in clinical pharmacology. Cosmides cited the fact that "50 schools of medicine now have NIGMS-sponsored programs with over 500 predoctoral and postdoctoral trainees," with the emphasis in these programs being "to provide the clinically oriented practitioner with training in basic pharmacological sciences."[63] Jean K. Weston of the AMA's Department of Drugs, who also attended the meeting, was skeptical of Cosmides' interpretation of the term *clinical pharmacology,* however. Weston suspected that when Cosmides used the term to describe the NIH's support of the field, he did so "in about as broad a sense as it can be used. . . . [U]sed in this fashion, the NIH can seem to be supporting a relatively large program in clinical pharmacology which, however, may well be doing mighty little to set up centers engaged in actively training clinical pharmacologists."[64]

William Kirby, himself a member of the DRB, reported on the AAMC's efforts to establish a task force to study present needs in clinical pharmacology, to encourage the "development of units of clinical pharmacology in all medical schools," and "to take leadership in setting standards, goals, and objectives for these programs." At the same time, though, Kirby cited the need for industry support to establish many of the proposed units of clinical pharmacology. Kirby noted that "if industry were disposed to contribute $50,000 per year for five years, the AAMC could take an active role in awarding grants to schools showing promise and interest in this field."[65] In doing so, Kirby highlighted the recognition by the DRB—and academic physicians more generally—that efforts to expand the field of clinical pharmacology required collaboration among academia, government, and industry. Reflecting this point, AMA and PMA representatives present at the meeting urged the DRB to assume a mediating role in that collaborative process in the hope that "the Drug Research Board could be a powerful force in helping to get clinical pharmacology solidly established."[66]

Over the course of the subsequent decade, the DRB worked hard to encourage the pharmaceutical industry and government to commit greater financial support to training in clinical pharmacology at the level of undergraduate medical education.[67] Early in his role as DRB chairman, for example, William Middleton proposed that the DRB establish a funding pool for clinical pharmacology, sustained by fixed annual contributions from the drug industry (Middleton proposed that the amount be "5% of the payroll of detail men for the first five years," increasing to 10 percent if the plan proved effective). The DRB would use the funding pool to award grants to qualified institutions and individuals to support the strengthening of undergraduate instruction and graduate training in clinical pharmacology.[68]

Although no such program was developed, the pharmaceutical industry responded positively to the DRB's charge of financial responsibility. Early in 1965, on the recommendation of the Commission on Drug Safety, the PMA established the PMA Foundation for Education and Research "to receive and administer funds supplied by the Association."[69] By 1970, the PMA Foundation had awarded nineteen two-year Faculty Development Awards to young faculty members in clinical pharmacology units, and had provided "special grants for clinical research and fellowships that enable[d] medical students to work in clinical pharmacology units."[70] Individual firms also increased their funding of clinical pharmacology. In the early 1960s, Merck & Co. established a fellowship in clinical pharmacology, which funded foreign, research-oriented clinicians to spend two years in the United States studying clinical pharmacology. The expectation was that after two years, the fellows would return to their home countries, teach clinical pharmacology, and eventually establish schools of clinical pharmacology. In addition to building the field, Merck generated an international pool of clinical pharmacologists whom the company could "call, not to do the work, but for advice," particularly on conducting research in those countries.[71] The Burroughs Wellcome Fund, an endowment of the drug firm Burroughs Wellcome, for example, by 1971 had supported twenty clinical pharmacology units "with grants of $15,000–25,000 per year for 5 years each."[72]

The DRB also worked to secure greater government support of clinical pharmacology. In this effort, the DRB achieved some success after the NIGMS established a pharmacology and toxicology program in 1964. By 1970, the program was providing "$10 million annually for research, of which $3–4 million is considered to be in noncategorical clinical pharmacology." During the same period, the NIH also increased its support of training in clinical pharmacology; by 1970, the NIH was awarding "$740,000 for training programs supported by the NIGMS, the National Heart and Lung Institute, and the National Cancer Institute."[73] Yet, as the AMA's Jean Weston had cautioned in 1965, the NIH in general, and the NIGMS in particular, used a very broad definition of clinical pharmacology in its categorization of funded research, one not generally shared by other groups working to expand the field. Therefore, these figures likely overstate the NIH's contribution to the development of clinical pharmacology.

Indeed, despite the moderate improvements in NIH support for research and training in clinical pharmacology, at the end of 1970 the DRB still felt that development of the field was being hindered by the lack of sustained federal support. Although the number of clinical pharmacology programs within medical schools in the United States had risen from twenty-seven in 1963 to thirty-six in 1970, the DRB still cautioned that "the number of clinical pharmacologists must be substantially increased and the discipline further developed in order to meet critical national needs."[74] In particular, as an academic consultant to the DRB noted, the field would benefit significantly from the establishment of an Institute of Clinical Pharmacology within the NIH.[75]

The DRB placed responsibility for confronting the workforce problem squarely on the shoulders of the government, "recommend[ing] that the federal government establish a new program that will solve the problem of support for clinical pharmacology and in so doing aid in recruiting more highly qualified persons into this field." Specifically, the DRB called for the establishment of "a substantial and long-range program that will fund faculty positions in clinical pharmacology. Such a salary support mechanism, with a continuing provision for renewal on the basis of favorable review," the DRB proposed, "would provide tangible evidence of a career opportunity . . . essential to effective recruitment."[76]

The advice of the DRB did not go entirely unheeded. As will be discussed in chapter 6, the issue of government support for clinical pharmacology reached the halls of Congress in 1975 when the pharmaceutical reformer Senator Edward Kennedy (D-MA) introduced a series of bills that called for the creation a National Center for Clinical Pharmacology within the Department of Health, Education, and Welfare. In writing these bills, Kennedy drew on the recommendations of the DRB.[77] In this way, the DRB's effort to expand the field of clinical pharmacology shows the important role played by the DRB in influencing the pharmaceutical policy agenda in the late 1960s and 1970s. At the same time, it highlights an important theme in the history of American pharmaceutical policymaking: each of the stakeholders in pharmaceutical policymaking in the 1960s—the federal government, the medical profession, and the pharmaceutical industry—recognized that to achieve a policy goal (in this case, expansion of clinical pharmacology) the stakeholders needed to work cooperatively with one another to effect policy change.

DRUG INFORMATION

The role played by the shared political interests of the drug industry and medical profession in circumventing pharmaceutical reformers' efforts to cement the FDA's authority can be seen in the debates over the continuing pharmaceutical education of physicians. Even after passage of the drug amendments and the resulting tightening of regulations around prescription drug advertising, pharmaceutical marketing remained a source of unanimous criticism among academic physicians and pharmaceutical reformers alike throughout the 1960s. The veracity of pharmaceutical marketing and the (in)appropriate role of pharmaceutical promotion in guiding therapeutic practice were prominent issues debated during Senator Nelson's hearings on the pharmaceutical industry. Surveys of physicians' prescription practices conducted during the 1950s and the testimonies of several physicians during the Kefauver hearings had indicated that the majority of practitioners regarded pharmaceutical marketing products as their primary source of information about new drugs and new dosage regimes.[78] As Senator Nelson began his hearings on the drug industry, there was little evidence that the prominence of pharmaceutical promotion in the continuing education of physicians had declined.

The extent and effectiveness of companies' pharmaceutical marketing campaigns in part explain physicians' reliance on pharmaceutical marketing products for their drug information. In the 1960s, as they do today, the largest pharmaceutical firms spent more on marketing than they did on any other area of the pharmaceutical enterprise. On average, the American drug industry spent 20 percent of annual sales on promoting—and, they argued, educating physicians about—their drug products.[79] The centrality of pharmaceutical marketing to physician practice, however, was also due to the paucity of pharmaceutical education provided by the medical profession.[80] Although academic and nonacademic physicians alike agreed that, with the wealth of new drugs reaching the market each year, the continuing education of physicians on prescription drug use was important, neither medical schools nor medical societies were willing to assume the intellectual and financial burden of keeping physicians informed about new drugs. Thus, although critics of the industry's marketing practices admonished the industry for masquerading marketing as education, the industry's contention that its marketing provided physicians with a critical source of drug information was not mere hyperbole. Drug marketing throughout the 1960s did in fact serve a valuable educational function, albeit one that lacked the balance and oversight of an academically oriented education program.[81]

The issue of expanding and improving physicians' access to reliable, accurate, and objective drug information became a focal point in the work of the Drug Research Board. In its first meeting in January 1964, the DRB identified as a critical area of study an assessment of the drug information sources currently available to physicians. In the view of the DRB's chairman, William Middleton, while the pharmaceutical industry was spending $250 million a year on the promotion of new drugs, academic medicine had "abrogated its position of leadership in graduate medical education insofar as drug use and abuse are concerned."[82] Though not all DRB members agreed that academic medicine was to blame, they did concur that although the AMA was "conducting some educational programs for physicians in drug use," drug information provided by the drug industry was now "a central source of drug education."[83]

In criticizing the lack of continuing education provided by medical schools and medical societies, the DRB acknowledged the "very real problems" encountered when devising such programs: "The conference technique has serious limitations, and it is estimated that only 5 percent of physicians regularly participate in formal programs of this kind." And circulation of the educational publications put out by the AMA—the *Medical Letter*, the *Physician's Desk Reference, New and Non-Official Drugs,* and the *Journal of the American Medical Association*—was generally limited to the AMA's membership rolls, which were declining by the 1960s. To help the medical profession "assess its information responsibilities," the DRB resolved at its first meeting to "bring together the forces of education for thought" on the problem of continuing pharmaceutical education.[84]

The work of the DRB to improve physicians' access to drug information focused on two areas in particular. The first involved the creation of a "therapeutic consultants" program in which trained experts in therapeutics would visit academic institutions and medical societies around the country providing educational programs and instructions to all physicians in the region. The academic detailing programs currently being experimented with by academic institutions bear striking a resemblance to the DRB's therapeutic consultants program of the 1960s. The key difference is that contemporary academic detailing programs are completely independent of the industry (including of industry-funded scientists).[85] The second component of the DRB's education program involved the production of a national drug compendium that would contain all necessary information— about dosage, indications, side effects, adverse reactions—about every drug available, which would be updated annually and distributed free of charge to all practicing physicians.

In each case, the DRB designated academic pharmaceutical experts as the appropriate producers and purveyors of drug information and deprecated the FDA's claims to being the authoritative—and legally mandated— source of pharmaceutical information. In doing so, the DRB protected the professional and political interests of the medical profession and the drug industry, as those groups perceived the FDA's attempts to assume responsibility for continuing pharmaceutical education as a threat to physician autonomy and authority.

The Therapeutic Consultants Program and the Effort to Create Expert Educators

In October 1964, the DRB created the Committee on Continuing Education. Chaired by Carl F. Schmidt, the research director of the U.S. Naval Air Development Center and a former professor of pharmacology at the University of Pennsylvania School of Medicine, the committee was charged with exploring what the DRB's role should be in expanding and improving physicians' access to pharmaceutical information. The committee was particularly troubled that medical schools were systematically reducing and in some cases discontinuing the teaching of therapeutics within the medical school curriculum just when that instruction was needed most. *Therapeutics* refers specifically to the *practice* of treating disease. Amid the rapid pace of pharmaceutical innovation, physicians were struggling to keep abreast of the latest developments in therapeutic practice. Without sufficient training in therapeutics and without access to accurate and reliable sources of pharmaceutical information, it was no wonder, the committee held, that physicians relied on the pharmaceutical industry for their information.

Despite the intellectual relationship of therapeutics to clinical pharmacology (which referred to the *study* of drug actions in humans and not to practice), the DRB realized that increasing the number of clinical pharmacologists and the amount of clinical pharmacology being taught to medical students would not be sufficient to provide all physicians with authoritative information on how to incorporate the wealth of new drugs into practice. Rather, what the nation's practicing physicians needed was access to accurate, up-to-date, and regularly available continuing pharmaceutical education.

Within eighteen months, the Committee on Continuing Education had determined that all existing methods of disseminating drug information to physicians—whether newsletters, workshops and conferences, or editorials—offered little hope of competing with the methods of pharmaceutical detailing. Acknowledging the "success of the face to face approach," the committee instead resolved to tackle the drug information problem by establishing an education program modeled on the work of pharmaceutical sales representatives.

To this end, the committee proposed a therapeutic consultants program in which medical schools (ten to begin with) would hire an academic physician or pharmacologist with expertise in therapeutics to serve on a full-time basis at the medical school. This therapeutic consultant would be responsible for bringing to physicians in the region "a wide range of authoritative information on the uses and limitations of new drugs."[86] The therapeutic consultants' educational efforts would be two-pronged. First, therapeutic consultants would offer regular seminars and workshops on specific aspects of pharmaceutical practice, which would be available to all physicians in the region. In this way, the work of the therapeutic consultants was to be modeled on the work of medical schools' existing continuing medical education programs. Second, therapeutic consultants would visit physicians in their offices and clinics, providing them with up-to-date and face-to-face information on prescription drugs. This, the most innovative aspect of the therapeutic consultants program, was modeled on the work of pharmaceutical detail men and the farmer education provided by states' agricultural extension officers.

To ensure their continued access to high-quality and authoritative drug information and preserve their status as experts, therapeutic consultants would attend regular seminar programs conducted by the NAS-NRC; they would have direct contact with leaders in medicine, industry, and the government; and the NAS-NRC would provide them with up-to-date unbiased information derived from material from all sources of drug information: the AMA, the FDA, the American Pharmacology Association, the PMA, and the United States Pharmacopeia (USP). Funding for the program, the committee proposed, might come from the AMA, the PMA, the FDA, or the NIH, with a projected annual budget of between $400,000 and $500,000. Control of the program, however, would rest with the DRB.[87]

In March 1967, the DRB approved the plans for the therapeutic consultants program and in the ensuing months, Carl Schmidt and Duke Trexler met with representatives from the Commonwealth Fund and the NIH's recently created Division of Regional Medical Programs (RMP) in an effort to secure funding for the program. Established amid considerable opposition from the AMA and uncertain institutional support, the RMP (a product of the Heart Disease, Cancer, and Stroke Amendments of 1965) was conceived as a way "to put the latest advances in medical treatment—beginning with those for heart disease, cancer and stroke—at the disposal of physicians throughout the country, and so bring such advances to hundreds of communities and thousands of people who otherwise would be denied them."[88] To aid with its funding requests, the DRB solicited sample applications from the Medical College of Virginia, the University of Florida Medical School, and Jefferson Medical College in Philadelphia.[89]

In spite of the enthusiasm for the therapeutic consultants program expressed by Robert Q. Marston, the director of the NIH Division of Regional Medical Programs and the Commonwealth Fund, and strong interest among the medical schools that submitted sample applications, the DRB's therapeutic consultants program never got off of the ground. The reason for the program's failure lies in part with the DRB's decision to tie the fate of the therapeutic consultants program to the NIH's RMP, whose institutional status remained unclear throughout the late 1960s and early 1970s. Although support for the continuing medical education of physicians was justified within the RMP's mandate, in practice, the RMP's programmatic and operational emphasis lay with the delivery of health care services rather than any provision to ensure physician education. Moreover, the brief history of the RMP (which was terminated by President Nixon in 1974) was beset with programmatic disagreements, conflicting and inconsistent goals (particularly between academic and nonacademic physicians), and insufficient federal funds.[90] The absence of broad-based support for the therapeutic consultants program among the AMA, leaders in academic medicine, and the PMA also accounts for the DRB's failure to move forward with the program.

Although the DRB's proposal for continuing pharmaceutical education was never translated into practice, there is much to be learned from examining the history of paths not taken. Despite its failure, the DRB's efforts to establish a continuing pharmaceutical education program highlights the fact that the provision and dissemination of accurate and unbiased pharmaceutical information represented a significant policy need in the 1960s. Despite this recognized need, the failure of DRB's efforts suggest that the policy need was not perceived by the stakeholders—most notably the federal government, the drug industry, and medical schools—to be sufficiently severe as to warrant substantial financial investment. In this instance, the history of the path not taken underscores the historical contingency of the current system of pharmaceutical education, making clear to contemporary policymakers that alternative models of pharmaceutical education have been—and arguably still are—possible.

The history of the DRB's abortive therapeutic consultants program also reveals the limits of the DRB's mandate: without the buy-in of institutional stakeholders, the DRB's efforts to effect practical (and not just policy) change were circumscribed. It is telling that recent efforts to establish "academic detailing" as an alternative source of therapeutic information to the still pervasive and persuasive pharmaceutical detailing, look remarkably like those of the 1960s. Yet in a significant departure from the programs of the 1960s, contemporary academic detailing programs use neither industry scientists nor industry-funded academic researchers.[91] Yet, if academic detailing is to succeed this time around, the subject of pharmaceutical information will need to garner much greater political and institutional support than it held in the 1960s.

The Battle over a National Drug Compendium

The second component of the DRB's pharmaceutical information program focused on efforts to produce a national compendium of drug information. Since the 1940s (and required by the FDA beginning in 1961), drug manufacturers had included an informational insert in all drug packages.[92] These inserts were intended to provide physicians and pharmacists with information about the drug—appropriate dosages, possible side effects and adverse reactions, potentially dangerous drug interactions—and thus were meant to be a source of continuing pharmaceutical education. According to the testimony of physicians during the Kefauver hearings and in the early meetings of the DRB, however, the inserts rarely reached the physician, being instead "discarded when the package is opened and dispensed." The inserts, more often than not, remained unread.[93] In 1964, one of the first acts of the DRB was to recommend to the FDA that the package inserts should be abolished in favor of a national drug compendium. The DRB believed that publication of an annually updated drug compendium, provided free of charge to all physicians and containing reliable, complete, and readily accessible information on all prescription drugs, would be an important step in improving physicians' access to drug information.

Between the summer of 1964 and winter 1965, the DRB held a series of meetings with representatives from the AMA, the PMA, and the FDA to determine the feasibility of and support for a national drug compendium. Although there was initial consensus that a compendium was needed, by the late winter and early spring of 1965, tensions were surfacing over questions of who should be the purveyor of drug information to physicians. The AMA believed that the "excellent lines of communication which the AMA has through its journals with the members of the health team" meant that the AMA was in the best position to "communicate readily any new or significant drug information to" physicians.[94] Some in the AMA leadership even questioned the need for a compendium, as the AMA was expanding its own pharmaceutical information program. As Jean Weston of the AMA's Department of Drugs expressed to the DRB's Duke Trexler that February, the AMA was unsure whether the compendium was really necessary, given the fact that the AMA was planning to publish two books that would contain extensive drug information, *New Drugs* and the *Reference Book on Drugs*.[95] According to Weston, *New Drugs* would "plug" the "educational hiatus which many believe exists for the practitioner in the area of new drugs," by providing the "busy medical practitioner" with concise, "objective and unbiased" information on "the vast majority of truly new single drugs which have received New Drug Application approval from the Food and Drug Administration over the past ten-year period." *New Drugs* would be produced under the auspices of the AMA's Council on Drugs and would be "brought up to date yearly."[96] Weston assured Trexler that with the AMA's drug education program "off the ground and running, there seems little need for a [compendium]."[97] Weston was confident that no other source of drug information—currently available or proposed for the future—could "more nearly meet the needs of the practicing physician" than *New Drugs* and the proposed reference book. Weston was in essence staking the AMA's claim to being the most authoritative—and thus, legitimate—educator of physicians.[98]

The task of the DRB, and in particular its Committee on Drug Compendium chaired by Chester S. Keefer, was to mediate and help resolve the disagreements among the AMA, the PMA, and the FDA.[99] To this end, Keefer's committee continued to meet and correspond with representatives from each group and, by the fall, could report that "the PMA still stands ready to finance the compendium," as long as the compendium replaced the legal requirement for package inserts and the FDA "still recognizes the need for the compendium" (the agency was undecided on whether the compendium could replace package inserts). The AMA was now firmly opposed to the project, fearing the loss of sales to its own new drug publications and claiming, because of its own publications, the redundancy of the compendium.[100] In December, the DRB wrote to Joseph Sadusk, the director of the FDA's Bureau of Medicine and a proponent of the compendium, urging the FDA to begin conversations with the PMA in order to move forward with the proposed compendium despite the AMA's resistance.[101]

Through the following summer, the AMA retained its recalcitrant attitude toward the proposed compendium and moved ahead with its own drug information program. The first edition of *New Drugs* was published toward the end of 1965 and immediately thereafter the Council on Drugs began the work of preparing the *Reference Book on Drugs*, which would contain "concise, authoritative, and useful information to the practitioner for all nationally distributed drugs," both single-entity and combination drugs. The *Reference Book*, in other words, would provide information on older drugs, and would be modeled—in terms of format and structure—on *New Drugs*.

The AMA thus remained insistent that an additional compendium was unnecessary. Moreover, Weston believed *its* publications would "meet all FDA (or any other) requirements as to the type of authoritative, valid, and full-disclosure information which they would like to see in the hands of every member of the health team," and thus could supplant the package insert. In May 1966, Weston went so far as to propose to the DRB, the FDA, and the PMA that, rather than produce a completely separate compendium, all groups should get behind the AMA's publications by providing continuing intellectual, financial, and administrative support and transforming the AMA's drug information program into a cooperative venture, albeit one ultimately controlled by the AMA. The FDA was against an AMA-controlled compendium, however, and the DRB questioned whether the AMA compendia could really achieve the broad-based pharmaceutical education the DRB regarded as essential. The DRB was concerned, for example, that the AMA publications would have limited distribution only to AMA members (whose numbers had been declining since the early 1960s).[102] By the summer of 1966, plans for a national drug compendium had stalled.

Despite the DRB's initial failure to get the compendium project off the ground, by early 1967, the FDA had renewed enthusiasm for the project, provoking a shift in the debate around—and the AMA's and PMA's stake in producing—a national drug compendium.[103] Part of the difficulty the DRB had faced in initially pushing its plan for a compendium came from the unwillingness of the FDA's then-commissioner, George P. Larrick, to commit either resources or (political) energy to a number of pharmaceutical policy proposals.[104] When Larrick retired at the end of 1965, he was replaced by James Goddard, a commissioner who was committed to reorienting the culture of the FDA away from what, during Larrick's tenure, had been perceived as "too friendly" an attitude toward the drug industry, and to transforming the FDA into a scientifically and politically activist agency.[105]

At the end of 1966, Goddard informed the DRB that the compendium had become a "number one priority" at the FDA and, citing its pharmaceutical expertise, Goddard called on the DRB to work with the agency to determine the content, format, and administration of the compendium.[106] Encouraged by Goddard's enthusiasm for the project, the DRB felt confident "that a turning point has been reached with respect to the compendium and that this project can be realized in the finite future."[107]

The reasons for the renewed interest in the compendium lay not only in the change of leadership at the FDA but also in a heightened political interest in the sources and quality of drug information. As part of the 1962 drug amendments, the FDA was required to review the efficacy of all drugs marketed between 1938 and 1962, some four thousand drugs. Since passage of the legislation, the FDA had failed to act on that requirement. When James Goddard became commissioner in 1966, he began to address the problem. Realizing the FDA had neither the necessary manpower nor the resources to undertake such a massive task, Commissioner Goddard asked the DRB if it would fulfill the drug efficacy requirement on behalf of the FDA. Despite some initial reluctance, the DRB agreed to oversee the efficacy review, and coordinated the recruitment of thirty advisory panels, composed of almost two hundred academic physicians deemed experts in critical areas of drug evaluation, to perform the evaluations; this review came to be called the Drug Efficacy Study (DES). The DES completed the evaluations in just three years, after which time the FDA decided, based on the DES's reports, which drugs were to be pulled from the market because they did not have sufficient evidence of efficacy, and which drugs required labeling changes to more accurately reflect the DES's findings.[108] By 1967, then, the DES was continuing apace and the reports of the DES's review panels indicated that a large number of existing package inserts would need to be changed in light of the DES findings.[109] This made discussion of alternative mediums for disseminating drug information particularly appropriate. Furthermore, Congress's interest in pharmaceutical reform had been reignited by Senator Gaylord Nelson's hearings on the pharmaceutical industry, and the issue of drug information now gained political traction. Indeed, two months after Goddard had solicited the DRB's assistance in developing a national drug compendium, Senator Nelson expressed his interest in the project.[110]

Beginning in January 1967, the DRB organized a series of monthly planning meetings in which it brought together representatives of the groups interested in developing a compendium. Principally this included the FDA, the PMA, and the AMA, but other professional organizations and agencies with a stake in the compendium, such as the United States Pharmacopeia (USP), were also invited to the meetings. Despite the FDA's renewed support for the compendium, there existed significant—and what proved to be persistent—disagreement over the information to be included and who would control the format and function of the compendium, with the AMA and the PMA standing on one side and the FDA on the other. In particular, the FDA wanted complete editorial control over the compendium, while the PMA and the AMA were staunchly opposed to such an arrangement.

At a November 1967 meeting, Goddard threatened the PMA and the AMA that if they were unable to move the compendium project forward, he would see to it "that Congress will push this compendium project through."[111] The AMA remained firmly committed to its own drug information program and took Goddard's threat to be a bluff. By January 1968, however, the AMA's Council on Drugs was frustrated with the FDA's agenda. The council's Maxwell Finland, for example, warned his colleagues "that we will never end up with one book that will be acceptable to the AMA, the PMA, and the FDA." Rather, he and his colleagues believed that while the AMA was interested in the "education of physicians," the FDA was interested only in a compilation of package inserts.

Therefore, the council feared that "Dr. Goddard's objectives and ours are absolutely incompatible."[112] Furthermore, the council argued, the FDA's strong-armed approach made "it essential that Congress and the public recognize the rigid controls that are being forced on the profession and, ultimately, their effect on the practice of medicine. This is not in the best interest of the physician or the patients. There is less hazard in trusting to the education of the physician than in adopting the attitude that it must be done this way or else."[113] In other words, the AMA's Council on Drugs argued that a government-published compendium, like the one proposed by the FDA, "was a highly improper intrusion by government into the private practice of medicine."[114]

Goddard's activist agenda provoked a storm of criticism from other leading academic physicians. Most notably, in a series of editorials in *Clinical Pharmacology and Therapeutics*, the Cornell clinical pharmacologist and Council of Drugs member Walter Modell accused Goddard and the FDA of attempting to censor the medical profession and the pharmaceutical industry.[115] Modell accused the FDA of trying "to discourage, to hobble, to stifle, to castrate" all other drug information publications in its effort to publish a single, FDA-controlled compendium that "will supersede all other works and to which all doctors will have to turn like Holy Writ when they seek help on drugs." Modell warned that in the eyes of the FDA—and thus in the eyes of the law—"no writing on therapy will be more expert than that of the group of nonexperts in the FDA who pass on the contents of drug package stuffers. The implications of this unprecedented FDA program are shattering." In pursuing its drug information program, Modell continued, "FDA operations cannot help but become dictatorial. And this can lead in only one direction—backward!"[116]

Building on long-held doubts about the intellectual capabilities of the agency, Modell went on to argue that "when the nonexpert ingroup of the FDA threatens to become the dictator of American medicine, we believe it will lead medicine away from its present eminence to its ultimate decline at a time in scientific understanding when we have every right to hope for even greater things. The best we can expect now is therapeutic nihilism."[117] To be sure, Modell wrote with a certain degree of hyperbole, and by the late 1960s, Modell (along with his fellow clinical pharmacologist Louis Lasagna) had become an outlier among leading academic physicians in his staunch and vociferous opposition to the FDA.[118] Although Modell took an extreme stance toward the FDA, his critique touched on more widely held concerns among the medical profession, particularly the unease that many academic physicians felt toward the FDA's ostensible incursions into the pharmaceutical education of physicians.

By 1968, the PMA was increasingly apprehensive about the FDA's efforts to make the compendium a government-controlled publication. Due to the government's preoccupation with reducing drug costs, industry executives feared that if the compendium was singularly an FDA initiative, it "might encourage generic prescribing to the disadvantage of brand name drugs of high repute."[119] The PMA's fears were not unfounded. In January 1967, Senator Nelson introduced a bill (S. 720) calling for the publication of a national drug compendium to be published regularly by the FDA and paid for by fees charged to drug firms for each new drug application made to the FDA.[120] Nelson's interest in a compendium was, as the PMA feared, in large part motivated by his commitment to lowering drug prices. As one congressional observer noted, if the government was going to be able to rein in drug costs, the government first needed a complete catalogue of available products. To this end, Nelson's bill also called for inclusion of a price supplement, which would list wholesale prices of drugs by both brand and generic name. Nelson's bill also coincided with the introduction by the Department of Health, Education, and Welfare of a bill that would designate the wholesale drug prices that the government would reimburse for under federally funded programs such as Medicare and Medicaid.[121] In light of this, the PMA's qualms that a government-controlled compendium would further the pharmaceutical reform agenda and push forward efforts to control pharmaceutical pricing were not misplaced.

The PMA was also reluctant to move forward with the compendium as long as the AMA remained opposed to it. As the PMA's president (and a former general counsel of the AMA), Joseph Stetler noted to Senator Nelson in November 1967, if the physicians "do not want this compendium . . . I don't see why we [the PMA] should put up $5 million to pay for a useless book." After all, as Stetler asserted, "we are talking about a tool for physicians, the best thing we could do is ask the doctor—What do you need or what do you want in the way of a compendium?"[122] Although the AMA's membership was in decline and by 1971 represented less than half of the nation's physicians, the AMA still wielded political power on issues of pharmaceutical policy.[123] As Stetler's comments indicate, the PMA still regarded the AMA as a valuable ally in the policy and regulatory arena, one that was to be courted and supported.

The involvement of the DRB in these discussions proved critical to protecting the interests of the industry and the medical profession. Although the DRB's compendium committee was "enthusiastic" about the AMA's drug information publications, it was "also unanimously of the opinion that the new AMA drug information book cannot be a substitute for the compendium as originally proposed in 1964 by the DRB." In particular, the DRB committee feared that the AMA's publications would "not meet the needs of the physician," as the DRB perceived them.[124] Yet the DRB joined the AMA and the PMA in opposing the FDA's plans for a government-controlled compendium, objecting to such a "bureaucratic undertaking" and recommending instead that the compendium be prepared either by a professional body such as the AMA or by "a non-profit organization representative of all groups with proprietary interests in the advancement of therapeutic practice."[125]

Senator Nelson's interest in a government-controlled drug compendium made clear to the DRB the political implications of its work. Although some academic physicians, including those who served on the DRB, viewed the involvement of Congress as having needlessly politicized the issue, others, such as Harry Dowling, regarded Congress's involvement as "a symptom of the fact that a compendium is needed, and that, as they so often do, politicians have sensed a need before every individual concerned became aware of it himself."[126] Despite congressional interest in the compendium, however, Nelson failed to secure passage of his bill and was forced to introduce a modified version of the drug compendium bill in February 1969. This time citing the recommendations of the DRB, Nelson's new bill (S. 950) proposed that the compendium be "published by an independent group in conjunction with governmental, industrial, and scientific organizations."[127] The difference between Nelson's first and subsequent drug compendium bills highlights the influential role the DRB played in the policy arena in the 1960s. Indeed, while the DRB served as forum for physician leaders, the industry, and FDA to discuss and attempt to resolve their differences and for the DRB's members to offer their expertise on matters of drug policy, Congress watched closely and responded favorably to the policy recommendations put forward by the DRB.

A national drug compendium—one that the FDA authorized as a legal replacement for package inserts—was never developed. Through the 1970s, Senator Nelson reintroduced his drug compendium bill during each new Congress, but his decision to couple the drug compendium bill with provisions that would further increase the FDA's authority over drug development and practice meant that each year the bill faced the steadfast opposition of the pharmaceutical industry and the medical profession (see chapter 6 for further discussion). Yet, although Nelson's efforts failed, the

AMA continued its drug information program and eventually produced its own version of a comprehensive compendium, *Drug Evaluations,* which had the support of the drug industry. First published in 1971 and revised and updated every two or three years by academic physicians the AMA deemed pharmaceutical experts, *Drug Evaluations* was made available free of charge to all members of the AMA.[128]

Although there are no figures available as to how widely *AMA Drug Evaluations* was used, and how informative physicians really found it, it reconfirmed the role of the medical profession—supported by the drug industry—as the primary providers of pharmaceutical education. Moreover, the subsequent development of several different compendia, each put out by a different institution or agency (such as the *USP Drug Information* and *American Hospital Formulary Service Drug Information*), reflected the lack of interest on the part of key stakeholders in the generation of a single source of drug information. This is reflective of the power struggles over who controls the production and dissemination of drug information, a struggle, invariably, among physicians, pharmacists, and the government, and one that continues to play out in pharmaceutical policy and practice.

REVISING INFORMED PATIENT CONSENT

The surest sign of the DRB's power to influence the regulatory environment of pharmaceuticals—and to preserve the interests of the industry and medical profession—in the post-Kefauver era involved the FDA's writing of the 1966 patient consent regulations. A component of the 1962 drug amendments had been the requirement that clinical investigators and drug firms provide evidence that patients enrolled in clinical drug trials had given their informed consent to partake in those trials. Prior to the amendments, and in response to enactment of the Nuremberg Code in 1948, ethical standards required that human research subjects *voluntarily* consent to participating in clinical research.[129] The FDA, however, required no formal documentation of voluntary consent, nor did the agency require that patients be fully informed about the nature of the research in which they were participating. As a result of the thalidomide disaster, in which roughly twenty thousand Americans (624 of them pregnant) had taken the experimental drug without knowing that it had yet to receive FDA approval, Congress and the FDA realized that voluntary consent did not offer sufficient protection to human research subjects. They argued, instead, that it was critical that every research subject be fully informed about the nature of the research they were participating in and of the risks of taking an experimental drug.[130]

Despite the inclusion of informed consent in the amendments, as Daniel Carpenter has noted, those amendments spoke only "briefly and vaguely on the subject."[131] Only after Henry Beecher's exposé of unethical research practices in human subjects research, published in the *New England Journal of Medicine* in 1966, did the FDA formalize the federal rules regarding informed consent and medical research in human subjects.[132] The FDA published its informed consent regulations in the *Federal Register* in August 1966. The FDA now required clinical investigators to include a signed statement from each human subject participating in a trial, acknowledging that he or she had been fully informed of the risks and was willing to accept those risks and participate in the trial.[133]

The FDA's 1966 ruling, however, unleashed a storm of protest among clinical investigators and clinical pharmacologists. Already frustrated by the increased reporting requirements and lengthened application process resulting from the drug amendments and the FDA's investigational new drug regulations in 1963, scores of investigators wrote to the FDA complaining about the danger the informed consent regulations posed to the future of clinical research and, thus, to the development of innovative new drugs.

Investigators railed, in particular, against paragraph (h) of the regulations, which required investigators to provide patients "with a fair explanation of all material information concerning the administration of the investigational drug, or his possible use as a control, as to enable him to make an understanding decision as to his willingness to receive said investigational drugs." The information to be conveyed to the patient should include, "the nature, duration, and purpose of the administration of the said investigational drug; the method and means by which it is to be administered; all inconveniences and hazards reasonably to be expected, including the fact, where applicable, that the person may be used as a control; the existence of alternative forms of therapy, if any; and the effects upon his health or person that may possibly come from the administration of the investigational drug. Said patient's consent shall be obtained in writing by the investigator."[134] As Morton Hamburger, an internist working at Cincinnati General Hospital and engaged in the clinical study of new antibiotics, wrote to the FDA in November 1966, "I can only say that if an investigator follows this section [paragraph (h)] to the letter and conscientiously adheres to its working it will be virtually impossible to test new antibiotics in cases where old ones have a good but not perfect record. I have been involved in clinical investigation since before World War II and can assure you that obtaining consent of patients under these conditions is simply not humanly possible."[135] Hamburger also sent a copy of his letter to Maxwell Finland in the hope that Finland would raise the issue of the patient consent regulations with the DRB.[136]

Hamburger's concern for what the informed consent regulations might mean for future clinical studies of antibiotics and other potential new drugs, and his decision to turn to the DRB for help, reflected a common sentiment among clinical investigators. That fall, the DRB received numerous complaints about the informed consent regulations from clinical investigators and from the academics among its ranks.[137] In separate letters that September, the DRB members Chester Keefer and William Castle wrote to the DRB chairman, William Middleton, urging him to make discussion of the FDA's informed consent regulations an urgent priority of the DRB. For Castle, the FDA's regulations "constitute[d] a most serious threat to the continuation of new drug testing for the benefit of the public. The prospect of substituting legal language for moral responsibility is self-defeating in principle and practice."[138]

Echoing the sentiment of other leading investigators, Keefer expressed to Middleton his hope that "the regulations might be amended in such a way that the investigator may use his best judgment and discretion when it comes to obtaining a patients [*sic*] consent in writing." Keefer continued, "I am inclined to believe that a statement by the investigator that is entered in the patient record stating that the patient had been informed about the use of an investigational drug with the proper qualifications. would be adequate. This decision should be based upon mature judgment and with the view that any signed statement is for the protection of the patient as well as the investigator." In this way, Keefer suggested that the authority to determine when patient consent was required should rest with the investigator and not with the FDA (which the current regulations dictated), because with their personal knowledge of the patient, the investigator (not the FDA) was best able to judge what was in the patient's best interests, including whether or not informed consent was possible or even necessary.[139]

For Keefer, the dual protections afforded by informed consent regulations further threatened the integrity of both the investigator-patient relationship and the research enterprise. Keefer feared that having patients *sign* a statement of consent increased the likelihood that patients dissatisfied with the procedures or results of clinical study would seek legal action against the investigator. As Keefer noted, "Every investigator knows that a signed statement by a patient does not protect him from law suit; in fact, in many instances it is taken as an invitation to one."[140]

Investigators' primary objection to the informed consent regulations, rested, however, on "the outstanding fact today . . . that all doctors of medicine and clinical investigators who are licensed by law to practice medicine are suffering more than a little from being governed by lawyers and government bureaucrats. These men attempt to analyze accomplished facts and look for reasons why something went wrong. They are rarely constructive." In other words, the investigators' opposition to the regulations was a variation on the medical profession's long-held opposition to any form of government intervention in medicine; fear that it was the first step toward socialized medicine. Keefer continued that, although federal statutes sought to make black and white the "moral choice" facing clinical investigators, most such "choices have to be made between shades of gray. This is a fact that is often overlooked by an overweening bureaucracy with a powerful and enormous administration super structure who are more interested in eroding individual initiative and promoting a supine citizenry of scientists and developing a monarchical rule with all of its excessives [sic]. . . . The scientists of the United States are being told how they should conduct their studies, and their experiments." Rather than placing all control in the hands of that bureaucracy (as the current patient consent regulations had done), Keefer argued, "The regulations need to be drawn so that sufficient flexibility is permitted for the scientist to exercise his best judgment in carrying out his studies with individual patients— studies which are designed with the hope and expectation of helping the patient." Nowhere did Keefer or any of the other investigators writing to the DRB acknowledge that allowing the investigator to "exercise his best judgment" had led to the unethical treatment of human research subjects exposed by Beecher.[141]

In October 1966, the PMA president, Joseph Stetler, also wrote to Middleton requesting that he include the FDA patient consent regulations on the DRB's next agenda.[142] In response, Middleton convened a special meeting of the DRB on October 20 to consider the "principles that should govern the solicitation of consent of patients invited to participate in clinical trials of new drugs." At that meeting, the DRB drew up a policy statement on the informed consent regulations in which it "affirm[ed] as desirable the policy of most investigators to gain the informed consent of most patients who are treated with research drugs" but also made clear the board's belief that "some notable exceptions to this policy must, however, be made by exercise of the judgment of the physician." In particular, the DRB called on the FDA to revise paragraph (h) of the regulations so that investigators would now be required to provide patients "with a fair explanation of *pertinent* information concerning the (2 words omitted) investigational drug, or his possible use as a control, as to enable him to make *a reasonable* decision as to his willingness to receive said investigational drug. (sentence omitted). Said patient's consent shall be obtained in writing by the investigator."[143] In this way, the DRB's revisions reaffirmed the sanctity of the clinical investigators' autonomy by removing any "attempts to dictate the substance of the physician's communication with his patient," and in reasserting the clinical investigators' authority to determine when informed consent should be given and exactly how much information should be shared with each patient.[144]

The DRB submitted its policy statement, along with detailed explanations for the proposed revisions, to Commissioner Goddard on November 10. The following month, DRB representatives met with Goddard, and on January 10, 1967, Goddard circulated a revised version of the informed consent regulations to the DRB, in which several of the DRB's recommendations had been incorporated. Most important as far as the DRB's efforts to preserve the clinical investigator's authority and autonomy, the revisions to paragraph (h) of the regulations now made clear "that the 'check list' of items to be included in the physician's discussion with the patient is now subject to the physician's judgment of the patient's condition and degree of understanding."[145]

Following a series of further meetings between Goddard and representatives from the DRB, the FDA published the final revisions of the patient consent regulations in the *Federal Register* on March 11, 1967. The DRB was satisfied that the FDA had "incorporated substantially all of the amendments that [had been] agreed upon" in a recent joint meeting of Goddard and the DRB. In this way, the DRB had played an instrumental role "in achieving the best possible compromise" between the interests of the medical profession and those of the FDA.[146]

In the 1967 iteration of the rulings, premised as they were on medical paternalism, the patient's own autonomy was conspicuously absent. In these regulations, as in medical practice more generally at that time, the physician was assumed to be the best protector of a patient's interests. A series of events in the late 1960s and early 1970s, however, severely undermined the assumptions on which medical paternalism was premised and forced a further revision of the informed consent regulations in which the patient's autonomy was prioritized. First, the activism of health feminists within the women's health movement challenged the notion that physicians were better able to judge whether a patient should assume the risk of taking an experimental drug than the patient herself. Health feminists held up the failure of the medical profession, the FDA, and pharmaceutical firms to adequately protect women from and to warn them about the dangers of taking oral contraceptives, diethylstilbestrol, and Depo-Provera as evidence of the oppressive and tragic consequences of medical paternalism, and demanded that women finally be granted the right to control their own bodies.[147]

Second, the revelations in 1973 that the U.S. Public Health Service (PHS) had for forty years lied to several hundred poor African American men participating in the Tuskegee syphilis study, drew stark attention to the fact that clinical investigators could readily disregard the ethical treatment of patients in the name of scientific study. The PHS had established the Tuskegee syphilis experiment in 1932 in Macon County, Alabama, with the goal of studying the natural progression of untreated syphilis. Although PHS officers recruiting men to the study had told participants that they would be receiving medical treatment for their syphilis, for the duration of the study the PHS withheld treatment from study participants even after researchers identified penicillin as a cure for syphilis after World War II.[148]

The activism of health feminists and the revelations about the Tuskegee syphilis experiment (together with a number of other public disclosures about unethical research practices), severely undermined the assumption, codified in the informed consent regulations of 1967, that physicians were best able to judge and protect the patient's interests. In response, the informed consent regulations—along with the ethical standards for the conduct of human subjects research—were revised. As of 1967, however, the DRB had been instrumental in constructing the regulations around patient consent. In that role, the DRB had managed to preserve the authority of clinical investigators and helped produce informed consent regulations that everyone—clinical investigators, drug firms, and the FDA—could live with.[149]

CONCLUSION

The 1962 drug amendments were a turning point in the history of drug regulation and in the history of drug industry–academic physician relations. In response to the new regulations, the drug industry drew on the relationships it had nurtured with the academic medical community since the interwar years and created a political alliance with academic physicians. The Drug Research Board, with its predecessor, the Commission on Drug Safety, allowed the industry and academic physicians to reassert their authority in a new regulatory context that threatened to undermine it. They did this by positioning themselves as pharmaceutical experts available to advise government on matters of drug policy and therapeutic practice. In this way, the DRB aimed to see government agencies—as part of their standard practice—"invite the biomedical community to participate in the management of drugs."[150] As an executive officer of the NAS-NRC proclaimed, "surely this is good political science because it broadens the base of democratic government, increases . . . the permeability of bureaucracy and fosters cooperation rather than conflict."[151] Moreover, it ensured industry and academic medicine seats at the policy table.

As pharmaceutical experts, the DRB was able to tackle one of the major problems confronting industry and academic medicine in the 1960s: the increasing authority of the FDA over pharmaceutical development and practice. Since World War II, the drug industry and the medical community had feared the expanding authority of the federal government in medicine. After passage of the 1962 drug amendments, however, pharmaceutical reformers attempted to transform the corporate system of drug development into one in which the government played a more central role. Indeed, in securing passage of the amendments, Senator Kefauver had succeeded in shifting the balance of power in the political economy of drug regulation further toward the federal government. The new regulations showed that the government was serious about correcting what critics of the industry had long viewed as the industry's exploitation of the America patient.

Through the work of the DRB, however, industry and academic medicine were able to undercut the FDA's new authority. The provision of this industry-academic expertise coincided with the FDA's tendency in the 1960s to consult with expert advisory committees in order to shore up its own authority within the scientific community.[152] Yet, as much as the FDA sought cooperation with academic medicine, academic physicians were acting out of their own interests when they agreed to provide that expertise to the agency. So too, as academic physicians and government officials were co-opting each other, the pharmaceutical industry was working with great success to co-opt both in an effort to preserve its own political interests.

The history of the DRB shows the importance of voluntary and purportedly independent expertise—in addition to explicit legislation and regulation—in shaping postwar American health care. Specifically, the DRB gave industry and academic medicine a vehicle for challenging the efforts of pharmaceutical reformers to increase the government's role in the corporate system of drug development. Nowhere was this clearer than in the efforts of pharmaceutical reformers, through the late 1960s and early 1970s, to introduce legislation that would make it mandatory for physicians to prescribe by generic name.

6 Generic Alliances and the Backlash against Regulatory Reform

> Pharmaceutical research is unusual as compared with all other
> kinds of applied chemical research, in that meaningful discovery
> involves issues of increasing political and social sensitivity. In
> fact, pharmaceutical innovation is now not only a scientific
> process, but also a socio-political one.
>
> —CHAS. PFIZER CO., *Annual Report*, 1975

In May 1967, Senator Gaylord Nelson launched what would become
a decade-long investigation into the American drug industry. Like his
reform-minded predecessor, Senator Estes Kefauver, Nelson regarded
mandatory generic prescribing as the solution to rising prescription drug
and health care costs. Over the course of the next decade, Nelson joined
with other pharmaceutical reformers—most notably Senators Joseph
Montoya, Russell Long, and Edward Kennedy—to push for legislation
that would reform physicians' prescription practices and add a prescription
drug benefit to Medicare. From the late 1960s through the 1970s, these
efforts to introduce generic prescription reform galvanized the political
alliance between the Pharmaceutical Manufacturers Association (PMA)
and the medical profession.[1]

At the same time, pharmaceutical reformers continued to push for measures that would otherwise increase the government's role in drug development. They attempted repeatedly to pass legislation that would allow
pharmacists to fill prescriptions with cheaper generic drug substitutions
for the brand-name drugs requested by physicians. These efforts to abolish
state antisubstitution laws, which prohibited such actions, threatened both
the autonomy of physicians and the profits of the pharmaceutical industry and thus met with vociferous opposition from both. Pharmaceutical
reformers also attempted to establish a national center of drug development within the Department of Health, Education, and Welfare (HEW),
seeking to make the government responsible for the preclinical and clinical
testing of all new drugs. In each instance, however, the pharmaceutical
industry was able to thwart these reform efforts to place the industry

163

under greater government control by mobilizing its political alliance with the American Medical Association (AMA) and academic physicians.

This industry-medical alliance marshaled the political strategies used to great effect during the 1960s. And by the mid-1970s, this alliance was pursuing a new strategy to prevent further pharmaceutical reform. In the early 1970s, the clinical pharmacologists Louis Lasagna and William Wardell introduced the notion of a "drug lag." They argued that as a direct result of the 1962 drug amendments the U.S. pharmaceutical industry had made significantly fewer pharmaceutical innovations. Moreover, they argued, because of America's stringent drug regulations, many new drugs were available to patients in European countries several years before they were available to patients in the United States. As a result, proponents of the drug lag argued, the public's health and America's technological and economic leadership were suffering.[2] The industry and its allies used the idea of the drug lag as evidence that the FDA had overstepped its authority and was overregulating drugs to the detriment of American patients. In doing so, they further undermined pharmaceutical reformers' efforts to increase the government's role in drug development and distribution, arguing that the FDA's authority should be reined in instead.

Yet, while the industry-physician alliance prevented federal reform, it proved less effective at the state level. Throughout the 1970s, the PMA and AMA promoted the brand-name drug as the economic foundation of the pharmaceutical enterprise. By the end of the decade, however, a coalition of pharmacists, consumer and patient groups, and state legislators succeeded in overturning the state antisubstitution laws of the 1950s and challenged the primacy of the brand-name drug in the pharmaceutical marketplace. This chapter contextualizes current debates among regulators, health policymakers, physicians groups, and pharmaceutical manufacturers about the safety, cost, and exchangeability of generic drugs.[3]

NOT ALL DRUGS ARE CREATED EQUAL

As a way of reducing prescription drug prices and thus applying the brakes to escalating health care costs, Senator Kefauver had pushed, during his subcommittee's hearings on the drug industry, for legislation that would require physicians to prescribe generically whenever a (cheaper) generic drug was available for use. The principal opponents of generic prescribing were the large research-based pharmaceutical manufacturers, whose brand-name drug sales (from which they garnered most of their profits) were threatened by mandatory generic prescribing, and physicians, who saw the legislation as another example of government intrusion into medical practice. They all argued that it was inaccurate and extremely dangerous to assume, as the reformers did, that generic drugs had the same therapeutic effect as their brand-name equivalents. Rather, the industry and medical profession contended, because generic drugs were not as rigorously evaluated as brand-name drugs and because they were usually produced by small drug firms whose reputation could not be guaranteed, you could be certain of neither their quality (and therefore safety) nor their efficacy.

Although Kefauver failed to secure passage of such legislation in 1962, Senator Gaylord Nelson (D-WI) continued the push for prescription drug reform. When Nelson launched his own investigation into the "Competitive Problems in the Pharmaceutical Industry" in 1967, he placed the issue of generic drug prescription at the center of his investigation.[4] As they had during the Kefauver hearings, brand-name manufacturers and their physician allies vigorously opposed passage of generic prescription legislation.[5] They did so on two grounds: first, that generic prescription legislation would abolish the physician's autonomy, and second, that generic drugs were not necessarily therapeutically equivalent to their brand-name counterparts.

In general, researchers and officials distinguished between three different types of drug equivalence. *Chemical equivalence* referred to drugs that contained identical amounts of the same active ingredient. *Biological equivalence* (or *bioequivalence*) was introduced by academic pharmacists and pharmacologists as a concept in the 1960s and referred to chemically equivalent drugs that, when administered in the same amounts, produced the same biological effects as measured by the degree to which the drug's active ingredient was made available within the bloodstream. Finally, *therapeutic* or *clinical equivalence* referred to those drugs that, when administered in equal amounts, produced the same therapeutic effects, usually measured by the degree to which the drug controlled a particular symptom or disease.[6]

Brand-name manufacturers had initially raised concerns about the therapeutic equivalence of generic drugs during the antisubstitution campaigns of the 1950s. But in the years since, pharmacists and pharmacologists working in government and academic laboratories had become engaged in the equivalence question and had found evidence that chemical equivalents (the then-current official criterion of a generic drug) did not always produce therapeutic effects equivalent to those produced by their brand-name counterparts. During the 1950s and early 1960s, for example, researchers at the Food and Drug Directorate of Canada's Department of National Health and Welfare had found that for several drug products, in vitro dissolution and disintegration tests—the existing pharmacopoeial standards of *chemical* equivalence—were an inadequate measure of biological availability and thus did not guarantee the therapeutic equivalence of the drug products.[7] These and similar studies had led officials at the United States Pharmacopeia (USP)—the organization responsible for setting drug standards in the United States—to worry "that a new kind of official standard is needed."[8]

Concerns about therapeutic equivalence were relevant not solely to generic drugs. By the mid-1960s, brand-name manufacturers were confronting the issue of equivalence as they evaluated different dosage forms of the same branded drug. At Merck & Co., for example, researchers had successfully tested the capsule form of their new anti-inflammatory drug Indocin in clinical subjects, finding no indication of significant side effects. Anticipating high demand for the drug, Merck sought to speed up production by using the tablet form of Indocin. Unlike the capsule form, however, tablet Indocin proved to be highly toxic, causing severe side effects (such as headaches and bleeding) in clinical subjects. Merck promptly abandoned development of tablet Indocin and marketed only capsulated Indocin (which received FDA approval in 1965). The experience made clear to Merck researchers that different dosage forms of the same drug did not necessarily produce the same clinical (or therapeutic) effects in patients. Although the *active* ingredient of the two forms of Indocin was chemically identical, the *inactive* ingredients that made up the final packaged forms of the drug were not and resulted in the two different dosage forms having *inequivalent* therapeutic effects. In response, Merck had, by 1965, begun to routinely evaluate the biological and therapeutic equivalence of all dosage forms of their new drugs.[9]

In their campaign against generic prescription reform, brand-name manufacturers mobilized evidence of the inequivalence of generic drugs. In their testimony before Nelson's subcommittee, representatives from brand-name manufacturers proclaimed the superiority of their products compared to the generic versions produced by smaller generic manufacturers. The PMA president C. Joseph Stetler, for example, cited a recent Parke-Davis study that had compared the equivalence of its own brand of chloramphenicol (Chloromycetin) against several generic versions of the drug and found that some of the generic drugs were absorbed into the blood stream of human volunteers at rates remarkably different from the Parke-Davis brand. Subsequently, the FDA withdrew nine of the generic chloramphenicol drugs from the market. Here, Stetler argued, was clear evidence that "although two products may contain, or are supposed to contain, the same amount of the same active ingredient, this provides no assurance that both products will produce the same clinical effect in any particular patient."[10]

Even when brand-name manufacturers lacked such comparative data, they held up the limits of the regulatory system as a guarantee of the superiority of brand-name drugs. Under the 1962 drug amendments, all new chemical entities (and therefore brand-name drugs) had to undergo rigorous clinical evaluation before the FDA could grant marketing approval. Generic drugs, however, named for the very fact that they were *not* new chemical entities, fell out of the purview of any such requirement and were granted approval merely on demonstration of their chemical equivalence to their brand-name counterpart. Thus, when Senator Nelson asked Ciba's president, Charles T. Silloway, to provide evidence to support Ciba's claim that its brand of reserpine (Serpasil) was much better than the reserpine manufactured by the generic firm American Pharmaceutical Corp., Silloway responded that although no clinical studies comparing the two versions of reserpine had been done, Ciba knew its version of the drug was superior "because ours consistently meets the standards of the USP and exceeds them, and because our product has been extensively clinically studied. Their product has not been."[11]

Nelson remained unconvinced, however. As he heard repeated testimony from representatives of hospital formulary committees and state welfare agencies who attested to the success of using generic drugs in their programs, Nelson labeled the brand-name manufacturers' assertions of generic inequivalence as "gobbledygook" and accused them of "broad-scale" propaganda "with the obvious purpose to destroy public confidence in the official standards and the general quality of drug products."[12] Physicians and consumer groups in favor of generic prescribing likewise lamented the brand-name manufacturers' campaign against generics. William Haddad, the chairman of the Citizens Committee for Metropolitan Affairs in New York, for example, accused the drug industry of perpetuating "false and malicious arguments that drugs sold under their generic names are unsafe." Dr. John Holloman, the president of the National Medical Association, the professional association of African American physicians, testified that he had never observed any differences in terms of safety and efficacy between generic and brand-name drugs. Like Haddad, Holloman accused the industry of propaganda—through its advertising and the words and deeds of its detail men—in telling "false, exaggerated and horrifying stories" about generic drug companies.[13]

The character and timing of brand-name manufacturers' arguments about the therapeutic inequivalence of generic drugs were significant on two fronts. First, at no point did brand-name manufacturers make the claim that generic drugs were universally unsafe. To do so would have been fallacious; after all, brand-name manufacturers were also in the business of marketing generic drugs. Rather, the PMA and its member companies very specifically and "emphatically disagree[d] with the assumption . . . that generic and therapeutic equivalency go hand in hand."[14] Second, at the same time that Nelson was pushing for generic prescribing legislation, the patents on the first generation of wonder drugs were beginning to expire. This meant that brand-name manufacturers were confronting a significant loss of revenue. Once the patents on the first generation of high-selling wonder drugs expired, generic drug manufacturers would be free to introduce generic versions of those drugs and compete with brand-name manufacturers for market share. The impending loss of revenue from the biggest-selling brand-name drugs and the concomitant growth in generic manufacturers' economic power contributed to the brand-name manufacturers' anxieties about Nelson's efforts to introduce mandatory generic prescribing.[15]

In their critique of generic equivalence, brand-name manufacturers found academic physicians as their allies. As the Johns Hopkins University clinical pharmacologist Louis Lasagna explained, "the science underlying [generic legislation] and the realistic appraisals of their economic impact are deficient." He noted, "After many years of blind reliance on United States Pharmacopeia [USP] standards for drug quality, biopharmaceutical experts have now realized our ancient standards for drug quality are inadequate." As an example, Lasagna held up the FDA's recent removal from the market of nine generic versions of chloramphenicol "when it became apparent that none of these met the criterion of reproducible and adequate blood levels in man. All of these preparations had been batch-tested by the FDA, and had presumably passed these tests." Legislation should not be passed, Lasagna concluded, "in scientific areas where we are abysmally ignorant."[16]

Even for those physicians who supported the concept of generic prescribing, their support came with qualifications. For example, the prominent clinical pharmacologist Walter Modell testified before Nelson's subcommittee that "if all drugs lived up to USP standards then there should be absolutely no difference between generically named drugs and [brand-]named drugs." However, Modell noted, this was not currently the situation. While "the large drug manufacturers take every precaution possible to insure that their drug lives up to proper standards . . . I think that there may be a tendency for smaller drug houses to cut corners because they can't afford the luxury of not cutting corners."[17]

In 1966, the matter of generic drugs had come before the Drug Research Board (DRB) as part of its work on the Drug Efficacy Study (DES) (see chapter 5 for details). As an evaluative study of all drugs marketed between 1938 and 1962, the DES necessarily included the evaluation of brand-name and generic drugs and thus dealt specifically with the matter of the therapeutic equivalence of generic drugs. Any recommendation that the DES made to the FDA regarding the efficacy of generic drugs thus stood to influence the legislative efforts of Senator Nelson and his fellow pharmaceutical reformers. This fact was not lost on the DES's Policy Advisory Committee (PAC) and its chairman, Alfred Gilman, who warned that Nelson's pending legislation signaled the government was "more concerned with the cost rather than the quality of medical care."[18]

According to Gilman, the problem of generics marked a double standard in the regulatory process. On the one hand, "the marketer of a patent-protected drug applies to the FDA for a change in formulation, no matter how slight, a supplementary NDA [new drug application] must be submitted and the proof of therapeutic equivalency required by the FDA is exacting and demanding." On the other hand, the marketer of a generic drug need only supply to the FDA proof of the drug's chemical equivalence to the brand-name drug for which approval had already been given. Thus by "rendering decisions on the efficacy of 'generic' drugs," and "accepting inadequate 'in vitro' tests as adequate evidence of therapeutic equivalency," the DES violated the 1962 drug amendments, Gilman believed. Without clinical data, "we have no idea of the efficacy in man of many of the generic drugs that we have declared to be effective." Until the FDA's evaluation of generic drugs was made more rigorous, the DES's PAC opposed any legislation that mandated generic prescribing.[19]

In coming to this position, Gilman and the PAC had consulted with representatives from the Defense Medical Material Branch (DMMB), which was responsible for procuring drugs for the armed forces and regularly used generic drugs instead of brand-name drugs. Nelson repeatedly held up the military's widespread use of generic drugs as evidence that generics were safe and effective. Despite their heavy procurement of generics, however, the DMMB representatives cited the difficulties they faced with regard to therapeutic effectiveness. In order to minimize the problem of therapeutic equivalence and finding the standards required by the USP inadequate, the DMMB had established its own tests to assess the quality of the drugs that were distributed to the military. When a drug company submitted a bid to the DMMB, the company had to provide detailed specifications with regards to the drug's therapeutic effectiveness. To further guarantee the efficacy of its drugs, the DMMB performed on-site inspections of firms submitting bids, and conducted tests in their in-house laboratories. In other words, the military evaluated the generic drugs it intended to use to a greater degree than that ensured by then-current regulatory standards.[20]

The PAC laid out its position on generic drugs in a "White Paper on the Therapeutic Equivalence of Generic Drugs." In it, the DES contended that the FDA should require a modified NDA for all generic drugs. Recognizing that it would not be feasible for all generic manufacturers to repeat all clinical studies on their drugs, the DES called for "proof of biological availability in man equivalent to that of the drug for which it claims to be a therapeutic equivalent." Any drug failing "to meet these requirements should not be allowed on the market."[21]

In September 1967, Gilman submitted these views to Senator Nelson's subcommittee. Repeating the assertions made in the white paper, Gilman argued "that the present practice constitutes a kind of double standard [for] originators of compounds and those who later market alleged 'equivalents.'" It was imperative, Gilman contended, that "all producers, and certainly the generic houses, should be required to submit proof of the performance of their drugs in human patients before they are permitted to market them. Once that is required, and this double standard is eliminated, I believe many of the problems facing us will be reduced." Gilman also challenged Nelson's premise that mandatory generic prescribing would significantly reduce health care costs, arguing instead that if the same regulatory "demands were placed on these so-called generic equivalents," the cost of developing generic drugs would rise and "then the price differential between generic and trade-marked drugs . . . would be very much less. In fact, many generics would disappear."[22] The DES's perspective was all the more important as it directly challenged the conclusions of the secretary of HEW's Task Force on Prescription Drugs. Composed of government officials, the majority of whom lacked any medical or scientific training, the task force was charged with determining the feasibility of expanding the Medicare program to include prescription drug coverage. This included an assessment of the benefits of using generic drugs.[23] As part of its evaluation, the task force initiated a program to determine whether any observed differences in biological equivalence could be related to differences in the physical or chemical characteristics of the products. Based on clinical studies of twenty-seven drugs, a review of the current literature on therapeutic drugs, and assessments of the use of generic drugs in foreign drug programs, state welfare programs, Veterans Administration hospitals, and military operations, the task force concluded that "lack of clinical [therapeutic] equivalency among chemical equivalents meeting all official standards has been grossly exaggerated as a major hazard to the public health."[24]

The task force's conclusion contradicted the DES's contention that there was *insufficient* evidence of therapeutic equivalence among chemically equivalent drugs to justify mandatory generic prescribing. As such, the task force's findings were a boon to Senator Nelson. Two years after publication of the task force's report, however, the secretary of HEW appointed a committee, chaired by the Harvard political economist John Dunlop to review the task force's findings and recommendations. Unlike the task force, the so-called Dunlop Committee was composed of non–government officials drawn from a variety of backgrounds, including physicians, academic and industry researchers, lawyers, and pharmacists. One of the committee's mandates was to evaluate the significance of chemical, biological, and therapeutic equivalence to the system of drug regulation. At the conclusion of its review, the committee challenged the task force's conclusions about the issue of generic equivalence. Following the lead of the DRB, the Dunlop Committee called on the government to require drug firms to establish that generic drug products were biologically or therapeutically equivalent to their brand-name counterparts before they received marketing approval.[25]

"ERODING THE PHYSICIAN'S CONTROL"

For academic physicians, then, Nelson's generic prescription legislation reflected a fundamental lack of understanding among policymakers and the public of the intricacies of pharmaceutical practice.[26] For the Boston physician and DRB member Dale Friend, the "widespread belief" among "a great many of our union leaders, many of the laity, a good many of our congressional leaders . . . that a solution to at least some part of the high cost of drugs to patients could be brought about by the simple expedient of using generic name drugs . . . causes me serious concern," not least because "most of it is based on a failure to understand the technicalities of drug therapy, and as a consequence, many are moving in the field to legislate the use of generic drugs and thus rather seriously interfere with the physician in his practice of Medicine."[27]

For the majority of nonacademic physicians, whose exposure to the scientific and regulatory debates over therapeutic equivalence were limited to the pages of the major medical publications, the key issue raised by generic prescription legislation was—as Friend implied—the threat it posed to their autonomy.[28] As one Memphis physician asserted to readers of the *Journal of the American Medical Association* in 1966, "the physician should be allowed to prescribe drugs from a pharmaceutical house that he knows is ethical and holds to high sanitary standards, even though it might cost his patient a little more money for the prescription at his pharmacy." For this physician, the "pending legislation before the U.S. Congress [that] would make . . . generic prescribing mandatory . . . is obviously not in the best interest of the patient." After all, he noted,

> The next time you attend a medical convention in any large city and are on your way from the airport to your hotel, raise your eyes above the street level. In second and third floor lofts you will see many small pharmaceutical companies in very dingy surroundings with obviously poor sanitary facilities. The pharmaceuticals manufactured in some of these loft factories are sometimes a combination of dust, ground-up cockroaches, and drug. Supervision by the local health department may be desultory and two years late. Almost every week we receive catalogs of cut-rate drugs from just such pharmaceutical companies.[29]

In the wake of Medicaid and Medicare's passage in 1965, the AMA leadership was particularly attuned to any legislative effort that sought, in their eyes, to grant the federal government any further control over medical practice. Mandatory generic prescribing looked to do just that. In a 1967 editorial in the *AMA News*, the AMA argued that physicians prescribed drugs by brand name so that they could be confident of the drugs' quality. Any "legislation that would nullify this knowledge [about quality] by removing the decision-making power from him," the AMA asserted, "clearly is not in the public interest."[30]

The medical community's concerns about physician autonomy were all the more pressing after Senators Russell Long (D-LA) and Joseph Montoya (D-NM) introduced amendments to the Social Security Act in 1967. These amendments called for the use of generic prescriptions for all patients receiving Medicaid benefits and adding a (generic) prescription drug benefit to Medicare.[31] John Adriani of the AMA's Council on Drugs wrote to Senator Long on several occasions offering his suggestions on the drug bill. Adriani, a Louisianan, was sympathetic to Long's goal of making prescription drugs more affordable and thus accessible to all those who needed them. Yet Adriani thought Long's proposal unworkable "for two main reasons. The first of these reasons is that doctors resent being told how to practice medicine, not only by laymen but also by other physicians. I know this from experience as one of the associate administrators at the hospital. I also know it from my own personal reactions. I want freedom of choice in the treatment and management of a patient who has entrusted his life and welfare to me." The second reason was that many physicians simply did not know the generic names of drugs. Rather than attempting to "tell a physician how he should practice medicine" by mandating the use of generic prescriptions, Adriani urged instead educating physicians on the generic names of drugs, and requiring manufacturers "to dispense the drug by its generic name." In other words, Adriani opposed legislative attempts to restrict the physician's right to prescribe whichever drug he or she wanted, but supported changing the way manufacturers labeled their drugs.[32]

Brand-name manufacturers later became vehement in their opposition to what they perceived as Adriani's attempt to abolish the brand name. And subsequently, as Adriani became increasingly vocal in his efforts to promote generic labeling, the AMA leadership distanced itself from Adriani's position. Yet Adriani's assertion that physicians would, on principle, oppose any attempt to encroach on their prescribing autonomy reflected the overwhelming sentiment of the medical profession. Adriani, for example, recounted the story of Louisiana's former commissioner of welfare who had, several years earlier, attempted "to force" generic prescriptions on physicians in Louisiana but "was taken care of via the route of medical politics." That commissioner was "now practicing law somewhere in West Louisiana."[33]

In spite of Adriani's pronouncements to Senator Long, in personal correspondence with his medical and industry colleagues, Adriani continued to express his misgivings about generic prescription legislation. Indeed, in May 1967, he wrote to Jean Weston, who had recently left the AMA's Department of Drugs to serve as executive director of the industry-sponsored National Pharmaceutical Council, that while a number of physicians were "sympathetic to the idea of generic prescribing . . . it is not practical under all circumstances. . . . We can't make a size 8 shoe fit everybody."[34] Two years later he restated his concern, referring to the pressing need "for a clarification of the matter on nomenclature—one name for one drug" while also maintaining that physicians should still be able to prescribe a brand-name drug if they choose to "because the integrity of the brand means much to me."[35]

Ultimately, the threat posed by mandatory generic prescribing to physicians' autonomy served as a rallying point for physicians fearful of the government's expanding reach into medical practice. To this end, the AMA repeatedly testified—and lobbied—against Nelson's generic prescription legislation.[36] As Donald O. Schiffman from the AMA's Department of Drugs asserted in 1973, "Until all similar drug preparations can be equated meaningfully in terms of their bioavailability to permit the interchange of different forms of a drug on a rational basis, legalistic maneuvering," which took away the physician's prescribing autonomy, "should be vigorously opposed by the medical community."[37] As Schiffman later warned, passage of any "laws allowing the pharmacist to exercise the right of autonomous product selection will open the door to a decrease in the physician's control over his patient's therapy. Without automatic and absolute control over the exact regimen of therapy, the physician cannot possibly utilize all of his training and ability to help the patient."[38]

DEFEATING GENERIC PRESCRIPTION LEGISLATION

The drug industry's campaign against generic prescription legislation did not rest solely on the work of the DRB or on the congressional testimonies of representatives from brand-name manufacturers, the AMA, and academic physicians. Rather, the industry mobilized a full-scale political campaign against generic legislation. As part of this, the PMA published two fifteen-page pamphlets that presented the industry's arguments against generic prescribing: *Compulsory Generic Prescribing—A Peril to the Health Care System* and *Drugs Anonymous?* Distributed in physicians' offices and by pharmacists, and to congressional members and staffers, the pamphlets warned of the dangers of making generic prescribing mandatory, asserting that such action "could and probably would bring about deterioration in the quality of medical care—through the wide sale of substandard products—by discouraging the struggle for excellence which has marked the astounding progress in the pharmaceutical field—and by impeding drug research on which future progress depends."[39]

During the summer of 1969, the news media accused the industry of pressuring the White House to withdraw its support for the appointment of John Adriani to the position of director of the FDA's Bureau of Medicine. Adriani, by then the chairman of the AMA's Council on Drugs, had accepted the position but the offer was withdrawn following his testimony to the Nelson subcommittee that May. In this testimony, Adriani had "said brand names should be abolished; they were aliases and deceptive and served no useful purpose."[40] Although the PMA denied applying any such pressure, Adriani was certain of their role. He regarded the experience—and the press's coverage of his withdrawn appointment—as "an important battle [that] has been won because the public at last is being made aware of the fact that the pharmaceutical lobby is powerful and could care less about the public."[41] Just a year earlier, the industry had also been accused of "pour[ing] money into Wisconsin in an attempt to defeat Senator Gaylord Nelson" in his reelection bid that fall.[42]

Despite the repeated efforts of Long, Montoya, and Nelson throughout the late 1960s and early 1970s, neither Long's nor Montoya's bill passed. Nelson's generic prescription legislation suffered the same fate. In each case, the prescription reform legislation rested on two problematic assumptions: that generic drugs were therapeutically equivalent (and, indeed, cheaper) than their brand-name counterparts, and that the act of prescribing was an appropriate site of legislative intervention. Given their shared foundation, it is no surprise that all failed to secure congressional passage. In the end, at least two factors account for their legislative failure.

First, concerns about the equivalence of generic drugs raised profound challenges to the drug regulatory system, forcing the FDA to reconsider the standards by which generic drugs were granted market approval. In the early 1970s, as more and more studies documented the inadequacy and clinical consequences of current generic drug standards (based as they were on chemical equivalence), the FDA began requiring generic drug manufacturers to submit evidence of the biological equivalence (bioequivalence) of their generic drugs to their brand-name counterparts before the FDA would grant marketing approval for the generics.[43] By February 1972, Nelson had seen the writing on the wall and, citing the work of the DRB and specifically its 1969 "White Paper on the Therapeutic Equivalence of Generic Drugs," revised his generic prescription bill. While still calling for the mandatory prescription of generic drugs, Nelson acknowledged the "inadequate information . . . made available to the physician, the pharmacist, or the consumer by pharmaceutical manufacturers" on the biological activity of chemically equivalent drugs. Although Nelson framed his statement as an attack on the industry's failure to adequately label prescription drugs, he was clearly responding to the concerns expressed by the DRB and the DES regarding the problem of therapeutic equivalence. By calling for the "inclusion of such biological performance data by manufacturers as part of their new drug application and to require the inclusion of such biological performance information in the labeling which accompanies the drug," Nelson acknowledged that chemical equivalence could no longer be regarded as an adequate measure of therapeutic efficacy.[44]

The second factor undermining prescription legislative proposals in the late 1960s was that prescription drugs made up only a small fraction of the ballooning health care costs. Certainly, in the late 1960s health care costs were rising and presented a serious financial burden to American senior citizens, the indigent, and the working poor. Yet generic prescription advocates had little political rope with which to work: prescription drug costs represented a relatively small percentage of total health care costs (around 10 percent), and prescription drug prices had actually declined slightly (0.1 percent) between 1965 and 1970, while total health care expenditures had increased 6.1 percent during the same time period. The majority of Americans' health care expenditures went to hospital costs and physician fees. In 1974, for example, hospital costs represented 39 percent and physician and other professional fees accounted for 26 percent of total health care expenditures, and between 1965 and 1970, fees for a semiprivate hospital room increased 13.9 percent while physicians' fees increased 6 percent.[45]

PHARMACEUTICAL REFORM IN THE 1970S

Despite Senator Nelson's failure to introduce mandatory generic prescribing, attempts to institute generic prescription reform—and pharmaceutical reform, more generally—were far from resolved. In the first half of the 1970s, health care costs—especially under Medicare and Medicaid—were expanding at unanticipated rates. This led to increased calls from policymakers, federal and state health care officials, and consumer and patient groups for legislation to reduce the cost of prescription drugs.[46]

The early 1970s also witnessed the burgeoning of a public interest movement in American politics. Environmental and consumer groups, in particular, successfully lobbied the government to pass environmental and consumer protection regulations, the most notable of which were passage of the National Environmental Protection Act (NEPA) and the Occupational Safety and Health Act (OSHA) in 1970. These regulations established two new federal agencies, expanding the federal government's regulatory oversight over American industries.[47] The pharmaceutical reform movement of the 1970s must be understood within the context of this broader public interest movement. Throughout the decade, consumer advocates like Ralph Nader joined with congressional pharmaceutical reformers to introduce legislation that would increase the patient-consumer's access to safe and affordable prescription drugs and rein in any perceived corporate largess that threatened consumers' interests. Such legislation would in turn increase the federal government's role in drug development and therapeutic practice. Senators Gaylord Nelson and Edward Kennedy— who each played a key legislative role in securing passage of NEPA and OSHA—were at the center of the 1970s pharmaceutical reform effort. Nelson's Subcommittee on Antitrust and Monopoly continued to hold investigative hearings on the pharmaceutical industry through the late 1970s, while Kennedy, as chair of the Senate Subcommittee on Health, held legislative hearings from 1973 through the late 1970s on a series of pharmaceutical reform bills.[48]

The pharmaceutical reforms of the 1970s shared with those of the 1960s two basic commitments. First, in order to reduce government and patient expenditures on drugs, the reforms aimed to reduce physicians' reliance on brand names and increase their use of generic prescribing. Second, these bills sought to increase physicians' access to reliable and "objective" pharmaceutical information by restricting drug firms' marketing practices; mandating the publication of a federal drug compendium; and expanding the field of clinical pharmacology. A third aspect of the 1970s reform effort, distinct from that of the 1960s, was an attempt to transfer responsibility for the preclinical and clinical testing of new drugs to the federal government. Congressional reformers packaged these measures into two key pieces of legislation—the Drug Utilization Acts of 1975 and 1977, and the Drug Regulation Reform Acts of 1978 and 1979. Elsewhere, federal officials introduced the maximum allowable cost (MAC) program to federal health care programs, and various state legislators—motivated by escalating Medicaid costs—worked to repeal the state antisubstitution laws of the 1950s.[49]

In addition to mobilizing the political strategies of the 1960s, the central feature of the industry's defense strategy in the 1970s was to shift the political critique from its own practices to the ability of the FDA to properly fulfill its regulatory responsibilities. The industry's critique also drew attention to the economic consequences of government regulation. The remainder of this chapter considers each of the 1970s pharmaceutical reform efforts in detail, and the strategies employed by the pharmaceutical industry and its allies in Congress and medicine to challenge them.

Limiting Federal Expenditures on Prescription Drugs

From December 1973 through the fall of 1974, Senator Edward Kennedy (D-MA), the chairman of the Senate Subcommittee on Health, held new hearings on the pharmaceutical industry. The goal of these hearings was to find "legislative solutions to the problems surrounding the way drugs are developed, marketed, and used in this country."[50] On the opening day of those hearings, the secretary of the Department of HEW Casper Weinberger proposed limiting reimbursement for drug purchases under federal programs to "the lowest price at which the drug is generally available, unless there is demonstrated difference in the therapeutic effect."[51] The MAC program was Secretary Weinberger's effort to rein in the federal government's prescription drug expenditures, with anticipated savings of at least $89 million a year in prescription drug costs to federal, state, and local governments.[52] Despite the problems identified by the DRB and the Dunlop Committee regarding the therapeutic equivalence of generic drugs, HEW's MAC program was predicated on the "critical assumption that uniform quality and therapeutic equivalence of drugs can be and is being assured."[53]

The PMA opposed the HEW policy on the grounds that "medically and scientifically, there is a uniform opinion that equivalency cannot be assumed today, and that is exactly what Weinberger's proposal is bottomed on."[54] Although the FDA now required firms to include evidence of the bioequivalence of their generic drug to the brand-name counterpart before marketing approval would be granted, the PMA president Joseph Stetler contended that the FDA was still in no position to guarantee the quality or effectiveness of different versions of the same drug. He blamed this on the agency's failure to adequately carry out its regulatory responsibilities. As evidence, Stetler cited the Department of Defense's rejection of 42 percent of drug samples submitted to it—the majority of which had been approved by the FDA—because they failed to meet the department's own quality control standards. Stetler blamed the failures in "quality control" on the FDA, noting that FDA inspections of drug plants had been decreasing in frequency. While the 1962 drug amendments required the FDA to inspect drug manufacturers at least once every two years, some drug manufacturers had not been inspected for five years, and others had never been inspected.[55] Until the FDA could guarantee the high quality, effectiveness, and biological equivalence of all marketed drugs, Stetler argued, enactment of the MAC program would jeopardize Americans' health care. Instead of guaranteeing Americans' access to "first-class medical care at the least cost," as Secretary Weinberger intended, Stetler maintained, the MAC program would force "Medicare and Medicaid beneficiaries to accept inferior products or . . . pay the cost of first-class medicines from their own household budgets."[56]

In addition to a critique of the FDA's regulatory ability, at the core of the PMA's opposition to the MAC program lay an argument about the economics of government regulation and innovation. As Stetler explained, "the lowest-priced generic is marketed by the manufacturer who does no research, who does no innovating, who probably has limited quality control." Unlike the research-based firm that "does all these very important things . . . that have made us the great industry we are," the generic manufacturer did not need to recoup the costs of research, innovation, and quality control, and therefore "he can sell cheaper." By reimbursing for only the cheapest drug on the market, Stetler argued, the MAC program "would be very tough on the company with expenditures for research," and would ultimately undermine the economic foundation of pharmaceutical innovation.[57]

Concerns about the impact of federal regulations on the innovativeness of the drug industry became a defining feature of the debates over pharmaceutical reform after 1975. When HEW officially introduced the MAC program in 1975, it counted as a "win" for pharmaceutical reformers. Yet that success was muted by the administrative difficulties encountered by the FDA as the agency worked to resolve the problems of assuring the bioequivalence of drugs included within the program. As a result, the first MAC program—for penicillin and ampicillin—did not become effective until June 1977, and subsequent MAC programs were introduced only slowly and sporadically, as and when the FDA was able to guarantee the therapeutic equivalence of participating drugs.[58] In the end, what congressional Democrats had once dismissed as "ballyhoo" and propaganda on the part of the brand-name drug manufacturers turned out to be a critical scientific and regulatory issue that stymied passage of prescription drug legislation through the mid-1970s.

Improving Drug Information

Despite their economic stake in the outcome of Kennedy's hearings on the pharmaceutical industry, generic drug manufacturers were conspicuously absent during the Kennedy hearings and the political and legislative debates that followed. Constrained by a lack of resources and by the nebulous character of the generic drug industry, the trade association of small generic firms, the National Association of Pharmaceutical

Manufacturers, held no political power. Advocacy for the MAC program, and pharmaceutical reform more broadly, was left instead to nascent consumer and patient advocacy groups such as Ralph Nader's Public Citizen, state and municipal health agencies seeking to reduce their health care costs, and the American Pharmaceutical Association, which represented a core segment of organized pharmacy (notably, however, all other pharmacy groups joined with organized medicine and brand-manufacturers in opposing the MAC program).

For Nader, the hearings held by Kennedy's Subcommittee on Health were a forum for challenging the fact that "every day millions of American patients and consumers are being gouged millions of dollars by overpriced drugs." As Nader and his colleague Sidney Wolfe, the director of the Public Citizen's Health Research Group, perceived it, two of the key mechanisms for preventing such gouging were to overturn the state antisubstitution laws that had been passed in the 1950s and to eliminate the pharmaceutical detail man as the physician's primary source of pharmaceutical information. Physicians' reliance on detail men for information about new drugs struck Nader as something of a paradox. After all, the medical profession was "fighting all attempts to encroach on its professionalism, and yet, in prescribing drugs, they take the words of highly articulate, persuasive pitchmen called detail men, who have nothing . . . beyond the mission of maximizing sales for their company. In other words," Nader continued, "here you have professional people relying on rank amateurs to advise them as to what drugs to prescribe for what ailments. If it was not so absurd, one could almost describe the process as having tens of thousands of physicians belonging to a 'Drug of the Month Club.' "[59]

Nader was not alone in lamenting the source of physicians' pharmaceutical information and general lack of pharmaceutical education. As they had in the 1960s, reform-minded physicians, FDA officials, and Democratic congressional reformers continued throughout the 1970s to criticize the marketing practices of pharmaceutical firms and to rail against the lack of "objective" continuing pharmaceutical education available to physicians. As a solution to the paucity of "objective" information about new drugs, Senator Nelson had, since 1967, introduced legislation calling for the publication of a national drug compendium. Nelson and FDA officials insisted that the compendium should be controlled and produced by the FDA (with drug firms footing the bill). As a result, Nelson's compendium bill faced vigorous opposition from the AMA, the PMA, and the DRB, which supported the concept of a national compendium but argued that an FDA-controlled compendium signaled the federal government's inappropriate intrusion in pharmaceutical practice and thus its encroachment on physicians' therapeutic autonomy. As chapter 5 detailed, this opposition continually stymied passage of Nelson's drug compendium bill through the early 1970s.

As the DRB had highlighted in the mid-1960s, however, an additional hurdle to providing physicians with suitable pharmaceutical education was the shortage of those best equipped to provide that education: clinical pharmacologists. With the support of academic physicians and drug firms, the DRB continued to advocate throughout the 1970s for greater government funding of education, training, and research in clinical pharmacology. In 1975, Senator Kennedy took up the issue. Joined by Senator Nelson and a handful of other pharmaceutical reformers, Kennedy introduced the Drug Utilization Improvement Act (S. 1282) before the Senate Committee on Labor and Public Welfare in 1975.[60] Among other provisions, Kennedy's bill called for the establishment of a National Center for Clinical Pharmacology within the Department of HEW. The purpose of the center, Kennedy asserted, was "to improve the education of each member of the health care team about the use of drugs; to collect reliable national data on the way drugs are used and on the extent of the problems caused by drug misuse; to develop mechanisms to monitor the ongoing use of drugs; and to improve the use of those drugs."[61] Yet, although the bill acknowledged the need to improve physicians' knowledge of clinical pharmacology, it made no provision for increasing federal funding of the field. Rather than see the increased education and training of physicians in clinical pharmacology as the way of "minimiz[ing] those drug problems that are caused by physician error or ignorance," (as the DRB had recommended), Kennedy's solution was to undercut the physician's authority and give greater authority to the secretary of HEW over the prescription practices of physicians.[62]

The Drug Utilization Improvement bill included other provisions aimed at increasing the government's control over the drug development process. In particular, Kennedy's bill required the publication of an FDA-controlled drug compendium, and included provisions that would eliminate abuses in and tighten regulations of firms' marketing practices. The bill sought, for example, to "prohibit the giving of any gift product, premium, prize, or other thing of value to a physician or pharmacist by the drug companies." For Kennedy, "this kind of promotional activity can have no purpose other than the improper influence on physician prescribing habits."[63]

The first iteration of Kennedy's bill did not make it out of committee, and two years later Kennedy reintroduced the Drug Utilization Improvement Act. Although similar to his earlier bill, Kennedy's 1977 bill incorporated a new perspective on tackling the problems in pharmaceutical education and research. Reflecting the DRB's earlier recommendations, this version of the bill sought to establish a National Center for Clinical Pharmacology specifically to boost federal funding of the field. As Kennedy noted when he introduced the revised bill, "clinical pharmacology has been a low priority of the Nation's medical schools [and] health sciences schools for too long. Medical students receive an inadequate education about how drugs are used, and the Federal Government provides too little support of the science of clinical pharmacology." Kennedy continued, "The National Center for Clinical Pharmacology will correct both deficiencies. It will provide research at the Nation's universities in clinical pharmacology as well as an intensive intramural Federal research program. It will also allow medical schools to get necessary funding support to develop curriculum with emphasis on clinical pharmacology for medical students."[64]

Despite its more moderate emphasis, Kennedy's proposal failed to win sufficient support that year or in the two subsequent congressional sessions when he and his fellow pharmaceutical reformers, Senator Gaylord Nelson and Representative Paul Rogers (D-FL), reintroduced the concept of a National Center for Clinical Pharmacology (together with provisions for a national drug compendium and restrictions on pharmaceutical marketing) as a provision in the Drug Regulation Reform Acts of 1978 and 1979. The Drug Regulation Reform Act also included a provision that would give the National Center for Clinical Pharmacology the authority to do research and development on "drugs of limited commercial value." This meant that "anytime the pharmaceutical industry is not pursuing a scientific lead the Government will have the option of doing it under this legislation." Kennedy hoped this would lead to rare diseases and "diseases of developing nations . . . get[ting] the special attention that they so desperately need."[65]

Because these bills sought to increase the authority of the Department of HEW over physicians, they faced significant opposition from the drug industry and physicians. Indeed, unlike the DRB's recommendations, which aimed to preserve the autonomy of clinical pharmacologists by keeping them outside the purview of a government department, the Drug Utilization Improvement Act and later the Drug Regulation Reform Acts sought to give the government, via the secretary of HEW, direct control over the development of clinical pharmacology, something that industry and medical leaders vociferously opposed. In effect, Kennedy had repackaged the DRB's recommendation into support for expanding the federal government's role in drug development.

Kennedy's failure to pass legislation that would establish a National Center for Clinical Pharmacology highlights two key themes in the history of American pharmaceutical policymaking. First, it reveals the extent to which the federal government, the medical profession, and the pharmaceutical industry recognized that to achieve a policy goal (in this case, expansion of clinical pharmacology), the stakeholders needed to work cooperatively with one another to effect policy change. Second, the DRB's work to build the field of clinical pharmacology and the failure of Senator Kennedy to translate the DRB's policy recommendations into effective legislation exposes the limits of that cooperation when questions of authority and professional autonomy are at stake. In the DRB's vision, ultimate authority to determine the nature and form of clinical pharmacology training and research should rest with academic leaders, while Kennedy's vision placed that authority within the federal government. The ever-present disconnect between the policy recommendations of expert committees and the political goals of legislators who seek to translate those recommendations into practice makes clear a third theme in the history of American pharmaceutical policymaking: although all stakeholders may agree in principle to work cooperatively, the often incompatible motivations and interests of the different stakeholders may work in practice to stymie policy change.

THE BACKLASH AGAINST REGULATORY REFORM

Through the 1960s and early 1970s, when the American economy was prospering, regulatory reformers in general found significant public support for increasing the government's regulatory powers over American corporations. This in part explains the legislative successes achieved by the public interest movement in the early 1970s. The declining U.S. economy in the mid-1970s, however, precipitated a change in the American public's perception of business and, thus, their regard for the government's regulatory authority over American corporations. Rather than taking business's profitability for granted, Americans realized that in a weak economy, business's growth could be vulnerable. As a result, more Americans became sympathetic to business's calls for reducing government regulation of business practices and sought to provide a political climate more conducive to economic recovery and business growth. At the same time, the 1970s saw the resurgence of conservatism in the American political economy, which had at its core a commitment—borne of the Chicago School of economics—to free markets and opposition to government regulation.[66]

In this context, the efforts of pharmaceutical reformers to expand government regulation of one of the largest sectors of the U.S. economy—and a sector, no less, that controlled the major share of the global pharmaceutical market—meant going against the changing tide of public opinion. Indeed, as HEW worked to implement the MAC program and as Congress debated the Drug Utilization Improvement Act and later, the Drug Regulation Reform Act, the drug industry and its physician allies mobilized a powerful economic critique of pharmaceutical regulation. In doing so, the industry and its allies situated their opposition to greater pharmaceutical regulation within the broader debate about the appropriate level of government oversight of the American economy.

Immediately following passage of the 1962 drug amendments, academic physicians and pharmaceutical executives alike had expressed concern that the administrative and economic demands of the new regulations would deter firms and researchers from pursing pharmaceutical research, leading to a decline in pharmaceutical innovation. By the mid-1970s, a series of economic studies published by the probusiness think tank the American Enterprise Institute (AEI) seemed to indicate that this was indeed the case.

In 1973, William Wardell, a clinical pharmacologist at the University of Rochester in New York published a comparative study of new drug approvals in the United States and Britain. Wardell found that between 1962 and 1971, four times as many new drugs (so-called new chemical entities) were introduced to the British market as to the U.S. market. Wardell concluded that a "drug lag" existed in the United States.[67] A year later, the University of Chicago economist Sam Peltzman published an assessment—funded by the AEI—of the economic costs of the 1962 drug amendments on the pharmaceutical industry and on consumers. Peltzman concluded that rather than providing economic benefits to consumers (as Senator Kefauver had originally intended), the drug amendments had instead resulted in fewer new drugs being introduced to the U.S. pharmaceutical market. Furthermore, Peltzman argued, the longer drug approval process necessitated by the amendments, and the subsequent delays in new drugs reaching the market, had in fact cost the American public an extra $300 million to $400 million a year.[68] In 1975, Wardell joined forces with his Rochester colleague, the prominent clinical pharmacologist Louis Lasagna. Extending Peltzman's analysis, Lasagna and Wardell argued that the "drug lag" was a direct result of the 1962 drug amendments. Because of the United States' overly stringent regulations (compared to the regulatory standards of European countries), new drugs were being introduced as much as two years earlier in Britain and 1.6 years earlier in Germany. As a result, Lasagna and Wardell argued, American patients were being denied access to important new drugs, especially in the fields of cardiovascular and respiratory disease and hypertension, and were paying more for the drugs to which they did have access. Excessive FDA regulations, Lasagna and Wardell surmised, were threatening the American public's health. Like Peltzman's study, Lasagna and Wardell's work was funded and published by the AEI.[69]

In the late 1950s, Lasagna had been one of the most vocal academic physicians who had called for reform of the pharmaceutical industry and specifically for the tightening of regulations around the approval of prescription drugs. Yet within a decade, Lasagna had done an apparent "180 degree turn" and become one of the loudest critics of the FDA and its regulation of the American drug industry.[70] Although Lasagna's opponents often accused him of being in the pocket of the drug industry (he had, for many years, served as a consultant to and collaborator with a number of drug firms), he maintained that, rather than opposing drug regulation per se, he instead found the FDA guilty of having acted overzealously in its interpretation of the 1962 drug amendments. For Lasagna, the issue was not so much that the drug amendments should be repealed but rather that the FDA's stringent requirements of what counted as sufficient evidence of efficacy needed to be loosened. Most notably, Lasagna argued that "a few well done controlled clinical trials can establish beyond a reasonable doubt that a drug has efficacy and that a modest amount of clinical experience can tell us reasonably well what the pattern of fairly common adverse drug reactions will be." In light of this, Lasagna recommended that "earlier release" of new drugs "be combined with a commitment on the part of the manufacturer to monitor the drug's usage after release so as to accumulate the evidence we really want to have." Lasagna and Wardell thus called on the FDA to reduce the degree of premarket testing required for new drug approvals and to introduce instead a new stage of drug testing, "postmarketing surveillance." Modeled on the regulatory processes in Britain and Germany, in which the majority of drug testing occurred after a drug had been introduced to the market, postmarketing surveillance would, Lasagna argued, permit the FDA to determine how "the drug [will] perform when it is used in actual practice, instead of by experts working in homogenous populations."[71]

The industry and its allies pointed to the drug lag as evidence that the FDA had overstepped its authority and was overregulating drugs to the detriment of American patients.[72] In defense of the existing drug regulations, however, FDA officials and congressional pharmaceutical reformers challenged the very premise on which the idea of the drug lag was based. During Kennedy's hearings, for example, Senator Nelson (a member of the Subcommittee on Health) held up data from the pharmaceutical analyst Paul deHaen that showed that the number of new chemical entities introduced to the American market had actually peaked in 1959—and declined significantly thereafter—several years before the drug amendments were enacted.[73]

FDA officials also challenged the basis on which Wardell and Lasagna made their international comparisons. In 1976, for example, the FDA commissioner Alexander Schmidt maintained that it was a mistake to "compare this country with its [regulatory] requirements with another country that has no such requirements." Schmidt was particularly troubled that drug lag advocates compared new drug introductions in the United States to those in Britain, where drug efficacy requirement regulations had been passed only two years earlier. Schmidt also pointed out that with the majority of large pharmaceutical firms being multinational corporations, it was up to the firm to "pick and choose where they develop drugs. . . . So when a company has to decide whether to develop a drug here or in a foreign country where it has a subsidiary and where it can cheaply, quickly, and easily develop the drug [as compared to the United States with its lengthy and thus expensive testing requirements], you can easily see where that drug company will go to experiment with the drug and first introduce it." For Schmidt then, if a drug lag existed (and he insisted it did not), the fault for it lay not with the regulatory system but with the economic choices made by corporate executives about where they would first introduce and market a new drug.[74]

Elsewhere, FDA officials pointed out that very few if any of those drugs available earlier in Europe than in the United States were regarded as significant therapeutic advances on existing drugs.[75] As Donald Kennedy, the FDA commissioner in 1978, noted, "to fail to make distinctions on the basis of quality rather than merely on quantity leads to absurd conclusions." For Kennedy, "the most notable reason" for the drug lag was "what the former president of Merck, Sharp and Dohme, Henry Gadsden, characterized as an 'apparent exhaustion of certain basic knowledge in which the [drug] industry's earlier breakthroughs were based.' "[76]

The drug lag was an issue around which the drug industry galvanized significant political support, not least because it resonated with growing national concerns about the vitality of the American economy.[77] The oil crisis of 1973 and 1974 and the economic recession that followed had brought an abrupt end to the American economy's unprecedented postwar growth. As the U.S. economy stagnated, the West German and Japanese economies—particularly in high-technology sectors such as pharmaceuticals—boomed. This raised concerns among U.S. economists, policymakers, and business leaders that the United States was at risk of losing its economic and technological leadership in the global economy. In response, business leaders launched a massive political and public relations campaign aimed at reeducating American lawmakers and the public on the economic dangers wrought by the overregulation of American industries.[78] Within this context, the apparently declining rates of pharmaceutical innovation among American manufacturers alongside the apparently increasing innovativeness of European firms served as immediate—and powerful—evidence that government regulations were detrimental not only to the country's economic well-being but also to the nation's health. Thus, when drug industry representatives and their medical allies argued that any further regulation by the FDA would potentially "drive research overseas," "stifle innovation" in the United States, and further threaten America's economic and pharmaceutical dominance, they effectively situated their critique within a broader backlash against government regulation of business.[79]

By focusing attention on the drug lag, the industry and its allies undermined Senators Kennedy and Nelson's efforts to introduce the Drug Utilization Improvement and Drug Regulation Reform Acts, and provided a basis on which to argue that the FDA's authority should be reined in. In particular, the industry and its medical allies joined with their congressional allies in calling for repeal of what they perceived to be the main cause of the drug lag: the efficacy provision of the 1962 drug amendments. To this end, from 1976 through the end of the decade, Representative Steven D. Symms (R-ID) introduced the Medicine Freedom of Choice Act, which would repeal the "proof-of-efficacy" provision of the 1962 drug amendments. Although it never made it out of committee, in successive congressional sessions Symms's bill garnered substantial support, with as many as 105 cosponsors to the bill. The congressional support for the Medicines Freedom of Choice Act (later renamed the Food and Drug Reform Act) reflected the degree of concern among congressional members in the late 1970s about the innovativeness and strength of the American pharmaceutical industry and of the American economy more generally.[80]

A PRESCRIPTION FOR STATE-BASED REFORM

Although pharmaceutical reformers struggled throughout the 1970s to secure passage of federal reform, the early 1970s saw the emergence of a state-based reform effort. As Ralph Nader and Sidney Wolfe testified before Kennedy's Subcommittee on Health in 1973, a key means of increasing consumers' access to cheaper prescription drugs was to overturn the state antisubstitution laws enacted during the 1950s (see chapter 3). As Nader and Wolfe perceived it, state legislatures had been "wooed" in the 1950s by "a highly effective promotional campaign" orchestrated by brand-name "drug companies and their physician allies in order to . . . preserve exclusive prescribing for brand-name drugs which are higher priced." Two decades later, however, "in the face of a large amount of testing showing that there really is not the difference between generic and brand-name drugs the large manufacturers would like us to believe exists," Nader and Wolfe were confident that "pharmacists and consumers will succeed in overthrowing many of these laws at the State level."[81]

In this effort, Public Citizen had as an ally the largest association of American pharmacists, the American Pharmaceutical Association (APhA), which in April 1970 had passed a resolution calling for repeal of the state antisubstitution laws. Although the APhA had supported passage of those antisubstitution acts in the 1950s, the APhA's about-face on the issue of substitution reflected the tensions and separations that had grown between organized pharmacy, organized medicine, and the PMA during the 1960s. The APhA had become increasingly frustrated by the tendency of physicians and industry representatives to suggest—in their congressional testimony and public speeches—that prescription drug costs were high in part because they incorporated the professional fees and markups applied by retail pharmacists. Because pharmacists' fees and pricing practices had been excluded from Kefauver's (and later Nelson's) investigation of the pharmaceutical industry, industry officials and physicians had been able to shift some of the blame for prescription drug prices to pharmacists without congressional recourse.[82]

To pharmacy leaders, this blame-shifting strategy reflected a lack of respect among physicians for pharmacists' professional abilities. William

Apple, the president of the APhA throughout the 1960s and 1970s, accused the AMA of "relegat[ing the pharmacist] to the role of a merchant." He explained, "I don't think the AMA fully appreciates the extent to which physicians are relying on pharmacists to help patients purchase their prescriptions more economically. I don't think the AMA is aware of the informal understandings that many physicians have with pharmacists regarding brand interchange." According to Apple, the pharmacy profession was "fighting for liberation" from medicine, the path to which depended on the profession "eliminat[ing] the old concept that the pharmacist is merely the handmaiden of the physician . . . [and] wip[ing] out the last vestiges of the view that the pharmacist is the final link—the end-of-the-line—in what is essentially a marketing system for prescription drug manufacturers."[83]

Pharmacists had been struggling since the early twentieth century to craft a professional identity for themselves.[84] The compounding pharmacist of the first half of the twentieth century had been superseded in the 1950s by the vertically integrated pharmaceutical firms that compounded and packaged their own drug products. In the same decade, regional and national supermarket chains had begun offering pharmacy services to their customers, supplanting the unique services once provided by the community pharmacist.[85] Throughout the 1960s, pharmacists—and their professional organizations—had been relatively content to accept their subordinate position within the health care team. In the early 1970s, however, recognition of the clinical importance of bioequivalence offered pharmacists a new foundation on which to fashion their professional identity. Indeed, as practicing physicians struggled to make sense of the ever-growing number of new drugs on the market, pharmacists argued that they—not physicians—possessed the appropriate pharmaceutical knowledge and expertise to make sense of the plethora of me-too drugs and identify the most appropriate version of a prescription drug for each patient.[86] The APhA hoped that through repeal of the antisubstitution laws and the assertion of pharmacists' authority in drug product selection, pharmacists would finally be regarded "as bona fide members of the health care team," with professional standing equal to that of physicians.[87]

The AMA and brand manufacturers lost the battle over substitution and pharmacists succeeded in securing a new professional role in prescription practice. By mid-decade, driven by rising medical costs, state legislatures around the country were acting on the APhA's recommendation to repeal the antisubstitution laws. In February 1975, for example, the New Jersey state senator Frank J. Dodd and assemblyman Martin A. Herman each introduced bills that would authorize pharmacists to substitute a generic drug for a specific brand-name drug prescribed by a physician. Signaling the state's escalating Medicaid costs, Senator Dodd argued, "We could save as little as $3 million or as much as $5.7 million," by authorizing generic substitution, a measure that "would stabilize the ever-increasing drug costs to Medicaid in the future."[88] The following month, the California assemblyman Barry Keene introduced a similar measure authorizing substitution amid claims that it "could save Californians $40 million in drug costs the first year and more in future years."[89] The California legislature passed the generic substitution bill later that year.[90] In February 1977, after two years of legislative apathy on the matter (not surprising, given that New Jersey is home to several of the world's largest brand-name manufacturers), the New Jersey legislature finally approved a bill authorizing generic substitution.[91] And by 1979, forty states and the District of Columbia had modified their antisubstitution laws so as to permit pharmacists to substitute generically equivalent drugs for the brand names prescribed.[92]

CONCLUSION

Although federal reform of the pharmaceutical industry remained tantalizingly out of reach to pharmaceutical reformers, by the end of the 1970s they had achieved a modicum of reform at the state level. That pharmaceutical reformers achieved success at the state level is in part explained by the political motivation of states to reduce the economic burden of rising Medicaid costs (of which prescription drug prices were a small part). At the same time, by the late 1970s the grounds on which brand-name manufacturers had previously opposed prescription reform had been severely undermined. Through the mid-1970s, brand-name manufacturers had opposed mandatory generic prescribing and substitution on the basis that the FDA could not adequately regulate generic drugs, and thus could provide no guarantee that a generic drug was therapeutically equivalent to its brand-name counterpart. For brand-name manufacturers and their physician-allies, this meant that "until all similar drug preparations can be equated meaningfully in terms of their bioavailability to permit the interchange of different forms of a drug on a rational basis, legalistic maneuvering designed to weaken or revoke drug anti-substitution laws should be opposed vigorously."[93] The flip side of this defense, though, was the possibility that once the "equivalence problem" was resolved and the FDA was able to guarantee the therapeutic equivalence of generic drugs, the rationale for opposing substitution and generic prescribing would be lost. And indeed, this is exactly what happened. Once the FDA began approving generic drugs on the basis that their manufacturers had demonstrated the biological equivalence of the generic to a brand-name counterpart, the PMA and AMA lost a major leg on which to stand in their opposition to substitution.

By the end of the 1970s, generic substitution posed much less of an economic risk to brand-name manufacturers than it had in the 1950s, when the antisubstitution laws were first passed. Although the repeal of the antisubstitution laws permitted pharmacists to substitute a generic drug for the brand-name drug prescribed by a physician, the new substitution laws did so only if the physician specifically *authorized* the pharmacist to make such a substitution. Under Missouri's new substitution law, for example, a prescription form was valid only if it contained "two signature lines at opposite ends at the bottom of the form," with "dispense as written" under one, and "substitution permitted" under the other. When writing a prescription, the physician was then required to sign on one line or the other according to his or her preference.[94] In Michigan, the pharmacist was prohibited from substituting unless the patient specifically requested a generic drug or unless the physician actively authorized the substitution.[95] And in California, as in the majority of other states, the physician was required to check a "no substitution" box on the prescription form if he or she did not want the pharmacist to substitute.[96] Thus, as long as physicians continued to specify the use of brand-name drugs in higher number than generic drugs (a product of brand-name firms' marketing efforts), repeal of the antisubstitution laws actually did little to challenge the economic foundation of the pharmaceutical enterprise.

The failure of pharmaceutical reformers to secure *federal* reform of the drug industry after two decades of concerted activism also highlights the effectiveness with which the pharmaceutical industry had transformed itself, over those decades, into a politically activist industry. As this chapter makes clear, the alliances the industry forged with the medical profession over issues of shared interest, particularly as they related to the government's role in drug development and medical practice, were critical to that transformation. The success achieved by pharmaceutical reformers at the state level is also suggestive of the limits of the industry's political alliances. Unlike Congress, state legislators could respond to the demands of local consumer, hospital, and pharmacy groups pressing for prescription reform because their demands were politically and economically tenable. After all, state health and welfare agencies were themselves part of the pharmaceutical reform movement as they struggled to balance the economic burden of rising health care costs.[97]

Epilogue

The substance and character of pharmaceutical politics changed little between the 1960s and 2009. Each episode of prescription drug policymaking was shaped by the same alignment of interest groups (brand-name manufacturers and organized medicine on one side; consumer and senior citizen groups, reformist congressional Democrats, and, increasingly, generic drug manufacturers on the other). The issues on which critics challenged the pharmaceutical industry and sought reform continued to be the high price of prescription drugs, the marketing practices employed by pharmaceutical firms, and the ability of regulators to ensure the safety of prescription drugs. Similarly, the industry's response to proposals for reform remained largely unchanged, with the political debate shaped by the same arguments about promoting innovation, protecting physician autonomy, and preserving the freedom of physicians to prescribe and patients to consume the pharmaceuticals they choose. In the 2009 and 2010 debate over health care reform, however, the pharmaceutical industry adopted a significantly different posture toward pharmaceutical reform. Rather than pursuing an oppositional stance to the Obama administration's proposals for overhauling the health care system, the pharmaceutical industry supported national health care reform, agreeing to $80 billion in pharmaceutical cost savings over the next ten years and agreeing to disclose all gifts and payments in excess of ten dollars to physicians and academic researchers as part of the Physician Payment Sunshine Act. To what extent has the pharmaceutical industry's apparent about-face altered the interlocking array of incentives and interests that characterized pharmaceutical politics since the 1960s?

This chapter considers two examples of prescription drug policy that illustrate the continuities in pharmaceutical politics since the 1970s: the 1984 Hatch-Waxman Act and the 2003 Medicare Prescription Drug

Improvement and Modernization Act. This chapter also examines the changing politics that led to passage of the 2010 Patient Protection and Affordable Care Act, and assesses what this recent shift in the pharmaceutical industry's response to reform means for ongoing efforts to reform the system of drug development and regulation in the United States.

First, let us consider passage of the Drug Price Competition and Patent Term Restoration Act of 1984 (also known as the Hatch-Waxman Act, named for the primary sponsors of the bill—Orrin G. Hatch [R-UT] and Henry A. Waxman [D-CA]). Widely hailed as the most important piece of drug legislation since passage of the 1962 drug amendments, the Hatch-Waxman Act introduced significant economic reform into the pharmaceutical industry. It did so by establishing a new regulatory pathway for generic drug approvals and providing incentives to generic drug manufacturers in order to facilitate the entry of generic drugs into the market after the patents of brand-name drugs expired. At the same time, however, the Hatch-Waxman Act also shored up the economic power of brand-name manufacturers by extending the patent term on prescription drugs by up to five years.[1]

In the early 1980s, brand-name manufacturers had begun calling for passage of legislation that would extend the patents on drugs by restoring time lost to the approval process. Brand-name manufacturers argued that the testing requirements imposed as part of the 1962 drug amendments had resulted in longer development and marketing approval times for new drugs, causing manufacturers to lose a significant portion of their patent-protected time to the approval process. These regulatory delays, brand-name manufacturers maintained, contributed to the drug lag.[2] Typically, brand-name manufacturers secured patents on their new drugs early in the development process, guaranteeing the patent holder seventeen years of market exclusivity. A study published by the Office of Technology Assessment in 1981, however, showed that on average, it took manufacturers seven to ten years to develop and test a drug after the patent had been awarded. The result was that by the time a patented drug reached the market, the company had only a few years left on the patent in which to reap the benefits of marketing exclusivity. Brand-name manufacturers argued that the shortened period of marketing exclusivity made it difficult for them to recoup their development costs and earn sufficient profits on new drugs—profits, they noted, that were used to fund future drug development.[3]

In response to the drug industry's calls, Representative Robert Kastenmeier (D-WI) and Senator John P. East (R-NC) introduced the bipartisan Patent Term Restoration bill to Congress in 1981 and again in 1982. By "restor[ing] the patent life that has been consumed during a particular product review and approval process," the bill's sponsors hoped to "restore fundamental fairness by fulfilling the intent of Congress that all inventions be accorded equal and adequate protection."[4] Using the same arguments that had served the industry so well since the late 1950s, the Pharmaceutical Manufacturers Association (PMA) and its congressional supporters (of which there were many—from both sides of the aisle) tied the fate of pharmaceutical patents to the innovativeness of the industry and, by extension, the availability of lifesaving drugs.[5] As Representative Kastenmeier noted, "the issue involved is not simply the growth of the economy, it is encouraging future investment of large sums of private capital in the high-risk area of breakthrough pharmaceutical and chemical technology. Such investments pay off not only in economic growth, but even more importantly in improvements in the health and well being of our people." Representative Harold Ford (D-TN) further explained that while the country confronted "soaring health care costs ... new drugs have alleviated human suffering and saved billions of dollars by providing effective alternatives to costly surgical procedures and hospitalization."[6]

Opposing the bill was an equally familiar alliance of pharmaceutical reformers: consumer groups like Ralph Nader's Public Citizen, senior citizens groups like the National Council of Senior Citizens (NCSC) and AARP, and a cadre of congressional Democrats committed to protecting patients' and consumers' interests, including Senator Edward Kennedy (D-MA) and Representative Albert Gore Jr. (D-TN).[7] The executive director of the NCSC, for example, warned, "This thing is so bad. To think of an additional giveaway to the drug companies at a time when drug prices are so high." Senator Kennedy likewise argued that the bill "in its present form ... is not in the public interest."[8] Pharmaceutical reformers feared that by further extending the patent term of brand-name drugs and delaying the entry of generic drugs onto the market, the bill would put "effective cost control" of prescription drug prices "further out of the reach of the consumers."[9]

Generic drug companies, represented by their trade association, the Generic Pharmaceutical Industry Association (GPIA) joined with pharmaceutical reformers in opposing the bill. William Haddad, the president of the GPIA (and a prominent consumer advocate during the Nelson hearings), challenged the very premise of the Patent Term Restoration bill, noting that many brand-name firms were, in fact, able to secure additional patents on their drugs by patenting not only the drug product but also the process used to manufacture the drug. The result, Haddad argued, was that "the top-selling drugs in America are realizing actual legal patent protection for an average of 18.5 years."[10]

For the next two years, the battle lines remained drawn between brand-name manufacturers and their allies favoring passage of the patent term extension bill, and generic manufacturers, consumer and senior citizen groups, and consumer-oriented congressional Democrats opposing it. During the summer of 1984, following several months of negotiation between the two sides, Representative Henry Waxman and Senator Orrin Hatch drew up a compromise bill, which promised to restore the time on patents lost to the approval process in exchange for measures that made it easier for generic drugs to enter the market after a patent had expired. President Ronald Reagan signed the Patent Term Restoration and Price Competition Act into law on September 24, 1984.

Thus, passage of the act continued the pharmaceutical politics of the previous three decades. Although pharmaceutical reformers and generic manufacturers gained substantially from the bill—the Hatch-Waxman Act is credited with stimulating the emergence of a vast generic drug industry, which in turn led physicians to significantly increase the number of prescriptions written for generic rather than brand-name drugs—brand manufacturers also scored a significant win. The Hatch-Waxman Act, after all, prevented enactment of the more stringent regulatory and marketing changes that were being demanded by pharmaceutical reformers. In the end, the compromise legislation enabled brand-name manufacturers to balance the losses incurred by expanded generic competition as long as they continued to innovate and secure new patents on new drugs and on new formulations of older drugs. The result was less an undermining than a reinforcement of brand-name manufacturers' economic interests.[11]

Pharmaceutical politics-as-usual was again on display in the early 2000s, as pharmaceutical reformers, industry, Congress, and the White House debated the addition of a prescription drug benefit to Medicare. In the 2000 presidential election, prescription drug prices had been at the center of political debate with both presidential candidates, Vice-President Albert Gore Jr. (D) and Governor George W. Bush (R-TX), advancing proposals for a Medicare drug benefit. Pharmaceutical companies, led by the Pharmaceutical Research and Manufacturers Association (PhRMA, the successor to the PMA), had responded by launching a $60 million campaign that urged policymakers: "don't interfere with our ability to save lives."[12] After Bush won the election and Republicans secured control of Congress, the debate focused on the form that a Medicare drug benefit would take. Building on Gore's campaign proposal, Democrats advocated adding a standardized drug benefit to the traditional Medicare program, which would establish the government as a large-scale purchaser of prescription drugs, thereby giving the government significant purchasing power with which to negotiate prescription drug prices. By contrast, the Bush administration and congressional Republicans favored a market-oriented approach in which the government would subsidize private insurance companies to offer drug coverage to Medicare beneficiaries. Purchasing power would thus be distributed among a variety of insurance companies (each significantly smaller than the federal government), thereby mitigating any one company's or the government's ability to negotiate significantly lower drug prices.[13]

The partisan debate over the Medicare drug benefit reprised the alliances in pharmaceutical politics since the 1960s. Brand-name manufacturers, led by PhRMA, and the American Medical Association (AMA) joined with Republicans in opposing the Democrats' plan on the grounds that it would lead inevitably to government price controls and incursions on physicians' autonomy. The House majority leader, Representative Richard K. Armey (R-TX), argued that the addition of a standardized drug benefit to Medicare "must and does rely on government price controls to control its massive costs. These price controls will make it unprofitable to develop new miracle drugs, and this will kill innovation."[14] As they had done since the 1950s, pharmaceutical companies argued that prescription drug prices reflected the industry's research costs, and warned that a government-run prescription drug benefit would, by reducing the industry's prices and thus profits, hinder the ability of pharmaceutical firms to conduct the expensive research needed to innovate new drugs.[15] Pharmaceutical companies also reminded legislators that by reducing the length and thus cost of patients' hospitalization, even the most expensive prescription drugs "are the most cost-effective part of our health care system."[16]

Patient advocacy groups to which the pharmaceutical industry had been providing financial support for the previous two decades joined with the industry in warning of the loss of innovation and increased patient suffering that would result from the Democrats' plan.[17] The AMA and congressional Republicans also attacked the Democrats' plan, warning that a government-run prescription drug benefit would undermine physicians' professional autonomy and patients' freedom to choose the type of medical care (including which type of prescription drug) they would receive. For Representative Armey, the Democrats' plan would "forc[e] all seniors into a government-chosen HMO [health maintenance organization] for drugs," leaving "government bureaucrats," instead of physicians, "decid[ing] which drugs are and are not covered. If they decide the drug you need is too expensive, they will force you to switch to a cheaper, less effective one."[18]

On the other side, an alliance of congressional Democrats, labor, consumer, and senior citizens groups, including the AFL-CIO, Public Citizen, and AARP, argued that the Bush plan—without the promise of price controls—would do little to resolve the problem of high prices. Citing the millions of senior citizens struggling to meet the cost of prescription drugs, this reform alliance maintained that high prescription drug prices were not, as the pharmaceutical industry claimed, attributable to the industry's high research costs. Rather, they were due to the "exorbitant profits" made by pharmaceutical companies. "It is simple greed," asserted Representative James Turner (D-TX). "The big drug makers are not about to let these profits slip away, and that is why they are spending billions of dollars on marketing and lobbying in this Congress. In fact," Turner continued, "nine out of the ten top drug makers spend more money on marketing than they do on research and development."[19]

Health insurance companies and HMOs were also prominent in the debate. The health insurance industry had been absent in the pharmaceutical reform debates of the 1960s and 1970s because prescription drugs were relatively minor costs to insurance companies in those decades. In 1970, for example, health insurance companies covered only 8 percent of the nation's total drug costs.[20] By 2000, however, the insurance industry had a substantial economic stake in the outcome of the Medicare drug benefit debate. Indeed, by 1999, insurers and HMOs were for the first time paying more for prescription drugs than they were for hospitalization.[21] The Bush administration's proposal for a Medicare drug benefit, which was predicated on the government subsidizing private insurance companies to provide prescription drug coverage to seniors, would force insurance companies to sell stand-alone drug coverage. Health insurance companies, however, opposed providing seniors with stand-alone drug coverage because of concerns that prescription drug costs for the elderly would grow faster than either insurance premiums or the proposed federal subsidies. As a result, the insurance industry was critical of Republican proposals to subsidize prescription drug coverage through private insurance plans, although in general the industry preferred a market-oriented drug benefit to any government-run plan.[22]

After three years of congressional debate and lobbying by the pharmaceutical and health insurance industries, AARP, and other senior citizen groups, President Bush signed the Medicare Prescription Drug Improvement and Modernization Act in September 2003, adding a prescription drug benefit to Medicare. Medicare Part D, the name for the drug benefit, assumed the market-oriented approach advocated by the Bush administration. As with earlier pharmaceutical reform efforts, the drug industry secured from Congress the passage of compromise legislation that ultimately reinforced rather than undermined the industry's economic interests. In addition to drug firms gaining access to forty million newly covered Medicare consumers, the 2003 act explicitly barred the federal government from using its purchasing power to negotiate lower drug prices. The government instead would have to accept the prices negotiated by groups with far less purchasing power—insurers, drugstore chains, and pharmacy benefit managers. The Bush administration was able to win the insurance industry's support for Medicare Part D by also passing Medicare Part C, which financially shored up the private-sector Medicare option known as Medicare Advantage and generated substantial income for the insurance industry.[23] For senior citizens, the benefits of Medicare Part D were less definitive. After the act's passage, Medicare beneficiaries struggled to make sense of the confusing array of prescription drug coverage available to them and continued to face debilitating prescription drug costs because of the "doughnut hole" in Medicare coverage.

Pharmaceutical politics-as-usual continue to shape prescription drug policy. The Patient Protection and Affordable Care Act, signed into law by President Barak Obama on March 23, 2010, is a testimony to the continuing power that pharmaceutical companies hold over the legislative process, and the pervasiveness of the industry's rhetoric in contemporary debates over prescription drug reform. On its surface, passage of the health care reform bill suggested that pharmaceutical politics might be changing. After all, the pharmaceutical industry and the AMA both supported the bill. PhRMA even went so far as to run an advertising campaign in the summer of 2009 urging Americans to support the health care reform bill. PhRMA's support came after the group negotiated with the White House and Senator Max Baucus (D-MT), the chair of the Senate Finance Committee, that the industry would, over the next ten years, come up with $80 billion in drug savings for seniors and federal health programs.[24] Below its surface, however, the politics of the health care reform bill were anything but different. In striking its deal with Democrats, PhRMA received commitments from Baucus and the White House that there would be no government price controls, no provision authorizing the reimportation of drugs from countries such as Canada and Mexico, and no reduction in the patent term of branded biologic drugs (a measure advocated by consumer groups and generic manufacturers as a way of encouraging generic competition in the expensive biological drug field). At the same time, the bill's provision that required most Americans to carry health insurance essentially guaranteed pharmaceutical companies a large market of newly insured pharmaceutical consumers.[25] The AMA also benefited from passage of the bill; in exchange for its support, it saw the "public option" dropped from serious policy discussion and a commitment that the new bill would not result in reduced Medicare payments to physicians.[26] In the end, the overhaul of the health care system promised by President Obama looked less like an "overhaul" than a reaffirmation of a market-oriented approach to health care in which corporate interests dominate.[27]

Despite the continuity of decades-old pharmaceutical politics, there are encouraging signs of change in the political culture of pharmaceuticals. For one thing, since the 1980s, pharmaceutical politics is no longer a partisan issue, with Republicans and Democrats automatically standing on opposite sides of pharmaceutical reform. In the debates that led to passage of the Hatch-Waxman Act in 1984, brand-name manufacturers found significant support on both sides of the congressional aisle. And although the debate over the Medicare prescription drug benefit was more traditionally partisan, the recent debate over the Obama health reform bill saw the pharmaceutical industry for the first time align itself with Democrats. This change in the partisan character of pharmaceutical politics in part reflects the drug industry's pragmatic approach to politics, realizing the benefits of finding favor on both sides of the aisle. This has been reflected in the industry's campaign contributions over the past two decades. Although historically, the industry has favored the typically probusiness Republican Party, during the 2008 election cycle pharmaceutical companies donated $20 million to federal candidates and the parties, of which 49 percent went to Democrats and 51 percent to Republicans. This compared to the 31 percent received by Democrats in 2000. Yet, as the chairman of the House Ways and Means Subcommittee on Health, Representative Pete Stark (D-CA), asserted, "people in the pharmaceutical industry have not suddenly changed their spots. They understand who will be writing legislation in the next few years. They want to be at the table." The pharmaceutical industry's increased support of Democrats was also a response to a shift in attitude among some Republicans. Senator John McCain (R-AZ), for example, throughout his 2008 presidential campaign, was strongly critical of the pharmaceutical industry and promised, if elected, to seek legislation that would allow the government to negotiate drug prices with pharmaceutical firms.[28]

Another change in the pharmaceutical political culture since the 1970s has been the arrival of new interest groups, which have reshaped the traditional alliances of pharmaceutical companies and pharmaceutical reformers. Most powerful among the new groups advocating for pharmaceutical reform have been health insurance companies and the states. The health insurance industry has been a powerful interest group in American health care politics since its expansion in the 1950s and 1960s.[29] Despite its general support for Medicare and Medicaid in the 1960s, the insurance industry was conspicuously absent during the pharmaceutical reform debates of that decade. Until the 1980s, insurance companies provided little in the way of prescription drug coverage and thus were relatively unburdened by prescription drug prices. Since feeling the brunt of high prescription drug prices, however, insurance companies have, on matters of pharmaceutical reform, had a substantial interest in legislation that would increase generic drug competition and drive down prescription drug prices while maintaining a market-oriented approach to health care reform.[30] Given the political power of the health insurance industry (according to the Center for Responsive Politics, the health insurance and pharmaceutical industries are two of the largest and most powerful industry-sector lobbies in Washington, D.C.), the industry's stake in prescription drug prices has added a loud and influential voice to discussions of pharmaceutical reform.[31]

State governments have also come to play an increasingly important role in pharmaceutical politics. Though they had always been advocates of pharmaceutical reform, not until the 1990s did states develop sufficient policy competence to secure effective state-based policy reforms and to push for changes in federal health policy.[32] This policy competence was borne out in the debates over the reimportation of prescription drugs in the early 2000s. Governors from states that were reeling under their enormous prescription drug expenditures (particularly those from Minnesota, Massachusetts, Oregon, Vermont, and Washington) took the lead in calling for legislation that would allow them to import cheaper drugs from countries such as Canada and Mexico.[33]

Though the pharmaceutical industry lobby succeeded in preventing passage of such legislation, an increasing number of states established preferred drug lists (PDLs). These lists were established by panels of physicians and pharmacists, which recommended coverage of specific drugs within a given drug class based on published clinical data, information provided by pharmaceutical firms, and the informed opinions of the committee's members. Physicians could prescribe any drug on the PDL to Medicaid beneficiaries, but to prescribe a nonpreferred drug to a Medicaid patient a physician needed prior authorization. Drug manufacturers could secure preferred status for an equivalent but more expensive drug if they paid supplemental rebates to states, thereby reducing the cost of the drug to that of the preferred drug. In 2003, a consortium of states interested in integrating comparative effectiveness research into PDL decision making established the Drug Effectiveness Review Project (DERP). Paid for by state and matching federal funds, DERP conducted systematic reviews of independent clinical trial data to determine the most effective drug within each major class. DERP made these systematic reviews available to state PDL committees and to the state policymakers they advised. Many states outside the consortium also used DERP reviews to inform their decisions about PDLs.[34]

Although the ability of state governments to directly influence the actions of federal legislators is limited, states can have an *indirect* influence on federal policymaking. Since 2007, states' use of drug effectiveness research has influenced congressional interest in comparative effectiveness research. When Congress passed the $787 billion economic stimulus bill in January 2009, it provided $1.1 billion for the federal government to compare the effectiveness of different treatments used for the same illness.[35] And as the example of the Physician Payment Sunshine Act (discussed below) shows, if several states begin enacting pharmaceutical reform, such as laws requiring firms to publicly disclose their payments to physicians, the pharmaceutical industry may look more favorably on—and even give its support to—federal reform. After all, a federal law with a single set of national requirements is easier (and less costly) for the industry to comply with and adapt to than are fifty different state laws each with its own set of requirements.[36]

The increased activism of state governments and the health insurance industry is reflective of the greater economic burden that annual increases in prescription drug prices place on patients, states, and insurance companies today as compared to the 1970s.[37] It is also a result of having better information about effectiveness and adverse effects as a result of the growing availability of independent systematic reviews of drug safety and efficacy. This harsher economic reality, combined with findings from independent science, has given the issue of pharmaceutical reform much greater political traction. Indeed, one of the challenges that pharmaceutical reformers faced as they tried to get their reforms through Congress in the

1960s and 1970s was that at the time there was not a compelling economic rationale for pushing through reforms that would, potentially, jeopardize the viability of an industry at the core of the American economy. In these decades, prescription drug prices were relatively stable and growing much more slowly than prices of other health care and consumer goods. Prescription drug prices today, however, reflect a substantially greater proportion of the country's national health care expenditures. And since at least 1993, expenditures on prescription drugs have increased faster than expenditures on other health care services and goods.[38] In 2000 and 2001, health expenditures ranked higher than all other state expenditures in most states, and expenditures on prescription drugs were increasing faster than expenditures on any other covered health care service. In 2002, for example, states spent $30 billion on prescription drug purchases, which accounted for a seventh of all health service expenditures.[39] As a result, those arguing for pharmaceutical reform in the hope of reducing prescription drug prices now have a much greater economic platform from which to argue.

Patients and consumers—another consistent presence in pharmaceutical politics—have also grown in both the extent and the effectiveness of their political organization. Although in the 1960s and 1970s, senior citizens were represented by a range of political organizations committed to protecting their interests, patient-consumers not of retirement age were represented primarily by a nebulous array of small disease-based foundations (such as the Rheumatoid Arthritis Foundation), Consumers Union, and the newly created Public Citizen. Since that time, the number of patient advocacy and disease-based organizations has grown exponentially. By 2000, there were more than three thousand such groups.[40] The increasing political presence of patients derived from the consumer, public interest, and women's health movements of the 1970s, and from the success achieved by HIV/AIDS activists in the 1980s in changing the drug approval process and influencing the way randomized controlled clinical trials are conducted.

Despite the increased political presence of patients, recent pharmaceutical politics has made clear that patients do not always speak with one voice. As the debates over the Hatch-Waxman Act in the early 1980s revealed, patients suffering from chronic conditions for which pharmaceutical treatments were available had a very different stake in pharmaceutical reform than those patients suffering from diseases for which no treatment was yet available. For the former group of patients, the most pressing concern was the cost of already available prescription drugs. For this reason, they did not support extending the patent term and thus the period of exclusivity for expensive brand-name drugs. Instead, they favored the passage of legislation that would make it easier for cheaper generic drugs to be introduced to the market. By contrast, prescription drug prices were not the primary concern for those patients suffering from diseases for which no treatment was currently available. Their priority, instead, was to incentivize pharmaceutical companies to invest in drug development in the hope that the industry would eventually develop a treatment for their disease. Today, many of the groups claiming to represent patients, such as Citizens for the Right to Know and Citizens for Better Medicare, are heavily bankrolled by pharmaceutical companies, raising serious questions about how much they truly represent the interests of patients.[41] In spite of this potential for conflict, numerous *legitimate* disease-based organizations, particularly those representing patients with so-called orphan diseases, have for years lobbied pharmaceutical firms to invest more research time and money in searching for cures for their diseases. In such instances, patients have a genuine interest in securing the help of the pharmaceutical industry.[42] As the recent debates over governments' use of comparative drug effectiveness research show, the conflicting commitments of patient-consumers continue to define pharmaceutical politics.[43]

The medical profession's stance toward pharmaceutical politics has also shown signs of change in recent years. Divisions have always existed among physicians regarding their attitude toward the pharmaceutical industry. During the 1950s, 1960s, and 1970s, numerous physicians criticized pharmaceutical firms for excessively marketing their products and expressed concern that the industry was putting profits above patients' interests. Yet, in these decades, the shared economic, intellectual, and political interests of physicians and pharmaceutical firms overrode physicians' concerns. And despite the decline in its membership, the AMA was still the major political voice of American physicians. Since the 1980s, however, those divisions have taken on greater political significance as the profession has become increasingly divided in its views, its commitments, and its political organization. Physicians are organized increasingly along specialty lines, and not all specialty organizations share the same political priorities or the same attitudes toward pharmaceutical reform.[44] As the history of pharmaceutical industry–medical profession relations makes clear, academic and nonacademic physicians have quite different stakes in supporting the policies preferred by the pharmaceutical industry. For academic physicians, these stakes include significant financial and intellectual support from the industry for their research and the development of disciplines like clinical pharmacology. Working with the industry also brings academic physicians the prestige and career advancement that come with being associated with new drug developments. For nonacademic physicians, the stakes are different but no less compelling, as the industry's financial support and gift giving helps supplement their clinical income. But as the previous chapters detailed, the medical profession's gains were not solely economic, as academic and nonacademic physicians alike had very real—albeit quite different—political stakes in limiting the government's role in medical practice.

Despite the increasing political and institutional heterogeneity of the medical profession, or perhaps because of it, the AMA is still the most politically influential physician group. After all, it remains the largest organization of physicians and spends more than any other interest group in the United States on lobbying, except for the U.S. Chamber of Commerce.[45] Until the mid-2000s, physician groups still tended to favor Republican politics and held firm against any reforms that would encroach on their professional autonomy or their economic interests. The result was that physician groups still tended to align politically with the pharmaceutical industry, although academic and nonacademic physicians did so for different reasons and for quite different payoffs.[46] In recent years, however a growing number of prominent physicians have taken an increasingly critical—and politically activist—stance against the pharmaceutical industry. Editors and former editors of leading medical journals such as Arnold Relman and Marcia Angell of the *New England Journal of Medicine* and Drummond Rennie, deputy editor of the *Journal of the American Medical Association*, have led the charge by publishing informative, albeit polemical, critiques of the industry's practices. In February 2008, the Association of American Medical Colleges (AAMC) and the Association of American Universities (AAU) published recommendations for the nation's medical schools and research universities to revise their conflict of interest policies and ban pharmaceutical and medical device manufacturers from offering free food, gifts, travel, and ghostwriting services to physicians, staff members, and medical students.[47] Two months later, the *New York Times* reported that a number of prominent academic researchers had stopped accepting payments from drug companies because they were troubled by the ethical conflicts inherent in their financial relationships with drug firms.[48] In light of the AAMC and AAU's recommendations, several of the country's largest medical schools have in recent years restricted pharmaceutical marketing activities on their campuses and rewritten their conflict of interest policies to limit the nature and degree of financial relationships permitted between their faculties and pharmaceutical and medical device manufacturers.[49] That a small but growing number of physicians and medical institutions are reevaluating their relationships with pharmaceutical firms suggests that an alliance that has been at the core of pharmaceutical politics for several decades is starting to fracture.

As the depth and breadth of the political pressure on the pharmaceutical industry mounts, and the economic and scientific rationale for reform grows ever stronger, there is some hope that attitudes within the pharmaceutical industry may begin to shift. Senator Charles Grassley's (R-IA) three-year investigation into the financial relationships between pharmaceutical and medical device manufacturers and academic researchers and physicians has put increasing pressure on pharmaceutical firms to publicly disclose their financial contributions to academic researchers and physicians.[50] Meanwhile, since 2008 several states, including Maine, Massachusetts, Minnesota, and Vermont, have enacted legislation that either bans pharmaceutical and medical device companies from giving gifts above a certain value to physicians (fifty dollars in the case of Minnesota) or requires firms to disclose all payments to physicians above a certain value (ten dollars in Massachusetts).[51]

The industry's recent concessions are signs of the industry's adaptation to the political culture. PhRMA's support of the Physician Payment Sunshine Act, which was signed into law as part of the Patient Protection and Affordable Care Act of 2010, represented a substantial shift in pharmaceutical politics. Although PhRMA had repeatedly opposed states' efforts to enact payment disclosure laws, in the summer of 2008 the industry endorsed legislation introduced by Senators Grassley and Herb Kohl (D-WI) that would establish a national registry of payments between companies and physicians. That legislation eventually became the Physician Payment Sunshine Act, which mandates financial transparency in the relationships between the pharmaceutical and medical device industry and academic researchers and physicians. The pharmaceutical industry's support of a federal disclosure law essentially forestalled a situation in which each of the fifty states had its own set of disclosure laws, with its own set of standards.[52]

The firing of Billy Tauzin as CEO of PhRMA just months after he had committed $80 billion in industry cost savings to the Democrats' health care overhaul, however, suggests the partial nature of the industry's change.[53] After all, the industry is in the midst of its own crisis: the patents on the blockbuster drugs of the 1980s and 1990s have expired or are about to expire, several experimental drugs that appeared in early clinical trials to hold much therapeutic promise have recently had their trials halted, and firms are struggling to build their innovation pipelines.

Therefore, pharmaceutical firms are—as they have been since the late 1950s—looking for ways to extend their existing patents, to expand the market for existing drugs, to restrict generic competition, and to capitalize on the innovativeness of university campuses.

As much as pharmaceutical firms have long appreciated that their interests are better served if the public holds them in high regard, the stark reality is that the public, comprised as it is of past, current, and future patients, is beholden to the pharmaceutical industry for its products. Indeed, one of the defining features of pharmaceutical politics is that even as policymakers have criticized the industry's claims about the expense of and threats to innovation, they have been equally reluctant to introduce legislation that might undermine the industry's ability to innovate.[54] At the same time, American health care politics is still characterized by distrust of government-run health care, as the vitriolic rhetoric of conservative Republicans and Tea Party activists during the health care debate of 2009 and 2010 revealed, despite the fact that the vast majority of senior citizens like Medicare. Until something changes in the broader political culture, the pharmaceutical industry and its allies will continue to benefit enormously from the strategies of alliance building and politicking that are predicated on opposition to government encroachment on professional autonomy and patient choice, and the preservation of market-oriented health care—strategies that have served the industry well for the past six decades. In the same way that pharmaceutical firms learned to adapt to the health care politics of the post–World War II era, so too they will learn to adapt to the new climate of physician skepticism and patient discontent. And it is likely that, even as pharmaceutical politics change, they will bear a strong resemblance to the pharmaceutical politics of the past sixty years.

Notes

1. A number of books have been published in recent years about the pharmaceutical industry. These often polemical accounts tend to paint the American drug industry as an evil empire of sorts, whose primary goal is to exploit vulnerable patients by duping the overworked physician into prescribing overly expensive—and oftentimes unnecessary—drugs. The most notable of these polemical books are Marcia Angell, *The Truth about the Drug Companies: How They Deceive Us and What to Do about It* (New York: Random House, 2005); Merrill Goozner, *The $800 Million Pill: The Truth behind the Cost of Drugs* (Berkeley: University of California Press, 2004); Ray Moynihan and Alan Cassels, *Selling Sickness: How the World's Biggest Pharmaceutical Companies Are Turning Us All into Patients* (New York: Nation Books, 2005); and Greg Critser, *Generation Rx: How Prescription Drugs Are Altering American Lives, Minds, and Bodies* (New York: Houghton Mifflin, 2005). For more evenhanded analyses, see Jerry Avorn, *Powerful Medicines: The Benefits, Risks, and Costs of Prescription Drugs* (New York: Alfred A. Knopf, 2004); and Howard Brody, *Hooked: Ethics, the Medical Profession, and the Pharmaceutical Industry* (Lanham, Md.: Rowman & Littlefield, 2006). A common feature of these accounts is that they view the drug industry's practices ahistorically. Typically, these authors see the early 1980s—when the Reagan administration undercut the regulatory authority of government agencies, including the FDA, and passed a series of proindustry patent and tax reforms—as the origins of the crisis in pharmaceutical consumption. This is an inaccurate reading of the history of prescription drugs.

2. The pharmaceutical reform movement coincided with the increasing political power of consumers in post–World War II America, and intersected with ongoing health policy reform efforts and the emergence of a public interest movement. On the political power of consumers, see Lizabeth Cohen, *A Consumers' Republic: The Politics of Mass Consumption in Postwar America*

(Cambridge, Mass.: Harvard University Press, 2003). On the public interest movement, see David Vogel, *Fluctuating Fortunes: The Political Power of Business in America* (New York: Basic Books, 1989), especially pp. 93–112. On the history of health policy reform in the United States, see Daniel M. Fox, *Power and Illness: The Failure and Future of American Health Policy* (Berkeley; University of California Press, 1995); and Colin Gordon, *Dead on Arrival: The Politics of Health Care in Twentieth-Century America* (Princeton, N.J.: Princeton University Press, 2003).

3. There is a growing body of literature on the history of prescription drugs that examines the social, cultural, and political context of the development and consumption of specific prescription drugs. Together, these books offer a detailed account of pharmaceutical innovation in the mid and late twentieth century. See, for example, Mickey C. Smith, *Small Comfort: A History of the Minor Tranquilizers* (New York: Praeger, 1985); Rein Vos, *Drugs Looking for Diseases: Innovative Drug Research and the Development of the Beta Blockers and Calcium Antagonists* (Dordrecht: Kluwer Academic Publishers, 1991); Louis Galambos and Jane E. Sewall, *Networks of Innovation: Vaccine Development at Merck, Sharp & Dohme, and Mulford, 1895–1995* (Cambridge: Cambridge University Press, 1995); Elizabeth S. Watkins, *On the Pill: A Social History of Oral Contraceptives, 1950–70* (Baltimore: Johns Hopkins University Press, 1998); Lara Marks, *Sexual Chemistry: A History of the Contraceptive Pill* (New Haven, Conn.: Yale University Press, 2001); John E. Lesch, *The First Miracle Drugs: How the Sulfa Drugs Transformed Medicine* (New York: Oxford University Press, 2006); Robert Bud, *Penicillin: Triumph and Tragedy* (Oxford: Oxford University Press, 2007); Elizabeth S. Watkins, *The Estrogen Elixir: A History of Hormone Replacement Therapy in America* (Baltimore: Johns Hopkins University Press, 2007); Jeremy A. Greene, *Prescribing by Numbers: Drugs and the Definition of Disease* (Baltimore: Johns Hopkins University Press, 2007); Andrea Tone and Elizabeth S. Watkins, eds., *Medicating Modern America: Prescription Drugs in History* (New York: New York University Press, 2007); Erica Dyck, *Psychedelic Psychiatry: LSD from Clinic to Campus* (Baltimore: Johns Hopkins University Press, 2008); David Herzberg, *Happy Pills in America: From Miltown to Prozac* (Baltimore: Johns Hopkins University Press, 2008); Nicolas Rasmussen, *On Speed: The Many Lives of Amphetamine* (New York: New York University Press, 2008); and Andrea Tone, *The Age of Anxiety: A History of American's Turbulent Affair with Tranquilizers* (New York, Basic Books, 2009).

4. AARP, "Rx Watchdog Report: Drug Prices Continue to Climb Despite Lack of Growth in General Inflation Rate," AARP Public Policy Institute, 2009; Duff Wilson, "Drug Makers Raise Prices in Face of Health Care Reform," *New York Times*, November 15, 2009, www.nytimes.com/2009/11/16/business/16drugprices.html?scp=1&sq=aarp&st=nyt; "The Drug Industry Cashes In," *New York Times*, November 17, 2009, www.nytimes.com/2009/11/18/opinion/18wed3.html?scp=4&sq=drug&st=nyt (both accessed July 18, 2010).

5. For an example of this critique, see Angell, *The Truth about the Drug Companies.*

6. "Statement of Ethel Percy Andrus," in *Administered Prices in the Drug Industry: Corticosteroids,* hearing before the U.S. Senate Committee on the Judiciary, Subcommittee on Antitrust and Monopoly, December 11, 1959 (Washington, D.C.: Government Printing Office, 1959), pp. 8262, 8272, 11701.

7. "Statement of Frank J. Wilson," in *Administered Prices: Corticosteroids,* December 12, 1959, pp. 8352.

8. In 2003, researchers at Tufts Center for the Study of Drug Development reported that the average capitalized cost of drug development (including the cost of failed innovations) was $802 million per approved drug. See Joseph A. DiMasi, R. W. Hansen, and Henry G. Grabowski, "The Price of Innovation: New Estimates of Drug Development Costs," *Journal of Health Economics* 22, no. 2 (2003): 151–185. Marcia Angell, in particular, has heavily criticized the economic methods used by DiMasi and his colleagues to estimate drug costs. By way of contrast, she cites a study by the consumer advocacy group Public Citizen, which calculated that the average cost of drug development is less than $100 million for each approved drug. See Angell, *The Truth about the Drug Companies,* pp. 37–73.

9. "Testimony of Austin Smith," in *Administered Prices: Drugs: General (PMA),* 1960, pp. 10615–10621, 10898–10901.

10. Ibid., pp. 10615–10621, 10898–10901.

11. Gardiner Harris, "Research Ties Diabetes Drug to Heart Woes," *New York Times,* February 19, 2010, www.nytimes.com/2010/02/20/health/policy/20avandia.html?ref=policy; Harris, "Diabetes Drug Maker Hid Test Data, Files Indicate," *New York Times,* July 12, 2010, www.nytimes.com/2010/07/13/health/policy/13avandia.html?scp=1&sq=paxil+glaxosmithkline+2004&st=nyt (both accessed July 13, 2010).

12. Once the world's biggest-selling diabetes drug, Avandia's sales peaked at $3.2 billion in 2006. Figure cited in Gardiner Harris, "Caustic Government Report Deals Blow to Diabetes Drug," *New York Times,* July 9, 2010, www.nytimes.com/2010/07/10/health/10diabetes.html?pagewanted=1&sq=sales%20avandia&st=cse&scp=10 (accessed July 19, 2010).

13. "Drugmakers Sued over Child Deaths," *Los Angeles Times,* March 10, 1953, p. 2.

14. "Some Drugs Held Peril to Patients," *New York Times,* February 26, 1960, p. 12.

15. Harry Nelson, "Antibiotic Sales Up Despite Peril," *New York Times,* October 13, 1960, p. 2.

16. Gardiner Harris, "Lawmaker Calls for Registry of Drug Firms Paying Doctors," *Los Angeles Times,* August 4, 2007, www.nytimes.com/2007/08/04/us/04drug.html?ref=charles_e_grassley; Harris, "Senators Seek Public Listing of Payments to Doctors," *New York Times,* September 7, 2007, www.nytimes.com/2007/09/07/washington/07doctors.html?scp=23&sq=charles+grassley+pharmaceutical&st=nyt (both accessed July 18, 2010).

17. On the creation of a "revolving door" among the pharmaceutical industry, academic institutions, and government agencies in the early twentieth century, see Jonathon Liebenau, *Medical Science and Medical Industry: The Formation of the American Pharmaceutical Industry* (Baltimore: Johns Hopkins University Press, 1987). As John Swann has described, collaborative research between the pharmaceutical industry and biomedical scientists "emerged as a general movement in the interwar period." John P. Swann, *Academic Scientists and the Pharmaceutical Industry: Cooperative Research in Twentieth-Century America* (Baltimore: Johns Hopkins University Press, 1988). See also Nicolas Rasmussen, "The Moral Economy of the Drug Company–Medical Scientist Collaboration in Interwar America," *Social Studies of Science* 34, no. 2 (2004): 161–185; and Rasmussen, "The Drug Industry and Clinical Research in Interwar America: Three Types of Physician Collaborator," *Bulletin of the History of Medicine* 79, no. 1 (2005): 50–80. For an example of the collaborative efforts of academic, industry, and government researchers during World War II, see Leo B. Slater, *War and Disease: Biomedical Research on Malaria in the Twentieth Century* (New Brunswick, N.J.: Rutgers University Press, 2009). For an in-depth analysis of the collaborative relationships that developed between pharmaceutical firms and academic researchers in Europe in the mid-twentieth century, see Viviane Quirke, *Collaboration in the Pharmaceutical Industry: Changing Relationships in Britain and France, 1935–1965* (New York: Routledge, 2007).

18. A number of books published in recent years have depicted the FDA as an agency captured by unscrupulous pharmaceutical firms. Most prominent among these accounts are Angell, *The Truth about the Drug Companies;* and Richard Epstein, *Overdose: How Excessive Government Regulation Stifles Pharmaceutical Product Innovation* (New Haven, Conn.: Yale University Press, 2007). Earlier historical studies of drug regulation and the FDA have tended toward oversimplification. See, for example, Peter Temin, *Taking Your Medicine: Drug Regulation in the United States* (Cambridge, Mass.: Harvard University Press, 1980); and Philip J. Hilts, *Protecting America's Health: The FDA, Business, and One Hundred Years of Regulation* (New York: Alfred A. Knopf, 2003). For a rich and theoretically grounded account of the FDA's complex history that clearly and persuasively undermines arguments that it has been "captured," see Daniel P. Carpenter, *Reputation and Power: Organizational Image and Pharmaceutical Regulation at the FDA* (Princeton, N.J.: Princeton University Press, 2010). For a detailed historical analysis of the science and politics of drug regulation, see Harry Marks, *The Progress of Experiment: Science and Therapeutic Reform in the United States, 1900–1990* (Cambridge: Cambridge University Press, 1997). For a comparative study of drug regulation in the United States and Germany after World War II, see Arthur A. Daemmrich, *Pharmacopolitics: Drug Regulation in the United States and Germany* (Chapel Hill: University of North Carolina Press, 2004).

19. Gardiner Harris, "FDA, Strong Drug Ties and Less Monitoring," *New York Times*, December 6, 2004, www.nytimes.com/2004/12/06/health/06fda .html?scp=38&sq=%22generic+drug%22+policy&st=nyt; Harris, "Potentially Incompatible Goals at FDA," *New York Times*, June 11, 2007, www.nytimes .com/2007/06/11/washington/11fda.html?pagewanted=1&sq=avandia%20 fda%20advisory%20committee%20&st=nyt&scp=5 (both accessed July 29, 2010).

20. Gardiner Harris, "Study Condemns FDA's Handling of Drug Safety," *New York Times*, September 23, 2006, www.nytimes.com/2006/09/23/health/ policy/23fda.html?scp=2&sq=gardiner+harris&st=nyt (accessed July 29, 2010); Roy Guharoy, Gregory Cwikla, Andrew Burgdorf, and Madan Joshi, "Prescription for a Stronger FDA," *Journal of Pharmacy Practice* 19, no. 5 (2006): 295–296.

21. Gardiner Harris, "FDA Limits Role of Advisers Tied to Industry," *New York Times*, March 22, 2007.

22. "Process for Recruiting Members and Evaluating Potential Conflicts of Interest," *GAO Reports*, September 30, 2008 (accessed through Lexis-Nexis).

23. Robert Pear, "Drug Companies Increase Spending on Efforts to Lobby Congress and Governments," *New York Times*, June 1, 2003, www .nytimes.com/2003/06/01/us/drug-companies-increase-spending-on-efforts- to-lobby-congress-and-governments.html?scp=1&sq=price%20control%20 phrma&st=nyt&pagewanted=1 (accessed July 29, 2010).

24. During the summer of 2009, as President Barack Obama and congressional Democrats traveled the country trying to raise support for health care reform, opponents of the administration's reform bill mounted a powerful propaganda campaign that accused the Obama administration of orchestrating a "government takeover" of health care and putting America on the path to "socialized medicine." See, for example, David Herszenhorn and Sheryl Gay Stolberg, "Health Plan Opponents Make Voices Heard," *New York Times*, August 4, 2009, www.nytimes.com/2009/08/04/health/policy/04townhalls. html?scp=4&sq=republican+socialized+medicine&st=nyt; Robert Pear and David M. Herszenhorn, "A Primer on the Details of Health Care Reform," *New York Times*, August 10, 2009, www.nytimes.com/2009/08/10/health/ policy/10facts.html?scp=11&sq=republican+socialized+medicine&st=nyt (both accessed July 29, 2010).

25. William M. Wardell and Louis Lasagna, *Regulation and Drug Development* (Washington, D.C.: American Enterprise Institute for Public Policy Research, 1975). For historical analysis of the "drug lag," see Arthur Daemmrich, "Invisible Moments and the Costs of Pharmaceutical Regulation: Twenty-Five Years of Drug Lag Debate," *Pharmacy in History* 45, no. 1 (2003): 3–17.

26. Robert Pear, "Medicare Debate Turns to Pricing of Drug Benefits," *New York Times*, November 24, 2003, www.nytimes.com/2003/11/24/us/ medicare-debate-turns-to-pricing-of-drug-benefits.html?scp=4&sq=medicare +prescription+drug+benefit+negotiate+price&st=nyt (accessed July 29, 2010).

27. A selection of the literature documenting the changing nature of American universities after the war includes Rebecca S. Lowen, *Creating the Cold War University: The Transformation of Stanford* (Berkeley: University of California Press, 1997); Henry Etzkowitz, *MIT and the Rise of Entrepreneurial Science* (New York: Routledge, 2002); Daniel Lee Kleinman, *Impure Cultures: University Biology and the World of Commerce* (Madison: University of Wisconsin Press, 2003); Daniel S. Greenberg, *The Politics of Pure Science* (Chicago: University of Chicago Press, 1999); and Greenberg, *Science for Sale: The Perils, Rewards, and Delusions of Campus Capitalism* (Chicago: University of Chicago Press, 2007).

28. In particular, see Louis P. Galambos, "Technology, Political Economy, and Professionalization: Central Themes of the Organizational Synthesis," *Business History Review* 57 (1983): 471–493; Brian Balogh, "Reorganizing the Organizational Synthesis: Federal–Professional Relations in Modern America," *Studies in American Political Development* 5 (1991): 119–172; Balogh, *Chain Reaction: Expert Debate and Public Participation in American Commercial Nuclear Power, 1945–1975* (Cambridge: Cambridge University Press, 1991); Chandra Mukerji, *A Fragile Power: Scientists and the State* (Princeton, N.J.: Princeton University Press, 1989); and Sheila Jasanoff, *The Fifth Branch: Science Advisors as Policymakers* (Cambridge, Mass.: Harvard University Press, 1990).

29. For detailed historical analyses of the tobacco industry and the science and politics of cigarette smoking, see Allan M. Brandt, *The Cigarette Century: The Rise, Fall, and Deadly Persistence of the Product That Defined America* (New York: Basic Books, 2007).

30. Mark P. Petticrew and Kelley Lee, "The 'Father of Stress' meets 'Big Tobacco': Hans Selye and the Tobacco Industry," *American Journal of Public Health* 101, no. 3 (2011): 411–418, online preprint, May 13, 2010.

31. Hill and Knowlton press release, "William Kloepfer, Jr., Joins Tobacco Institute as Vice President–Public Relations," October 23, 1967, Legacy Tobacco Documents Library, http://legacy.library.ucsf.edu/tid/lap90c00/pdf?search=%22hill%20knowlton%20press%20release%201967%20kloepfer%22; "For Senator Clements' Report at Spring Meeting," Legacy Tobacco Documents Library, http://legacy.library.ucsf.edu/tid/qbt92f00/pdf?search=%22senator%20clements%20report%20spring%22 (both accessed July 18, 2010).

32. "Staff Notes for the Communications Committee," Tobacco Institute, August 17, 1970, Legacy Tobacco Archives, http://legacy.library.ucsf.edu/tid/bet76b00/pdf?search=%22pharmaceutical%20stress%22 (accessed July 16, 2010). See chapters 3 and 4 for details of the pharmaceutical industry's public relations strategies.

33. Barbara Brown to William W. Shinn, July 27, 1977, Legacy Tobacco Documents Library, http://legacy.library.ucsf.edu/tid/wjl21c00/pdf?search=%22william%20w%20shinn%20july%2027%201977%22 (accessed May 18, 2011).

34. In 1970, the largest pharmacy organization, the American Pharmaceutical Association, passed a resolution commending pharmacists who had stopped selling cigarettes and encouraged other pharmacists to follow suit. In response, the chairman of the scientific advisory board of the Council for Tobacco Research, Sheldon C. Sommers, published an article that challenged the existence of a causal relationship between smoking and disease. Sheldon C. Sommers, "In Defense of Cigarettes," *American Druggist*, September 7, 1970, pp. 83–89.

35. For example, the American lead, chemical, and petroleum industries mounted substantial political and public relations campaigns throughout the second half of the twentieth century in reaction to government efforts to restrict the production and use of environment toxins by these industries. Gerald Markowitz and David Rosner, *Deceit and Denial: The Deadly Politics of Industrial Pollution* (Berkeley: University of California Press, 2002).

36. Read alongside Herman and Ann Somers' *Doctors, Patients, and Health Insurance*, which details the consolidation of the health insurance industry, and Jennifer Klein's *For All These Rights*, which describes the emergence of employee-based health insurance during the mid-twentieth century, *Pills, Power, and Policy* offers a more complete picture of the corporatization of American health care in the second half of the twentieth century. Herman Somers and Ann Somers, *Doctors, Patients, and Health Insurance: The Organization and Financing of Medical Care* (Washington, D.C.: Brookings Institution, 1961); Jennifer Klein, *For All These Rights: Business, Labor, and the Shaping of America's Public-Private Welfare State* (Princeton, N.J.: Princeton University Press, 2006). On the influence of corporate interests on American medicine, see Paul Starr, *The Social Transformation of American Medicine: The Rise of a Sovereign Profession and the Making of a Vast Industry* (New York: Basic Books, 1982).

CHAPTER 1

1. Francis Boyer, excerpt from a 1968 talk before Smith, Kline & French medical staff, Othmer Library of Chemical History, Chemical Heritage Foundation, Glenn E. Ullyot Collection, 2006.502.001, box 2, folder 2.

2. Alfred D. Chandler Jr., *Shaping the Industrial Century: The Remarkable Story of the Evolution of the Modern Chemical and Pharmaceutical Industries* (Cambridge, Mass.: Harvard University Press, 2005), pp. 177–201.

3. Peter Temin, *Taking Your Medicine: Drug Regulation in the United States* (Cambridge, Mass.: Harvard University Press, 1980), pp. 66–70.

4. Louis Galambos, Roy P. Vagelos, Michael S. Brown, and Joseph L. Goldstein, *Values and Visions: A Merck Century* (Whitehouse Station, N.J.: Merck & Co., 1991), pp. 28–30.

5. John P. Swann, *Academic Scientists and the Pharmaceutical Industry: Cooperative Research in Twentieth-Century America* (Baltimore: Johns Hopkins University Press, 1988).

6. Michael Bliss, *The Discovery of Insulin* (Chicago: University of Chicago Press, 1982); Rima D. Apple, *Vitamania: Vitamins in American Culture* (New Brunswick, N.J.: Rutgers University Press, 1996); John E. Lesch, *The First Miracle Drugs: How the Sulfa Drugs Transformed Medicine* (Oxford: Oxford University Press, 2006).

7. Temin, *Taking Your Medicine*, pp. 58–87.

8. Swann, *Academic Scientists and the Pharmaceutical Industry*.

9. For a detailed account of the OSRD, see Lawrence Owens, "The Counterproductive Management of Science in the Second World War: Vannevar Bush and the Office of Scientific Research and Development," *Business History Review* 68 (1994): 515–576. On biomedical research during World War II, see Harry Marks, "War and Peace," in *The Progress of Experiment: Science and Therapeutic Reform in the United States, 1900–1990* (Cambridge: Cambridge University Press, 1997), pp. 98–128; and Nicolas Rasmussen, "Of 'Small Men,' Big Science, and Bigger Business: The Second World War and Biomedical Research in the United States," *Minerva* 40 (2002): 115–146. On penicillin, see Robert Bud, *Penicillin: Triumph and Tragedy* (Oxford: Oxford University Press, 2007); and Gladys Hobby, *Penicillin: Meeting the Challenge* (New Haven, Conn.: Yale University Press, 1985). On antimalarial drugs, see Leo B. Slater, *War and Disease: Biomedical Research on Malaria in the Twentieth Century* (New Brunswick, N.J.: Rutgers University Press, 2009).

10. Temin, *Taking Your Medicine*, pp. 66–70.

11. Ibid., pp. 41–42; James Harvey Young, "Sulfanilamide and Diethylene Glycol," in *Chemistry and Modern Society: Essays in Honor of Aaron J. Ihde*, ed. John Parascandola and James C. Wharton (Washington, D.C.: American Chemical Society, 1983), pp. 105–125; Charles O. Jackson, *Food and Drug Legislation in the New Deal* (Princeton, N.J.: Princeton University Press, 1970); James Harvey Young, *Pure Food: Securing the Federal Food and Drugs Act of 1906* (Princeton, N.J.: Princeton University Press, 1989); Harry Marks, "Revisiting 'The Origins of Compulsory Drug Prescriptions,'" *American Journal of Public Health* 85, no. 1 (1995): 109–116.

12. Marks, *The Progress of Experiment*.

13. Galambos et al., *Values and Visions*, pp. 25–27; Chandler, *Shaping the Industrial Century*, p. 184.

14. Galambos et al., *Values and Visions*; Louis Galambos and Jane E. Sewall, *Networks of Innovation: Vaccine Development at Merck, Sharp & Dohme, and Mulford, 1895–1995* (Cambridge: Cambridge University Press, 1995).

15. Karl Folkers interview conducted by Leon Gortler, July 6, 1990, Merck Archives, Whitehouse Station, N.J., and Chemical Heritage Foundation, Philadelphia, Pa. (hereafter referred to as Folkers Oral History); Max Tishler interview conducted by Leon Gortler and John A. Heitman, November 14, 1983, Merck Archives, Whitehouse Station, N.J., and Chemical Heritage Foundation, Philadelphia, Pa. (hereafter referred to as Tishler Oral History).

16. See Robert Kargon and Elizabeth Hodes, "Karl Compton, Isaiah Bowman, and the Politics of Science in the Great Depression," *ISIS* 76 (1985): 301–318; Patrick J. McGrath, *Scientists, Business, and the State, 1890–1960* (Chapel Hill: University of North Carolina Press, 2002).

17. Owens, "The Counterproductive Management of Science in the Second World War."

18. Biographical note, Vannevar Bush Papers, Library of Congress, Washington, D.C. (hereafter referred to as Bush Papers).

19. Galambos et al., *Values and Visions*, p. 12.

20. On CMR projects, see Nicolas Rasmussen, "Of 'Small Men,' Big Science, and Bigger Business."

21. John T. Connor interview conducted by Leon Gortler, May 1, 1989, Merck Archives, Whitehouse Station, N.J. (hereafter referred to as Connor Oral History), p. 3.

22. Ibid., p. 5.

23. Galambos et al., *Values and Visions*, p. 19.

24. As director, Bush received a salary of $10,000, which he donated to the Carnegie Institution. George W. Merck to Vannevar Bush, March 29, 1951, Bush Papers, General Correspondence, box 72, folder 1751.

25. A.N. Richards to Bush, May 7, 1949, Bush Papers, General Correspondence, box 97, folder 2225.

26. George W. Merck to Bush, November 23, 1949, Bush Papers, General Correspondence, box 72, folder 1751.

27. Bush to George W. Merck, January 23, 1950, Bush Papers, General Correspondence, box 72, folder 1751.

28. Bush to George W. Merck, March 3, 1950, Bush Papers, General Correspondence, box 72, folder 1751.

29. James J. Kerrigan, "Organization Manual: A Message from the President," July 11, 1952, Bush Papers, General Correspondence, box 72, folder 1746.

30. Ibid.

31. Bush to A.N. Richards, March 31, 1952. Bush Papers, General Correspondence, box 97, folder 2225.

32. Ibid.

33. Vannevar Bush, "Memorandum on Planning Activities of Merck & Co.," December 8, 1952, Bush Papers, General Correspondence, box 72, folder 1746.

34. Bush to A.N. Richards, November 12, 1952, Bush Papers, General Correspondence, box 97, folder 2225.

35. Ibid.

36. Vannevar Bush, "Memorandum on Planning Activities of Merck & Co.," December 8, 1952, Bush Papers, General Correspondence, box 72, folder 1746.

37. Connor Oral History, p. 20.

38. J. M. Carlisle, "Memorandum to Randolph Major: Committee to Advise on Methods of Improving and Extending Company's Present Policy with Respect to Grants and Fellowships for the Support of Education," September 16, 1948, A. N. Richards Papers, box 19, folder 28; George R. Hazel to Randolph Major, May 17, 1950, A. N. Richards Papers, box 16, folder 36; L. Earle Arnow to Randolph Major, May 15, 1950, A. N. Richards Papers, box 16, folder 36. In 1948, Merck awarded approximately $90,000 in research grants. John T. Connor, memorandum: "Minutes of a Meeting Held on May 6, 1948, at the University Club, NYC, to Discuss the Policy of Merck & Co., Inc with Respect to Grants and Other Financial Support of External Research and Educational Activities," A. N. Richards Papers, box 17, folder 3.

39. Daniel Lee Kleinman, *Politics on the Endless Frontier: Postwar Research Policy in the United States* (Durham, N.C.: Duke University Press, 1995). As the Cold War continued, however, university administrators from leading research institutions such as the Massachusetts Institute of Technology and Stanford moved away from the "endless frontier" model of basic research and toward an entrepreneurial research model, which saw these institutions combining basic research, teaching, and industrial innovation. See Henry Etzkowitz, *MIT and the Rise of Entrepreneurial Science* (New York: Routledge, 2002); and Rebecca S. Lowen, *Creating the Cold War University: The Transformation of Stanford* (Berkeley: University of California Press, 1997).

40. Swann, *Academic Scientists and the Pharmaceutical Industry.*

41. Hans Molitor to Randolph Major, February 6, 1951, A. N. Richards Papers, box 17, folder 9.

42. Ibid.

43. W. L. Sampson to H. W. Chadduck, December 18, 1950, A. N. Richards Papers, box 17, folder 7.

44. R. M. Hayward to Randolph Major, February 7, 1951, A. N. Richards Papers, box 17, folder 9.

45. Hans Molitor to Randolph Major, February 6, 1951, A. N. Richards Papers, box 17, folder 9.

46. A. N. Richards to Chester S. Keefer, August 3, 1954, A. N. Richards Papers, box 16, folder 31.

47. Galambos et al., *Values and Visions,* p. 185.

48. Keith Wailoo, "The Corporate Conquest of Pernicious Anemia: Technology, Blood Researchers, and the Consumer," in *Drawing Blood: Technology and Disease Identity in Twentieth-Century America* (Baltimore: Johns Hopkins University Press, 1997), pp. 99–133.

49. Folkers Oral History, pp. 35–38 (Chemical Heritage Foundation version); Galambos et al., *Values and Visions,* p. 72.

50. Folkers Oral History, pp. 35–38 (Chemical Heritage Foundation version).

51. Galambos et al., *Values and Visions,* p. 72.

52. James J. Kerrigan, memorandum: "National Vitamin Foundation—Research Grants," December 8, 1950, A. N. Richards Papers, box 16, folder 42.

53. Various memorandums by Hans Molitor detailing his European trip, dated February 23 through March 29, 1955, A.N. Richards Papers, box 16, folder 47.

54. Hans Molitor, memorandum, March 3, 1955, A.N. Richards Papers, box 16, folder 47 (emphasis in original).

55. Hans Molitor, memorandum, February 23, 1955, A.N. Richards Papers, box 16, folder 47.

56. Galambos et al., *Values and Visions*, p. 185.

57. Connor Oral History, p. 6.

58. Galambos et al., *Values and Visions*, p. 74; Chandler, *Shaping the Industrial Century*, p. 184.

59. For a detailed history of this collaborative venture, see Nicolas Rasmussen, "Steroids in Arms: Science, Government, Industry, and the Hormones of the Adrenal Cortex in the United States, 1930–1950," *Medical History* 46 (2002): 299–324.

60. James J. Kerrigan to Vannevar Bush, September 11, 1952, Bush Papers, General Correspondence, box 62, folder 1464.

61. Galambos et al., *Values and Visions*, pp. 28–30.

62. Galambos and Sewall, *Networks of Innovation*, pp. 33–43.

63. Ibid., p. 51.

64. Galambos et al., *Values and Visions*, p. 135.

65. http://nobelprize.org/nobel_prizes/medicine/laureates/1956/richards-bio.html (accessed February 8, 2008).

66. A.N. Richards referred to D.W. Richards as the company's "chief medical adviser" in a letter to Chester Keefer, August 3, 1954, A.N. Richards Papers, box 16, folder 31.

67. A.N. Richards, "Notes," 1954, A.N. Richards Papers, box 18, folder 1.

68. A.N. Richards, "Notes," undated but probably sometime during 1954, A.N. Richards Papers, box 17, folder 50. See also Galambos et al., *Values and Visions*, p. 30.

69. D.W. Richardson, "Medical Coordinating Committee, Minutes of Meeting Held December 4, 1953," December 21, 1953, A.N. Richards Papers, box 17, folder 14.

70. D.W. Richards to A.N. Richards, August 5, 1953 or 1954 (year not noted), A.N. Richards Papers, box 16, folder 24.

71. D.W. Richards to A.N. Richards, November 8, 1954, A.N. Richards Papers, box 16, folder 22.

72. D.W. Richards to A.N. Richards, December 6, 1954, A.N. Richards Papers, box 16, folder 22.

73. D.W. Richards, memorandum: "Organization of an 'Ideal' Medical Division for Merck & Co., Inc.," July 28, 1955, A.N. Richards Papers, box 16, folder 48.

74. Ibid.

75. Ibid.

76. See chapter 3. For a detailed discussion of the medical profession's ongoing critique of pharmaceutical advertising, see Nancy Tomes, "The Fielding H. Garrison Lecture: The Great American Medicine Show Revisited," *Bulletin of the History of Medicine* 79, no. 4 (2005): 627–663; and Jeremy Greene and Scott Podolsky, "Keeping Modern in Medicine: Pharmaceutical Promotion and Physician Education in Postwar America," *Bulletin of the History of Medicine* 83, no. 2 (2009): 331–377.

77. A.N. Richards, "Notes," September 24, 1954, A.N. Richards Papers, box 18, folder 1.

78. D.W. Richards, "Notes on Duties and Responsibilities of Corporate Medical Consultants Derived from Meeting of February 18, 1955," A.N. Richards Papers, box 18, folder 7.

79. D.W. Richards to John T. Connor, September 28, 1959, A.N. Richards Papers, box 16, folder 38. In this letter, D.W. Richards explained to John Connor, Merck's president, "I feel a little depressed that medicine is not to be represented at any such Company level, either now or in the future."

80. For example, see Hans Molitor to George W. Merck, August 30, 1954, A.N. Richards Papers, box 16, folder 38. When Molitor suggested that there was a lack of medical people in Merck's top management, the vice-chairman of Merck's board strongly disagreed, citing the role of the two Richardses as evidence to the contrary: "Certainly the two Richards[es] have as much influence with us as in any institution that I know of." John S. Zinsser to George W. Merck, September 28, 1954, A.N. Richards Papers, box 16, folder 38.

81. Galambos et al., *Values and Visions*, p. 185.

82. Jeremy A. Greene, "Releasing the Flood Waters: Diuril and the Reshaping of Hypertension," *Bulletin of the History of Medicine* 79, no. 4 (2005): 749–794; sales figure cited in Jeremy A. Greene, *Prescribing by Numbers: Drugs and the Definition of Disease* (Baltimore: Johns Hopkins University Press, 2007), p. 43.

83. Swann, *Academic Scientists and the Pharmaceutical Industry*. In the handful of scholarly monographs on the history of postwar drugs, academic researchers often feature as collaborators with industry researchers in those developments. See, for example, Mickey C. Smith, *Small Comfort: A History of the Minor Tranquilizers* (New York: Praeger, 1985); Lara Marks, *Sexual Chemistry: A History of the Contraceptive Pill* (New Haven, Conn.: Yale University Press, 2001); Elizabeth S. Watkins, *The Estrogen Elixir: A History of Hormone Replacement Therapy in America* (Baltimore: Johns Hopkins University Press, 2007); and Greene, *Prescribing by Numbers*. Viviane Quirke describes the development of collaborative research networks among French and British researchers and pharmaceutical companies through the 1960s in *Collaboration in the Pharmaceutical Industry: Changing Relationships in Britain and France, 1935–1965* (New York: Routledge, 2007).

84. Jules Backman, "Economics of the Drug Industry," paper presented at the Pharmaceutical Manufacturers Association Annual Meeting, April 4–6,

1960. Printed in *Pharmaceutical Manufacturers Association Year Book, 1960–1961* (Washington D.C.: Pharmaceutical Manufacturers Association, 1961), pp. 52–65.

85. Temin, "The Therapeutic Revolution," in *Taking Your Medicine,* pp. 58–87.

86. Paul de Haen, "Compilation of New Drugs, 1940 through 1975," *Pharmacy Times,* March 1976, 40, cited in Milton Silverman, Philip R. Lee, and Mia Lydecker, *Pills and the Public Purse: The Routes to National Drug Insurance* (Berkeley: University of California Press, 1981), p. 10.

87. Quirke, *Collaboration in the Pharmaceutical Industry.*

CHAPTER 2

1. This concern over the workforce shortage in the field of pharmaceutical development must be considered in the context of the efforts made by scientific, military, and political leaders at this time to boost recruitment in all scientific fields in the name of national security. For example, see David Kaiser, "Cold War Requisitions, Scientific Manpower, and the Production of American Physicists after World War II," *Historical Studies in the Physical and Biological Sciences* 33 (2002): 131–159.

2. See Kenneth M. Ludmerer, *Time to Heal: American Medical Education from the Turn of the Century to the Era of Managed Care* (Oxford: Oxford University Press, 1999), pp. 139–161. Although Ludmerer sees the postwar years as a period of expansion for medical schools, my research shows that that growth was not shared equally by all aspects of the medical research enterprise. For a detailed analysis of the federal government's increasing investment in medical research after World War II, see Stephen P. Strickland, *Politics, Science, and Dread Disease: A Short History of United States Medical Research Policy* (Cambridge, Mass.: Harvard University Press, 1972).

3. John E. Deitrick and Robert C. Berson, *Medical Schools in the United States at Mid-Century* (New York: McGraw-Hill, 1953), p. 17. This volume is the formal report of the Survey of Medical Education, which was organized in 1947 and operational through 1951. Deitrick served as director of the survey and Berson served as its associate director.

4. Edwin J. Cohn, "Training for Research in the Medical Sciences," December 6, 1947, A. N. Richards Papers, box 20, folder 40.

5. Thomas S. Gates to William Feirer, March 3, 1944, University of Pennsylvania Archives, UPA 4, box 24, folder: Research—III 1940–1945.

6. Deitrick and Berson, *Medical Schools in the United States at Mid-Century,* pp. 86–89.

7. Oscar R. Ewing, *The Nation's Health: A Ten-Year Program. Report to the President by the Federal Security Administrator* (Washington, D.C.: Government Printing Office, 1948).

8. Edward H. Green to George W. Merck, June 23, 1947. A. N. Richards Papers, box 17, folder 3.

9. Deitrick and Berson, *Medical Schools in the United States at Mid-Century*, pp. 91–95.

10. Ibid., pp. 89–90, 112.

11. William G. Rothstein, *American Medical Schools and the Practice of Medicine: A History* (Oxford: Oxford University Press, 1987), pp. 235–236.

12. Harry M. Weaver, "The Costs of Conducting Programs of Research," *Journal of Medical Education* 27, no. 5 (1952): 316–325.

13. Deitrick and Berson, *Medical Schools in the United States at Mid-Century*, pp. 36–45; quotation from p. 44.

14. Cohn, "Training for Research in the Medical Sciences."

15. Ibid.

16. See Strickland, *Politics, Science, and Dread Disease*, pp. 55–74. For a discussion of the business community's involvement in passage of the National Science Foundation Act (including the work of pharmaceutical executives), see Daniel Lee Kleinman, "Layers of Interests, Layers of Influence: Business and the Genesis of the National Science Foundation," *Science, Technology, and Human Values* 19, no. 3 (1994): 259–282.

17. John A. D. Cooper, "Undergraduate Medical Education," in *Advances in American Medicine: Essays at the Bicentennial*, ed. John Z. Bowers and Elizabeth F. Purcell (New York: Josiah Macy Jr. Foundation, 1976), pp. 276–277; Lee Powers, Joseph F. Whiting, and K. C. Oppermann, "Trends in Medical School Faculties," *Journal of Medical Education* 37 (1962): 1065–1091, in particular see p. 1086; Rothstein, *American Medical Schools and the Practice of Medicine*, pp. 236–239.

18. Cohn, "Training for Research in the Medical Sciences."

19. Edward Reynolds to George W. Merck, May 4, 1948, A. N. Richards Papers, box 16, folder 34.

20. Ibid.

21. John G. Gage to A. N. Richards, January 12, 1949, A. N. Richards Papers, box 16, folder 21.

22. Reynolds to George W. Merck, May 4, 1948.

23. George W. Merck to A. N. Richards, January 25, 1946, A. N. Richards Papers, box 19, folder 12.

24. H. W. Chadduck to A. N. Richards, March 31, 1949, A. N. Richards Papers, box 16, folder 41.

25. "Survey of Business Practices: Postwar Trends in Corporate Giving," *Business Record*, May 1947, p. 133.

26. Ibid.

27. Chadduck to A. N. Richards, March 31, 1949.

28. Frank A. Howard to Randolph Major, April 12, 1950, A. N. Richards Papers, box 16, folder 36.

29. Ibid.

30. Ibid. See also Deitrick and Berson, *Medical Schools in the United States at Mid-Century*, pp. 102–103; and Rothstein, *American Medical Schools and the Practice of Medicine*, p. 294.

31. In 1946, *Chemical and Engineering News* published a list, compiled by the National Research Council, of research scholarships and fellowships supported by the chemical and pharmaceutical industries in the United States. As of 1946, 302 companies reported a total of 1,800 fellowships, scholarships, or research grants to academic institutions. For example, Abbott Laboratories supported 20 fellowships at $5,000 each for five years, Lederle Laboratories provided 13 fellowships, each with annual stipends of $1,000–$1,200, and Pfizer awarded two fellowships of $4,700 each. This was contrasted to the 56 firms supporting 95 fellowships and grants in 1929. See Callie Hull and Mary Timms, "Research Supported by Industry through Scholarships, Fellowships, and Grants," *Chemical and Engineering News* 24 (1946): 2346.

32. G. H. A. Clowes to George W. Merck, September 15, 1947, A. N. Richards Papers, box 16, folder 34.

33. C. Sidney Burwell to George Merck, July 2, 1947, A. N. Richards Papers, box 16, folder 34.

34. Hans Molitor, memorandum, July 30, 1947, A. N. Richards Papers, box 17, folder 3.

35. Clowes to George W. Merck, September 15, 1947.

36. Ibid.

37. George W. Merck, "Memorandum: Merck's Contributions to Harvard," June 20, 1947, A. N. Richards Papers, box 17, folder 3.

38. Chadduck to A. N. Richards, March 31, 1949.

39. John G. Gage to George W. Merck, October 1, 1947, A. N. Richards Papers, box 17, folder 3.

40. Chadduck to A. N. Richards, March 31, 1949.

41. Randolph T. Major to George W. Merck, July 22, 1947, A. N. Richards Papers, box 17, folder 3.

42. Burwell to George Merck, July 2, 1947.

43. National Research Council announcement of Merck Fellowships in Natural Sciences, undated but probably 1947, A. N. Richards Papers, box 19, folder 19.

44. A. N. Richards, "Memorandum to Directors: Report on Merck Fellowship Program," November 21, 1950, A. N. Richards Papers, box 19, folder 27.

45. George W. Merck to A. N. Richards, January 25, 1946.

46. Vannevar Bush, "Renewal of Our Scientific Talent," in *Science, the Endless Frontier: A Report to the President on a Program for Postwar Scientific Research* (Washington, D.C.: Government Printing Office, 1945), p. 24.

47. Ibid., p. 26.

48. Kleinman, "Layers of Interests, Layers of Influence"; Daniel Lee Kleinman, *Politics on the Endless Frontier: Postwar Research Policy in the United States* (Durham, N.C.: Duke University Press, 1995).

49. Arthur S. Cain and Lois G. Bowen, "Role of the Postdoctoral Fellowship in Academic Medicine: Report on a Survey of National Fellowship Programs in the Medical Sciences," *Journal of Medical Education* 36 (1961): 1360–1507, pp. 1383, 1489.

50. George W. Beadle to George W. Merck, October 17, 1950, A. N. Richards Papers, box 19, folder 25.

51. Max Tishler to Randolph T. Major, September 24, 1954, A. N. Richards Papers, box 19, folder 29.

52. Randolph T. Major, "Draft Minutes of Scientific Committee of the Board of Directors of Merck, April 18, 1950," A. N. Richards Papers, box 18, folder 21.

53. Karl Folkers to Randolph T. Major, September 26, 1952, A. N. Richards Papers, box 17, folder 10.

54. Ibid.

55. John G. Gage to R. E. Snyder, July 15, 1955, A. N. Richards Papers, box 17, folder 19.

56. L. Earle Arnow to Randolph T. Major, September 28, 1954, A. N. Richards Papers, box 19, folder 29.

57. Gage to Snyder, July 15, 1955.

58. Beadle to George W. Merck, October 17, 1950.

59. Paul Weiss to A. N. Richards, August 5, 1952, A. N. Richards Papers, box 16, folder 22.

60. Ibid.

61. C. R. Addinall, "Memorandum: Merck International Fellowships," February 2, 1952, A. N. Richards Papers, box 19, folder 26 1952.

62. For example, see Kaiser, "Cold War Requisitions, Scientific Manpower, and the Production of American Physicists after World War II."

63. Cain and Bowen, "Role of the Postdoctoral Fellowship in Academic Medicine," p. 1497.

64. Hans Molitor to Randolph T. Major, April 17, 1950, A. N. Richards Papers, box 19, folder 28.

65. Ibid.

66. Ibid.

67. Ibid.

68. P. K. Frolich to John T. Connor, May 12, 1954, A. N. Richards Papers, box 17, folder 15.

69. R. G. Dunning, "Minutes of Scientific Policy Council, Meeting June 14, 1954," A. N. Richards Papers, box 17, folder 28.

70. George W. Merck, dedication address of the Merck Research Laboratories, April 25, 1933, A. N. Richards Papers, box 17, folder 4.

71. Karl Folkers to P. K. Frolich, June 10, 1949, A. N. Richards Papers, box 17, folder 4.

72. W. H. Engels to P. K. Frolich, June 10, 1949, A. N. Richards Papers, box 17, folder 4.

73. John T. Connor to Randolph Major, July 25, 1949, A. N. Richards Papers, box 17, folder 4.

74. Hans Molitor, "Memorandum: Resolution of Publications Policy," June 3, 1949, A. N. Richards Papers, box 16, folder 41.

75. Cain and Bowen, "Role of the Postdoctoral Fellowship in Academic Medicine," p. 1388.

76. John P. Swann, *Academic Scientists and the Pharmaceutical Industry: Cooperative Research in Twentieth-Century America* (Baltimore: Johns Hopkins University Press, 1988); Hull and Timms, "Research Supported by Industry through Scholarships, Fellowships, and Grants"; Mead Johnson & Co., *Service in Medicine Program Annual Report, 1961*, I. S. Ravdin Papers, University of Pennsylvania Archives, UPT 50 R252, box 175, folder 14.

77. David A. Hounshell and John Kenly Smith, *Science and Corporate Strategy: Du Pont R&D, 1902–1980* (Cambridge: Cambridge University Press, 1988), pp. 365–383.

78. See, for example, Daniel Lee Kleinman and Steven P. Vallas, "Science, Capitalism and the Rise of the 'Knowledge Worker': The Changing Structure of Knowledge Production in the United States," *Theory and Society* 30 (2001): 451–492; and Kleinman, *Impure Cultures: University Biology and the World of Commerce* (Madison: University of Wisconsin Press, 2003).

79. Cain and Bowen, "Role of the Postdoctoral Fellowship in Academic Medicine," p. 1476.

80. On the increasing importance of clinical pharmacologists within the FDA, see Daniel P. Carpenter, *Reputation and Power: Organizational Image and Pharmaceutical Regulation at the FDA* (Princeton, N.J.: Princeton University Press, 2010), pp. 135–146.

81. Norman Topping to John McK. Mitchell, November 9, 1955, University of Pennsylvania Archives, UPA 4 GA94, box 0139, folder: School of Medicine, Department of Pharmacology 1955–1960.

82. American Drug Manufacturers Association, "Fellowship in Clinical Investigation," November 23, 1957, Louis Lasagna Papers, University of Rochester Archives, D302, box 1:10.

83. Ibid.

84. Topping to Mitchell, November 9, 1955. On the transformation of research universities into service institutions after World War II, see Rebecca S. Lowen, *Creating the Cold War University: The Transformation of Stanford* (Berkeley: University of California Press, 1997); and Henry Etzkowitz, *MIT and the Rise of Entrepreneurial Science* (New York: Routledge, 2002).

85. C. J. Lambertsen to Isidor S. Ravdin, July 6, 1959, University of Pennsylvania Archives, UPA 4 GA94, box 0139, folder: School of Medicine, Department of Pharmacology 1955–1960.

86. Ibid.

87. Louis Lasagna, "Gripemanship: A Positive Approach," in *Pharmaceutical Manufacturers Association Yearbook, 1959–1960* (Washington, D.C.: Pharmaceutical Manufacturers Association, 1960), pp. 71–72.

88. The status of clinical pharmacology in the 1960s is discussed in chapter 5.

89. Kaiser, "Cold War Requisitions, Scientific Manpower, and the Production of American Physicists after World War II."

90. For the history of the minor tranquilizers, see Andrea Tone, *The Age of Anxiety: A History of America's Turbulent Affair with Tranquilizers* (New York: Basic Books, 2009); on the history of antipsychotics such as chlorpromazine (Thorazine), see David Healy, *The Creation of Psychopharmacology* (Cambridge, Mass.: Harvard University Press, 2002); on the polio vaccines, see David M. Oshinsky, *Polio: An American Story* (Oxford: Oxford University Press, 2005); for a history of the development of chlorothiazide (Diuril), see Jeremy A. Greene, "Releasing the Flood Waters: Diuril and the Reshaping of Hypertension," *Bulletin of the History of Medicine* 79, no. 4 (2005): 749–794; and Greene, *Prescribing by Numbers: Drugs and the Definition of Disease* (Baltimore: Johns Hopkins University Press, 2007), pp. 19–80.

CHAPTER 3

1. This quotation is taken from a speech made by Eugene Beesley, the chairman of the PMA, at the central region meeting of the PMA on February 12, 1962. Eugene N. Beesley, "Preparing for Tomorrow," in *Pharmaceutical Manufacturers Association Year Book, 1962–1963* (Washington, D.C.: Pharmaceutical Manufacturers Association, 1963), p. 201.

2. William L. Laurence, "Victory Predicted in Arthritis Fight," *New York Times*, May 4, 1949, p. 34.

3. William L. Laurence, "More Relief Found in Arthritis Cases," *New York Times*, June 1, 1949, p. 33. For historical accounts of the discovery of cortisone and its medical impact, see Harry M. Marks, "Cortisone, 1949: A Year in the Political Life of a Drug," *Bulletin of the History of Medicine* 66 (1992): 419–439; and David Cantor, "Cortisone and the Politics of Drama, 1949–1955," in *Medical Innovations in Historical Perspective*, ed. John V. Pickstone (New York: St. Martin's Press, 1992), pp. 165–184.

4. Alfred D. Chandler Jr., *Shaping the Industrial Century: The Remarkable Story of the Evolution of the Modern Chemical and Pharmaceutical Industries* (Cambridge, Mass.: Harvard University Press, 2005); Peter Temin, *Taking Your Medicine: Drug Regulation in the United States* (Cambridge, Mass.: Harvard University Press, 1980).

5. Jules Backman, "Economics of the Drug Industry," paper presented at Pharmaceutical Manufacturers Association Annual Meeting, April 4–6, 1960, printed in *Pharmaceutical Manufacturers Association Year Book, 1960–1961* (Washington D.C.: Pharmaceutical Manufacturers Association, 1961), pp. 52–65.

6. Figure cited in William C. Connor, "Comments," in *Pharmaceutical Manufacturers Association Year Book, 1960–1961*, p. 43.

7. *FDC Reports*, April 14, 1958, p. 8; "Testimony of Austin Smith," in *Administered Prices: Drugs: General (PMA)*, hearings before the U.S. Senate Committee on the Judiciary, Subcommittee on Antitrust and Monopoly,

1959–1961 (Washington, D.C.: Government Printing Office, 1960), February 23, 1960, p. 10618.

8. Milton Silverman and Philip R. Lee, *Pills, Profits, and Politics* (Berkeley: University of California Press, 1974), p. 26. See also Office of the Secretary, U.S. Department of Health, Education, and Welfare, *The Drug Makers and the Drug Distributors: The Task Force on Prescription Drugs Background Papers* (Washington, D.C.: Government Printing Office, 1968), p. 9.

9. Rarely, though, did this translate into seventeen years of commercial activity because some of those seventeen years (up to ten years in some cases) would be taken up by the FDA's drug approval process.

10. For a description of drug patents and drug nomenclature, see Silverman and Lee, *Pills, Profits, and Politics*, pp. 35–39.

11. William Brady, "Are Wonder Drugs Really Wonderful?" *Los Angeles Times*, December 30, 1953, p. B2.

12. *FDC Reports*, August 8, 1953, p. W5.

13. *FDC Reports*, June 10, 1950, p. W6.

14. "3 Drugs Combined in New TB Therapy," *New York Times*, October 24, 1952, p. 25.

15. *FDC Reports*, October 11, 1952, p. W6.

16. The canonical work on the history of patent medicines and their sellers is that of James Harvey Young. For example, see James Harvey Young, *The Toadstool Millionaires: A Social History of Patent Medicines in America before Federal Regulation* (Princeton, N.J.: Princeton University Press, 1961). More recently, Nancy Tomes has provided a cogent analysis of proprietary drug advertising through the twentieth century; see Nancy Tomes, "The Fielding H. Garrison Lecture: The Great American Medicine Show Revisited," *Bulletin of the History of Medicine* 79, no. 4 (2005): 627–663.

17. This was part of a speech Beesley gave regarding the industry's public relations activities in 1961, in which he reflected on the industry's failure in the 1950s to seriously tackle the industry's public relations needs. Eugene Beesley, "The Fourth Dimension in Our Future," in *Pharmaceutical Manufacturers Association Year Book, 1961–1962* (Washington, D.C.: Pharmaceutical Manufacturers Association, 1962), pp. 135–139.

18. AMA Research Committee report published in the July 19, 1952, issue of *Journal of the American Medical Association*. Quotation is taken from *FDC Reports*, July 19, 1952, pp. 11–13.

19. *FDC Reports*, December 6, 1952, p. W15.

20. AMA Research Committee report published in the July 19, 1952, issue of *Journal of the American Medical Association*. Quotation is taken from *FDC Reports*, July 19, 1952, pp. 11–13.

21. See, for example, *FDC Reports*, January 24, 1953, pp. W6–W7. For a detailed sociological analysis of the debates over substitution in the 1950s, see Neil J. Facchinetti and W. Michael Dickson, "Access to Generic Drugs in the 1950s: The Politics of a Social Problem," *American Journal of Public Health* 72, no. 5 (1982): 468–475.

22. "Michigan Bill Would Permit Using 1 USP, NF Item for Another," *American Druggist*, February 18, 1952, p. 16.

23. Ibid.; *FDC Reports*, April 4, 1953, pp. W8–W10.

24. "State Conventions Act on Substitution as Makers Charge Practice Is Epidemic," *American Druggist*, July 2, 1952, pp. 5–6.

25. *FDC Reports*, December 5, 1953, p. W4.

26. "Abbott Wins First in Series of Suits to Stop Substitution: Execs Pilot Drive," *American Druggist*, May 11, 1953, p. 5; "Abbott Wins Second Substitution Case: Substitution Bill Signed," *American Druggist*, August 2, 1953, p. 9.

27. "Klumpp: Manufacturers May Go to Court to Halt Substitution," *American Druggist*, May 26, 1952, p. 22.

28. "American Druggist Survey Is the First to Explore All Aspects of Substitution," *American Druggist*, July 6, 1953, pp. 5–16.

29. *FDC Reports*, December 5, 1953, pp. W3–W4. The firms that established the National Pharmaceutical Council were Abbott, Ciba, Hoffman–La Roche, Lederle, McNeil Laboratories, William S. Merrell, Pfizer, G.D. Searle, Smith, Kline & French, Squibb, Upjohn, and Winthrop-Stearns.

30. Theodore G. Klumpp, "E Pluribus Unum: An Address Delivered at the Mid-Winter Luncheon of the Drug, Chemical, and Allied Trades Section of the New York Board of Trade, Inc., New York City, January 26, 1954," Archives Center, National Museum of American History, Smithsonian Institution, Sterling Drug, Inc., Collection (hereafter, Sterling Drug Collection), record group 4, subgroup 3, series 4, folder 04–00–03–004–0001.

31. *FDC Reports*, December 5, 1953, pp. W3–W4.

32. D.G. Baird, "Why Parke, Davis Is Advertising to Build Prestige for Pharmacists," reprint from *Sales Management*, September 15, 1946, Archives Center, National Museum of American History, Smithsonian Institution, Parke-Davis Collection (hereafter, Parke-Davis Collection), NL box 31, folder NLd 1946.

33. *FDC Reports*, December 17, 1956, pp. 13–14.

34. Klumpp, "E Pluribus Unum."

35. *FDC Reports*, December 17, 1956, pp. 13–14.

36. "86% of Manufacturers Say Substitution on Their Products Is Negligible Today," *American Druggist*, July 15, 1957, pp. 5–6.

37. Facchinetti and Dickson, "Access to Generic Drugs in the 1950s."

38. Ibid.

39. Parke-Davis & Co. Advertising Collection, National Museum of American History, Smithsonian Institution, Washington, D.C.

40. The phrase "drug price bug" comes from *FDC Report*, December 8, 1958, pp. 3–4.

41. Figures cited in Silverman and Lee, *Pills, Profits, and Politics*, p. 327. The 1954 Census of Manufacturers reported the industry's 1954 sales volume as $1.664 billion, from which the trade press estimated the following year's sales to be $1.9 billion. *FDC Reports*, September 17, 1956, pp. 3–10.

42. Firms cited are those for which financial data were available. *FDC Reports*, April 14, 1958.

43. *FDC Reports*, April 9, 1956, pp. 3, 9.

44. For details, see Paul A. Offit, *The Cutter Incident: How America's First Polio Vaccine Led to the Growing Vaccine Crisis* (New Haven, Conn.: Yale University Press, 2005).

45. Senator Morse and Senator Hubert Humphrey, "The Salk Vaccine," *Congressional Record* 101, pt. 6 (1955): 7115–7119.

46. Ibid.

47. Ibid.

48. Julian E. Zelizer, *On Capitol Hill: The Struggle to Reform Congress and Its Consequences, 1948–2000* (Cambridge: Cambridge University Press, 2004), pp. 36- 52. On Humphrey's congressional activism in the early 1950s, see Carl Solberg, *Hubert Humphrey: A Biography* (New York: W. W. Norton, 1984), pp. 133–159.

49. Morse and Humphrey, "The Salk Vaccine." On Holifield as a member of the liberal coalition, see Zelizer, *On Capitol Hill*, p. 49.

50. *FDC Reports*, May 19, 1958, pp. 3–5.

51. "Price Fixing and Profiteering on Polio Vaccine," *Congressional Record* 104, pt. 13 (1958): 16751–16755.

52. *United States Census of Manufacturers: 1954* (Washington, D.C.: Government Printing Office, 1957–1958).

53. *FDC Reports*, September 17, 1956, pp. 3–10; *FDC Reports*, April 9, 1956, p. 11.

54. *FDC Reports*, September 12, 1955, p. 17.

55. Victor L. Anfuso, "The Monopoly in the Antibiotic Field," *Congressional Record* 101, pt. 8 (1955): 10641–10642.

56. Robert Bud, "Antibiotics, Big Business, and Consumers: The Context of Government Investigations into the Postwar American Drug Industry," *Technology and Culture* 46 (2005): 329–349.

57. *Annual Report of the Federal Trade Commission for the Fiscal Year Ended June 30, 1957* (Washington D.C.: Government Printing Office, 1958), p. 66.

58. *FDC Reports*, January 6, 1958, pp. 3–5.

59. The companies included in the complaint were Pfizer, Lederle, Bristol Labs (and its parent company, Bristol-Myers), Squibb, and Upjohn. *FDC Reports*, August 4, 1958, pp. A4–A16.

60. For information on the antimonopoly movement throughout the twentieth century in general, and the efforts of economic reformers over the course of the century to increase Americans' purchasing power, see Meg Jacobs, *Pocketbook Politics: Economic Citizenship in Twentieth-Century America* (Princeton, N.J.: Princeton University Press, 2005).

61. The economist Gardiner C. Means is best known for his work with Adolf A. Berle, especially their classic book, *The Modern Corporation and Private Property* (New York: Commerce Clearing House, 1932). In the early

1930s, as advisor to Secretary of Agriculture Henry A. Wallace, Means distinguished between market prices, which were made "as the result of the interaction of buyers and sellers" and thus responded flexibly to supply and demand, and administered prices, which were "set by administrative action and held constant for a period of time." Administered prices, Means argued, were relatively inflexible. See Gardiner C. Means, *Industrial Prices and Their Relative Inflexibility*, Senate Document 13, 74th Congress, 1st session (Washington, D.C.: Government Printing Office, 1935).

62. Jacobs, *Pocketbook Politics*, especially pp. 246–261; Bud, "Antibiotics, Big Business, and Consumers"; Daniel Scroop, "A Faded Passion? Estes Kefauver and the Senate Subcommittee on Antitrust and Monopoly," *Business and Economic History On-Line*, 2007, www.thebhc.org/publications/BEHonline/2007/scroop.pdf.

63. *FDC Reports*, May 19, 1958, pp. 3–5.

64. Richard McFadyen, "Estes Kefauver and the Drug Industry" (Ph.D. dissertation, Emory University, 1973), p. 75.

65. "Price Fixing and Profiteering on Polio Vaccine."

66. U.S. Department of Health, Education, and Welfare, *Health United States 1975*, DHEW Publication no. (HRA) 76–1232, pp. 11–16.

67. Ibid, pp. 72–73. All annual price index values calculated in constant dollars.

68. "Brand-Name Drugs Called Big Expense," *New York Times*, May 14, 1958, p. 33.

69. "Price Fixing and Profiteering on Polio Vaccine."

70. *FDC Reports*, August 25, 1958, pp. 3–4.

71. Ibid.

72. Colin Gordon, *Dead on Arrival: The Politics of Health Care in Twentieth-Century America* (Princeton, N.J.: Princeton University Press, 2003), pp. 20–31, 224–243.

73. Senator Smathers and Senator Magnuson, "Study and Investigation of Present Prices of Drugs," *Congressional Record* 105, pt. 15 (1959): 19053–19054.

74. See, for example, *FDC Reports*, September 12, 1955, p. 17.

75. For a detailed discussion of the medical profession's ongoing critique of pharmaceutical advertising, see Tomes, "The Fielding H. Garrison Lecture." On pharmaceutical "detail men," see Jeremy A. Greene, "Attention to 'Details': Etiquette and the Pharmaceutical Salesman in Postwar America," *Social Studies of Science* 34, no. 2 (2004): 271–292.

76. McFadyen, "Estes Kefauver and the Drug Industry," pp. 56–60.

77. Harry F. Dowling, "Twixt the Cup and the Lip," *Journal of the American Medical Association* 165, no. 6 (1957): 657–661.

78. *FDC Reports*, November 11, 1957, pp. 13–14.

79. APMA Public Relations Committee, *A Primer of Public Relations for the Pharmaceutical Industry* (New York: American Pharmaceutical Manufacturers Association, 1953), p. 12.

80. Ibid., p. 24.

81. Klumpp, "E Pluribus Unum."

82. Ibid.

83. *FDC Reports,* November 7, 1955, pp. 12–14.

84. *FDC Reports,* March 5, 1956, pp. 7–9.

85. *FDC Reports,* July 6, 1959, pp. 3–5.

86. *FDC Reports,* May 6, 1957, p. 17.

87. Theodore G. Klumpp, "Medical Progress and the Pharmaceutical Industry," commencement address, University of Chattanooga, Chattanooga, Tennessee, June 6, 1960, p. 12, Sterling Drug Collection, record group 4, subgroup 3, series 4, folder 04–00–03–004–0002.

88. *FDC Reports,* May 6, 1957, p. 17.

89. *FDC Reports,* December 16, 1957, pp. 3–6.

90. *FDC Reports,* May 19, 1958, p. 22.

91. *FDC Reports,* April 8, 1957, pp. 12–13.

92. Ibid. For details of HIF research, see Odin W. Anderson, *The Evolution of Health Services Research: Personal Reflections on Applied Social Science* (San Francisco: Jossey-Bass, 1991). See also Eugene Beesley, "The Role of the Health Information Foundation," in *Pharmaceutical Manufacturers Yearbook, 1959–1960* (Washington, D.C.: Pharmaceutical Manufacturers Association, 1960), pp. 77–81.

93. *FDC Reports,* October 24, 1955, pp. 11–13.

94. Parke-Davis & Co. Advertising Collection, National Museum of American History, Smithsonian Institution, Washington, D.C.

95. "Pfizer Annual Report to Stockholders—1957," *New York Times,* March 23, 1958, section 10. The front page of the report included the notation "Advertisement." See also *FDC Reports,* March 25, 1957, pp. 2–4.

96. See, for example, Theodore G. Klumpp, "Partners in Progress," speech delivered to unnamed group of physicians, September 23, 1958, Sterling Drug Collection, record group 4, subgroup 3, series 4, folder 04–00–03–004–0001. See also Klumpp, "Medical Progress and the Pharmaceutical Industry."

97. For the history of the American medical profession's struggle against national health insurance, see Ronald L. Numbers, *Almost Persuaded: American Physicians and Compulsory Health Insurance, 1912–1920* (Baltimore: Johns Hopkins University Press, 1978); and Gordon, *Dead on Arrival.*

98. *FDC Reports,* December 16, 1957, pp. 7–10.

99. *FDC Reports,* December 23, 1957, pp. 9–13.

100. *FDC Reports,* April 21, 1958, pp. 15–16.

101. *FDC Reports,* June 18, 1956, pp. 13–16.

102. *FDC Reports,* March 17, 1958, pp. 1–4.

103. "Testimony of Austin Smith," p. 10618. See also McFadyen, "Estes Kefauver and the Drug Industry," p. 82.

104. "The Not-So-Long Arm of the Law," *Consumer Reports,* October 1958, pp. 503–509; "The High Price of Rx Drugs," *Consumer Reports,* November 1958, pp. 597–599.

105. Smathers and Magnuson, "Study and Investigation of Present Prices of Drugs."

106. William B. Graham, "Address of the Chairman of the Board," in *Pharmaceutical Manufacturers Association Year Book, 1960–1961,* pp. 3–8.

107. George F. Smith, "Address of the President," in *Pharmaceutical Manufacturers Association Year Book, 1959–1960,* pp. 3–9.

108. Nancy Tomes, "Merchants of Health: Medicine and Consumer Culture in the United States, 1900–1940," *Journal of American History* 88 (2001): 519–547.

CHAPTER 4

1. John T. Connor, "1959: The Year the Public Comes to Call," address delivered at the midwinter luncheon of the Drug, Chemical, and Allied Trade Section of the New York Board of Trade, New York City, January 29, 1959, Merck Archives, Whitehouse Station, N.J. This chapter is based on Dominique A. Tobbell, "Who's Winning the Human Race? Cold War as Pharmaceutical Political Strategy," *Journal of the History of Medicine and Allied Sciences* 64, no. 4 (2009): 429–473.

2. Senator Estes Kefauver, "Introduction," in *Administered Prices in the Drug Industry,* hearings before the U.S. Senate Committee on the Judiciary, Subcommittee on Antitrust and Monopoly (Washington, D.C.: Government Printing Office, 1959), December 7, 1959, p. 7838.

3. On the history of U.S. drug regulation, see Charles O. Jackson, *Food and Drug Legislation in the New Deal* (Princeton, N.J.: Princeton University Press, 1970); Peter Temin, *Taking Your Medicine: Drug Regulation in the United States* (Cambridge, Mass.: Harvard University Press, 1980); James Harvey Young, *Pure Food: Securing the Federal Food and Drugs Act of 1906* (Princeton, N.J.: Princeton University Press, 1989); Harry M. Marks, "Revisiting 'The Origins of Compulsory Drug Prescriptions,'" *American Journal of Public Health* 85, no. 1 (1995): 109–116; and Daniel P. Carpenter, *Reputation and Power: Organizational Image and Pharmaceutical Regulation at the FDA* (Princeton, N.J.: Princeton University Press, 2010).

4. Austin Smith, "Remarks of Austin Smith, M.D. (President Elect)," in *Pharmaceutical Manufacturers Association Year Book, 1959–1960* (Washington D.C.: Pharmaceutical Manufacturers Association, 1960), p. 39.

5. Ibid., p. 19.

6. William B. Graham, "Address of the Chairman of the Board," in *Pharmaceutical Manufacturers Association Year Book, 1960–1961* (Washington D.C.: Pharmaceutical Manufacturers Association, 1961), pp. 5–6.

7. Jessica Wang, *American Science in an Age of Anxiety: Scientists, Anticommunism, and the Cold War* (Chapel Hill: University of North Carolina Press, 1999), p. 253.

8. Colin Gordon, *Dead on Arrival: The Politics of Health Care in Twenti-eth-Century America* (Princeton, N.J.: Princeton University Press, 2003), p. 144.

9. Robert Bud, "Antibiotics, Big Business, and Consumers: The Context of Government Investigations into the Postwar American Drug Industry," *Technology and Culture* 46 (2005): 329–349; Richard Harris, *The Real Voice* (New York: Macmillan, 1964), pp. 1–49.

10. U.S. Senate, Committee of the Judiciary, Subcommittee on Antitrust and Monopoly, *Administered Prices, Drugs: Report of the Committee of the Judiciary, Subcommittee on Antitrust and Monopoly* (Washington, D.C.: Government Printing Office, 1961), p. 48.

11. For a detailed description and analysis of the work of detail men in the mid-twentieth century, see Jeremy A. Greene, "Attention to 'Details': Etiquette and the Pharmaceutical Salesman in Postwar America," *Social Studies of Science* 34, no. 2 (2004): 271–292.

12. Jeremy A. Greene and Scott Podolsky, "Keeping Modern in Medicine: Pharmaceutical Promotion and Physician Education in Postwar America," *Bulletin of the History of Medicine* 83, no. 2 (2009): 331–377.

13. Since the 1902 Biologics Control Act, manufacturers of biologics such as vaccines and antisera had been required to be licensed by the federal government.

14. Harris, *The Real Voice*, pp. 119–123.

15. Ibid.

16. The quotation, a comment Robert S. Meyer made during a press conference, was cited in the trade press following the publication of a survey of five hundred scientists about where they get their information about scientific knowledge, research, and development. The survey was conducted by Meyer's firm, Herner, Meyer & Co., and commissioned by the National Institutes of Health. *FDC Reports*, November 11, 1957, p. 19.

17. Senator Hubert H. Humphrey, "The Human Approach to Foreign Relations," *Congressional Record* 103, pt. 6 (1957): 8429–8432.

18. Ibid.

19. Carl Solberg, *Hubert Humphrey: A Biography* (New York: W.W. Norton, 1984), pp. 150–198.

20. M.H. Trytten letter to A.N. Richards, June 11, 1956, A.N. Richards Papers, box 19, folder 22.

21. *FDC Reports*, June 16, 1958, p. 18.

22. For a historical account of Soviet pharmaceutical research during World War II, see Mary Schaeffer Conroy, *Medicines for the Soviet Masses during World War II* (New York: University Press of America, 2008). For the postwar period, see Mary Schaeffer Conroy, "The Soviet Pharmaceutical Industry and Dispensing, 1945–1953," *Europe-Asia Studies* 56, no. 7 (2004): 963–991; and Conroy, "The Soviet Pharmaceutical Industry, Past and Present," paper presented at "Modern Medicines: The Perspectives in Pharmaceutical History,"

American Institute for the History of Pharmacy, Madison, Wisconsin, October 18, 2008. For detailed data on the nature of health care in the Soviet Union during the Cold War, see Michael Kaser, *Health Care in the Soviet Union and Eastern Europe* (Boulder, Colo.: Westview Press, 1976).

23. Kaser, *Health Care in the Soviet Union and Eastern Europe*, pp. 12–15. Much of Kaser's comparative data is from the early 1970s, but his analysis suggests that the comparisons should be similar for the previous decades. In 1973, for example, the Soviet Union had 27.9 physicians per 10,000 population; the European Economic Community had half that (13.9 physicians per 10,000 population).

24. Of the drugs produced by the Soviet industry, many were of poor quality and produced in insufficient quantities to meet the population's health needs. As a result, throughout the Cold War era the Soviet Union suffered from severe drug shortages, which contributed to high rates of mortality and morbidity from infectious diseases such as tuberculosis and malaria. For vital statistics for the Soviet Union and Eastern Europe, see Kaser, *Health Care in the Soviet Union and Eastern Europe*, pp. 27–29.

25. In 1968, for example, Comecon (the economic organization of Communist states) exported $51 million, or 2 percent of its total production, of pharmaceuticals to non-Comecon countries; see ibid., pp. 21–22, 267–268. V. K. Afanas'ev, K. A. Ermolina, V. N. Kadurina, L. I. Lavrent'eva, and L. F. Matveeva, *Zhivi, "Akrikhin!"* (Staraia Kupavna: TOO "Print," 1996), a study of the Akrikhin pharmaceutical factory, cites Egypt as a recipient of Soviet pharmaceuticals.

26. Dwight D. Eisenhower, "State of the Union Address, 1958," posted at www.pbs.org/wgbh/amex/presidents/34_eisenhower/psources/ps_state58 .html (accessed on March 20, 2007).

27. " 'Health for Peace' Bill: It Encourages but Cannot Require the Administration to Take Action," *Science* 132, no. 3420 (1960): 131–132.

28. "Statement of Honorable George A. Smathers," in *Administered Prices: Introduction to the Drug Hearings*, December 7, 1959, p. 7843.

29. "Testimony of John T. Connor," in *Administered Prices: Drugs: Merck Corticosteroids*, December 9, 1959, p. 8035. For more details on Merck & Co.'s efforts to establish a manufacturing plant in India and on Connor's mobilization of Cold War rhetoric during the Kefauver hearings, see Jeremy A. Greene, *Prescribing by Numbers: Drugs and the Definition of Disease* (Baltimore: Johns Hopkins University Press, 2007), pp. 45–47.

30. "Testimony of Dr. William B. Walsh," in *Administered Prices: Drugs: General (PMA)*, April 20, 1960, pp. 10862–10863.

31. For details concerning the Eisenhower administration's decision to donate a Navy vessel to Project HOPE, see Zachary A. Cunningham, "Project HOPE as Propaganda: A Humanitarian Nongovernmental Organization Takes Part in America's Total Cold War" (M.A. thesis, Ohio University, March 2008), pp. 38–44.

32. Graham, "Address of the Chairman of the Board," p. 5.

33. "Testimony of Dr. William B. Walsh."

34. Graham, "Address of the Chairman of the Board," pp. 5–6. In December 1962, the drug industry donated about $10 million worth of drugs and medicine to the federal government to facilitate the release of more than one thousand Americans imprisoned in Cuba for their role in the Bay of Pigs invasion. See "Red Cross Praises Ransom Participants," *Chicago Tribune*, December 23, 1962, p. 2; John T. Connor, "Government and Industry Relationships: Their New Impact on Medicine," talk presented at Texas Medical Association conference, Austin, Texas, January 19, 1963, Merck Archives, folder: Connor, John T. 9. People.

35. "Individual Views of Senator Alexander Wiley," in *Administered Prices, Drugs: Report of the Committee of the Judiciary, Subcommittee on Antitrust and Monopoly*, pp. 369–370.

36. Ibid., pp. 370–371.

37. Ibid., p. 372.

38. "Letter from Dr. Edward W. Boland," in *Drug Industry Antitrust Act*, hearings before the Senate Subcommittee on Antitrust and Monopoly (Washington, D.C.: Government Printing Office, 1961), reprinted in *Drug Industry Antitrust Act*, hearings before the Antitrust Subcommittee (Subcommittee no. 5) of the Committee on the Judiciary, House of Representatives, 87th Congress, 2nd session (Washington, D.C.: Government Printing Office, 1962), May 24, 1962, p. 809. See also similar testimony provided by Dr. Charles G. King, Dr. Richard H. Freyberg, and Dr. Roger Adams.

39. "Statement of Dr. Philip Hench," in *Drug Industry Antitrust Act*, hearings before the Antitrust Subcommittee (Subcommittee no. 5) of the Committee on the Judiciary, House of Representatives, May 24, 1962, p. 516.

40. Ibid.

41. Responsibility for the National Research Council's (NRC) antimalarial research program was transferred to the Committee on Medical Research (CMR) of the OSRD in the fall of 1941. For a detailed discussion of the NRC and CMR malaria research programs, see Leo B. Slater, "Preparing for War," in *War and Disease: Biomedical Research on Malaria in the Twentieth Century* (New Brunswick, N.J.: Rutgers University Press, 2009), pp. 84–108.

42. "Testimony of Dr. Lowell T. Coggeshall," in *Drug Industry Antitrust Act*, hearings before the Senate Subcommittee on Antitrust and Monopoly, 1961, reprinted in *Drug Industry Antitrust Act*, hearings before the Antitrust Subcommittee (Subcommittee no. 5) of the Committee on the Judiciary, House of Representatives, May 24, 1962, pp. 819–823.

43. Ibid.

44. "Statement of Dr. Vannevar Bush," in *Drug Industry Antitrust Act*, hearings before the Antitrust Subcommittee (Subcommittee no. 5) of the Committee on the Judiciary, House of Representatives, May 24, 1962, pp. 716–717.

45. See Nicolas Rasmussen, "Of 'Small Men,' Big Science, and Bigger Business: The Second World War and Biomedical Research in the United States," *Minerva* 40 (2002): 115–146.

46. "S. 1552: Statement of Dr. Vannevar Bush," in *Drug Industry Antitrust Act*, hearings before the Senate Subcommittee on Antitrust and Monopoly, December 7, 1961, p. 2198.

47. See, for example, "Testimony of Louis Lasagna," in *Administered Prices, Drugs: Corticosteroids*, December 10, 1959, pp. 8136–8163; "S. 1552: Statement of Dr. Harry Dowling," in *Drug Industry Antitrust Act*, hearings before the Senate Subcommittee on Antitrust and Monopoly, July 25, 1961, pp. 409–427; "S. 1552: Statement of Dr. Maxwell Finland," in *Drug Industry Antitrust Act*, hearings before the Senate Subcommittee on Antitrust and Monopoly, July 25, 1961, pp. 428–457; and "S. 1552: Statement of Dr. Walter Modell," in *Drug Industry Antitrust Act*, hearings before the Senate Subcommittee on Antitrust and Monopoly, July 20, 1961, pp. 305–332. Greene and Podolsky, "Keeping Modern in Medicine."

48. See, for example, "Statement of Ethel Percy Andrus, American Association of Retired Persons and National Retired Teachers Association," in *Administered Prices, Drugs: Corticosteroids*, December 11, 1959, pp. 8261–8280; "Statement of Frank J. Wilson, National Association of Retired Civil Employees," in *Administered Prices, Drugs: Corticosteroids*, December 12, 1959, pp. 8351–8356; and "Statement of Mildred Brady, Consumers Union," in *Administered Prices, Drugs, General: Generic and Brand Names*, May 11, 1960, pp. 11531–11542.

49. Harry Marks makes a similar argument regarding the drug industry's efforts to secure the support of the medical profession in the controversial passage of the 1951 Durham-Humphrey Amendment of the Food, Drug, and Cosmetic Act; see Marks, "Revisiting 'The Origins of Compulsory Drug Prescriptions.'"

50. Austin Smith, "Report of the President," in *Pharmaceutical Manufacturers Association Year Book, 1960–1961*, p. 14.

51. William S. Apple, "The Time of Our Greatest Opportunity," talk presented at the annual meeting of the Pharmaceutical Manufacturers Association, April 4–6, 1960, in *Pharmaceutical Manufacturers Association Year Book, 1960–1961*, pp. 30–31.

52. Ibid.

53. John H. Talbott, "Editorial: New Drive for Compulsory Health Insurance," *Journal of the American Medical Association* 172, no. 4 (1960): 344–345.

54. Larson's speech was presented at the PMA's Medical Section meeting on March 3, 1962. Leonard W. Larson, "Mutual Problems of the A.M.A. and P.M.A.," in *Pharmaceutical Manufacturers Association Yearbook, 1962–1963* (Washington, D.C.: Pharmaceutical Manufacturers Association, 1963), p. 345 (emphasis in original).

55. Ibid., p. 346.

56. "S. 1552: Statement of the American Medical Association," in *Drug Industry Antitrust Act*, hearings before the Senate Subcommittee on Antitrust and Monopoly, July 5, 1961, p. 45.

57. "S. 1552: Statement of Louis S. Goodman," in *Drug Industry Antitrust Act*, hearings before the Senate Subcommittee on Antitrust and Monopoly, July 18, 1961, p. 217. For a detailed discussion of the difficulty in assessing drug efficacy, see Louis S. Goodman, "The Problem of Drug Efficacy," in *Drugs in Our Society*, ed. Paul Talalay (Baltimore: Johns Hopkins University Press, 1963), pp. 49–67.

58. See "S. 1552: Statement of Eugene N. Beesley, Chairman of the Board, PMA," in *Drug Industry Antitrust Act*, hearings before the Senate Subcommittee on Antitrust and Monopoly, 1961, reprinted in *Drug Industry Antitrust Act*, hearings before the Antitrust Subcommittee (Subcommittee no. 5) of the Committee on the Judiciary, House of Representatives, May 24, 1962, p. 693; Morton Mintz, *The Therapeutic Nightmare: A Report of the Roles of the United States Food and Drug Administration, the American Medical Association, Pharmaceutical Manufacturers, and Others in Connection with the Irrational and Massive Use of Prescription Drugs That May Be Worthless, Injurious, or Even Lethal* (Boston: Houghton Mifflin, 1965), pp. 71–75; and John Swann, "Sure Cure: Public Policy on Drug Efficacy before 1962," in *The Inside Story of Medicines*, ed. Gregory J. Higby and Elaine C. Stroud (Madison, Wis.: American Institute for the History of Pharmacy, 1997), pp. 223–262. See also Carpenter, *Reputation and Power*, pp. 118–227.

59. See, for example, John T. Connor, "State of the Company Program: Merck, Sharp & Dohme—West Point—February 21, 1962," Merck Archives.

60. Howard Margolis, "The Drug Hearings: To No One's Surprise, Kefauver and the AMA Do Not Agree on What Should Be Done," *Science* 134, no. 3472 (1961): 89–90.

61. Philip J. Hilts, *Protecting America's Health: The FDA, Business, and 100 Years of Regulation* (New York: Alfred A. Knopf, 2003), pp. 117–128.

62. Margolis, "The Drug Hearings."

63. On the position of the AMA and the relationship between the AMA and the PMA during the Kefauver hearings, see Mintz, *The Therapeutic Nightmare*, pp. 71–92.

64. Ronald L. Numbers, *Almost Persuaded: American Physicians and Compulsory Health Insurance, 1912–1920* (Baltimore: Johns Hopkins University Press, 1978); Gordon, *Dead on Arrival*, pp. 136–171; Marks, "Revisiting 'The Origins of Compulsory Drug Prescriptions.'"

65. Harris, *The Real Voice*, p. 57.

66. John W. Finney, "Senate Panel Cites Mark-ups on Drugs Ranging to 7,079%," *New York Times*, December 8, 1959, p. 1; Joseph A. Loftus, "Big Profit Found in Tranquilizers: One 6 Times Costlier Than in Paris," *New York Times*, January 22, 1960, p. 14; "Inquiry Finds Drug Production Controlled by a Few Companies," *New York Times*, February 25, 1960, p. 21.

67. Bert C. Goss, "The Drug Industry's Public Relations," talk presented at the PMA annual meeting, April 4–6, 1960, in *Pharmaceutical Manufacturers Association Year Book, 1960–1961*, pp. 45–51 (emphasis in original).

68. Harry J. Loynd, "Let's Get Our Signals Straight," in *Pharmaceutical Manufacturers Association Year Book, 1961–1962* (Washington, D.C.: Pharmaceutical Manufacturers Association, 1962), pp. 223–228.

69. Howell J. Harris, *The Right to Manage: Industrial Relations Policies of American Business in the 1940s* (Madison: University of Wisconsin Press, 1982); Elizabeth A. Fones-Wolf, *Selling Free Enterprise: The Business Assault on Labor and Liberalism, 1945–1960* (Urbana: University of Illinois Press, 1994). See also Meg Jacobs, *Pocketbook Politics: Economic Citizenship in Twentieth Century America* (Princeton, N.J.: Princeton University Press, 2005).

70. Fones-Wolf, *Selling Free Enterprise*, p. 5.

71. Theodore G. Klumpp, "Medical Progress and the Pharmaceutical Industry," commencement address, University of Chattanooga, Chattanooga, Tennessee, June 6, 1960, p. 4, Archives Center, National Museum of American History, Smithsonian Institution, Sterling Drug, Inc., Collection (hereafter, Sterling Drug Collection), record group 4, subgroup 3, series 4, folder 04–00–03–004–0002. The PMA's chairman, Eugene Beesley, mobilized similar data in his testimony against S. 1552: "More than 4.4 million Americans living today would be dead if the Nation's mortality rate had remained at the 1937 level. Since 1944 the death rate from influenza has dropped 90 percent; the rate from tuberculosis, 83 percent; acute rheumatic fever, 83 percent; syphilis, 79 percent. Since 1940 the death rate among mothers in childbirth has declined by over 90 percent." "S. 1552: Statement of Eugene N. Beesley, Chairman of the Board, PMA," p. 691.

72. Klumpp, "Medical Progress and the Pharmaceutical Industry," pp. 7–8.

73. Ibid., pp. 10–11.

74. Ibid., pp. 6–7, 13–14.

75. Nancy Tomes, "Merchants of Health: Medicine and Consumer Culture in the United States, 1900–1940," *Journal of American History* 88 (2001): 519–547.

76. Gordon, *Dead on Arrival*, pp. 165–166.

77. Arthur Kemp and Walter R. Livingston, "Medical Care Costs in an Extended Inflation: A Discussion of the Development of the Voluntary Insurance Mechanism, the Medical Care Price Index, Inter-relationship of Price Indexes and Quality Changes, and the Real Cost of Medical Care," *Journal of the American Medical Association* 174 (1960): 1209–1215, figures from p. 1213.

78. "Drug Men Bet on Bolder, Deeper Research," *Business Week*, January 9, 1960, pp. 90–98, quotation from p. 92.

79. Ibid, p. 95.

80. Ibid, p. 98.

81. Harry F. Dowling, "Some Observations on Physicians and the Pharmaceutical Industry in the United States," paper delivered in Montreal, Canada, January 1962, Harry Dowling Papers, National Library of Medicine, MS C 372, box 3, folder: Talks date?

82. "Statement of Austin Smith," in *Administered Prices: Drugs: General (PMA)*, February 23, 1960, p. 10676.

83. *Administered Prices, Drugs: Report of the Committee of the Judiciary, Subcommittee on Antitrust and Monopoly*, p. 30.

84. Ibid., pp. 6–64, 105–154. See also "Statement of Dr. A. Dale Console," in *Administered Prices, Drugs, General*, April 13, 1960, pp. 10367–10392; and "Statement of Dr. Frederick Meyers," in *Administered Prices, Drugs, General*, April 13, 1960, pp. 10392–10413.

85. Dowling, "Some Observations on Physicians and the Pharmaceutical Industry in the United States."

86. "Statement of Dr. Frederick Meyers," p. 10397.

87. *Pharmaceutical Industry Advertising Program*, Archives Center, National Museum of American History, Smithsonian Institution, N.W. Ayers Advertising Agency Collection, collection no. 59, series 4, box 67, folder 7.

88. The advertising series ran for several years after the Kefauver hearings ended, as pressure in Congress to enact more radical reform of the corporate system of drug development continued through the 1960s (see chapter 5).

89. *Pharmaceutical Industry Advertising Program*.

90. Harry J. Loynd, "Address of the Chairman of the Board," in *Pharmaceutical Manufacturers Association Year Book, 1961–1962*, pp. 3–9.

91. William Kloepfer, "Report of the Director of Public Information," in *Pharmaceutical Manufacturers Association Year Book, 1961–1962*, pp. 81–83.

92. G. Fred Roll, "Report of the Public Relations Section," in *Pharmaceutical Manufacturers Association Year Book, 1961–1962*, pp. 75–76.

93. "Special Issue: Drug Industry," *Parke, Davis Review* 18, no. 7 (1961), National Museum of American History, Parke-Davis Collection, XT box 38, XTd 1961.

94. Ibid. Emphasis in original.

95. Harris, *The Real Voice*, p. 144.

96. For the history of the thalidomide tragedy, see Arthur Daemmrich, "A Tale of Two Experts: Thalidomide and Political Engagement in the United States and West Germany," *Social History of Medicine* 15, no. 1 (2002): 137–158. For details of the FDA's handling of thalidomide, see Carpenter, *Reputation and Power*, pp. 228–297.

97. For detailed examinations of the legislative history of Kefauver's bill and the administration's cooptation of that bill, see Richard E. McFadyen, "Estes Kefauver and the Drug Industry" (Ph.D. dissertation, Emory University, 1973); and Harris, *The Real Voice*.

98. Lizabeth Cohen, *A Consumers' Republic: The Politics of Mass Consumption in Postwar America* (Cambridge, Mass.: Harvard University Press, 2003).

99. Connor, "State of the Company Program"; "John T. Connor: An Interview Conducted by Leon Gortler, May 1, 1989," pp. 37–38, Merck Archives.

100. Connor, "Government and Industry Relationships"; Swann, "Sure Cure," pp. 223–261; Carpenter, *Reputation and Power*, pp. 118–227.

101. Connor, "Government and Industry Relationships."

CHAPTER 5

1. Leonard W. Larson, "Together for the Best Medical Care," in *Pharmaceutical Manufacturers Association Year Book, 1960–1961* (Washington, D.C.: Pharmaceutical Manufacturers Association, 1961), p. 38. Excerpts from this chapter have previously been published in Dominique A. Tobbell, "Allied against Reform: Pharmaceutical Industry–Academic Physician Relations in the United States, 1945–1970," *Bulletin of the History of the Medicine* 82, no. 4 (2008): 878–912, copyright © 2008, The Johns Hopkins University Press.

2. For the history of the American medical profession's struggle against national health insurance, see Ronald L. Numbers, *Almost Persuaded: American Physicians and Compulsory Health Insurance, 1912–1920* (Baltimore: Johns Hopkins University Press, 1978); and Colin Gordon, *Dead on Arrival: The Politics of Health Care in Twentieth-Century America* (Princeton, N.J.: Princeton University Press, 2003).

3. Harry Marks, "Revisiting 'The Origins of Compulsory Drug Prescriptions,'" *American Journal of Public Health* 85, no. 1 (1995): 109–116.

4. John T. Connor, "Government and Industry Relationships: Their New Impact on Medicine," address delivered to the 1963 Conference for Physicians, Texas Medical Association, Austin, Texas, January 19, 1963, Merck Archives, Whitehouse Station, N.J. See also Daniel P. Carpenter, *Reputation and Power: Organizational Image and Pharmaceutical Regulation at the FDA* (Princeton, N.J.: Princeton University Press, 2010), pp. 167–171, 195–197.

5. Louis Lasagna, "Gripemanship: A Positive Approach," in *Pharmaceutical Manufacturers Association Year Book, 1959–1960* (Washington, D.C.: Pharmaceutical Manufacturers Association, 1960), pp. 69–70.

6. Harry F. Dowling, "Statement before Subcommittee on Antitrust and Monopoly, Committee on the Judiciary, of the U.S. Senate," September 14, 1960, pp. 7–11, Harry F. Dowling Papers, National Library of Medicine (hereafter Dowling Papers), box 3, folder: Talks 1948, 1950, 1960–1963; Louis S. Goodman to Maxwell Finland, June 20, 1961, Dowling Papers, box 10, folder: Kefauver sub-committee hearing corr. and data 1960–1962; Maxwell Finland to Senator Estes Kefauver, July 31, 1961, Dowling Papers, box 10, folder: Kefauver sub-committee hearing corr. and data 1960–1962.

7. "Who Likes the New Drug Regulations?" *Medical News*, July 13, 1963, pp. 34–35.

8. "Drug Industry Situation Uncertain but Hopeful," *Medical News*, March 14, 1964, p. 35.

9. "Who Likes the New Drug Regulations?"

10. Connor, "Government and Industry Relationships"; George Y. Harvey, notes on meeting between chairman, Citizen's Advisory Committee, and FDA Commissioner George Larrick, February 21, 1963, William Middleton Papers, National Library of Medicine (hereafter Middleton Papers), box 25, folder: DRB Correspondence and miscellaneous data 1963–1.

11. William M. M. Kirby, "Impact of the New Drug Regulations on Teaching and Research in Medical Schools," talk presented at the Seventy-fourth Annual Meeting of the Association of American Medical Colleges, Chicago, University of Pennsylvania Archives, I. S. Ravdin Papers, UPT 50 R252, box 175, folder 1.

12. "S. 1552: Statement of the American Medical Association," in *Drug Industry Antitrust Act*, hearings before the Senate Subcommittee on Antitrust and Monopoly, 87th Congress, 2nd session (Washington, D.C.: Government Printing Office, 1962).

13. Harry F. Dowling to Maxwell Finland, September 24, 1962, Dowling Papers, box 7, folder: FDA-Outside comments on new regulations 1962–1967 (emphasis in original).

14. For example, see Lowell T. Coggeshall, "Drug Safety and Drug Control: An Address by L. T. Coggeshall, M.D., Chairman of the Commission on Drug Safety, at the Annual Meeting of the Division of Medical Sciences, NAS-NRC, April 9, 1963," National Academies Archives, Medical Sciences, folder: DRB, 1963. On the FDA's increasing recruitment of clinical pharmacologists, see Carpenter, *Reputation and Power*, pp. 135–147.

15. Lasagna, "Gripemanship."

16. For details, see chapter 4.

17. Daniel L. Shaw, "Physician-Industry-FDA Relationships: III," in *Pharmaceutical Manufacturers Association Year Book, 1965–1966* (Washington, D.C.: Pharmaceutical Manufacturers Association, 1966), p. 580.

18. Ibid., pp. 581–582. Sadly for us, Shaw did not name the "academic prigs" he had in mind.

19. William W. Coon to Duke C. Trexler, February 3, 1969, National Academies Archives, series 2 DES Panels; folder: Membership—Comments on Topics for Final Report.

20. Sidney Merlis, "Physician-Industry-FDA Relationships: I," in *Pharmaceutical Manufacturers Association Yearbook, 1965–1966*, p. 569. Merlis's speech was delivered at the Research and Development Section meeting of the Pharmaceutical Manufacturers Association, November 10, 1964.

21. Shaw, "Physician-Industry-FDA Relationships: III," p. 582.

22. Thomas M. Durant to William Middleton, December 12, 1963, Middleton Papers, box 25, folder: DRB Correspondence and miscellaneous data 1963.

23. Shaw, "Physician-Industry-FDA Relationships: III," p. 582.

24. This was actually a continuation of the price-fixing allegations first made by the FTC against the tetracycline manufacturers in 1958. Samuel Mines, *Pfizer ... An Informal History* (New York: Pfizer, 1978), pp. 198–212.

25. *Drug Safety*, hearings before the Subcommittee on Intergovernmental Relations of the Committee on Government Operations, House of Representatives (Washington, D.C.: Government Printing Office, 1964); *Interagency Coordination in Drug Research and Regulation*, hearings before the Subcommittee on Reorganization and International Organizations of the Committee on Government Operations, United States Senate (Washington, D.C.: Government Printing Office, 1962–1963).

26. Elizabeth Siegel Watkins, *On the Pill: A Social History of Oral Contraceptives, 1950–1970* (Baltimore: Johns Hopkins University Press, 1998), pp. 73–102.

27. *Competitive Problems in the Drug Industry*, hearings before the Senate Select Committee on Small Business, Monopoly Subcommittee (Washington, D.C.: Government Printing Office, 1967–1977), May 15, 1967, p. 1. (Hereafter referred to as Nelson hearings.)

28. *Pharmaceutical Industry Advertising Program*, Archives Center, National Museum of American History, Smithsonian Institute, N. W. Ayers Advertising Agency Records, collection no. 59 (hereafter referred to as N. W. Ayers Records), series 4, box 67, folder 7. Part of this public relations strategy included the president of the PMA making an annual "Report to the Nation" each winter. Some twenty thousand copies of the president's speech would be mailed to the media, business leaders, and public officials. For details of the PMA's public relations campaign, see William Kloepfer, "Report of the Director of Public Information," in *Pharmaceutical Manufacturers Association Year Book, 1961–1962* (Washington, D.C.: Pharmaceutical Manufacturers Association, 1962), pp. 81–85.

29. John F. Modrall, "Comments," in *Pharmaceutical Manufacturers Association Year Book, 1962–1963* (Washington, D.C.: Pharmaceutical Manufacturers Association, 1963), p. 98.

30. Ibid., pp. 99–101.

31. On the origins of the revolving door among drug companies, academic institutions, and government agencies, see Jonathon Liebenau, *Medical Science and Medical Industry: The Formation of the American Pharmaceutical Industry* (Baltimore: Johns Hopkins University Press, 1987).

32. The full membership list of the Commission on Drug Safety was Lowell T. Coggeshall (vice-president of the University of Chicago and member of the board of directors of Abbott Laboratories), Paul R. Cannon (editor of the *Archives of Pathology*), Thomas Francis Jr. (chairman of the Department of Epidemiology, University of Michigan), Hugh Hussey (director of the Division of Scientific Activities, AMA), Chester S. Keefer (Wade Professor of Medicine, Boston University School of Medicine), Theodore G. Klumpp (president and director, Winthrop Laboratories), John T. Litchfield (director of research, Lederle Laboratories), Maurice R. Nance (medical director, Smith, Kline & French Laboratories), Leonard A. Scheele (senior vice-president, Warner-Lambert Pharmaceutical Company), Leon H. Schmidt (director, National Primate Center, University of California, Davis), Austin Smith

(president, PMA), Thomas B. Turner (dean of the School of Medicine, Johns Hopkins University), Josef Warkany (professor of research pediatrics, University of Cincinnati, Children's Hospital Research Foundation), and Duke C. Trexler.

33. "Objectives of the Commission (As Stated by Dr. Coggeshall, July 31, 1962)," National Academies Archives, CDS, folder: Commission Establishment.

34. Ibid.

35. Eugene N. Beesley, "Address of the Chairman of the Board," in *Pharmaceutical Manufacturers Association Year Book, 1963–1964* (Washington D.C.: Pharmaceutical Manufacturers Association, 1964), p. 6.

36. Duke C. Trexler, "Activities of the Commission on Drug Safety (1962–1964) and of the Drug Research Board, National Academy of Sciences–National Research Council," talk presented at Fourth International Congress, International Federation for Hygiene and Preventive Medicine, Vienna, Austria, May 24–26, 1965, National Academies Archives, CDS, folder: Vienna—Grant Correspondence.

37. Ibid.

38. Ibid.

39. Lowell T. Coggeshall to Senate Subcommittee on Drug Safety, June 19, 1964, National Academies Archives, CDS, folder: Coggeshall—Senate Hearing June 19, 1964.

40. Lowell T. Coggeshall, "Strengthening the Forces of Drug Safety," in *Pharmaceutical Manufacturers Association Yearbook, 1964–1965* (Washington, D.C.: Pharmaceutical Manufacturers Association, 1965), p. 328.

41. On the government's national security strategy of maintaining an elite reserve labor force of scientists after World War II, see Chandra Mukerji, *A Fragile Power: Scientists and the State* (Princeton, N.J.: Princeton University Press, 1989).

42. F. Douglas Lawrason, "Report of the Liaison Committee with the NRC, VA, and USPHS," in *Pharmaceutical Manufacturers Association Year Book, 1963–1964* (Washington, D.C.: Pharmaceutical Manufacturers Association, 1964), p. 399.

43. NAS-NRC Division of Medical Sciences, "Appendix 7.2 of Meeting Minutes, September 29, 1963," National Academies Archives, Medical Sciences, folder: DRB, 1963.

44. In the DRB's first year, its members with industry ties included K. K. Chen of Indiana University School of Medicine (previously a research scientist at Eli Lilly & Co.), William B. Castle of Boston City Hospital (a longtime consultant to Merck & Co.), Chester Keefer of Boston University School of Medicine (another longtime consultant to Merck), and Carl F. Schmidt of the U.S. Naval Air Development Center (a former consultant to Merck). Pharmaceutical networks continued to dominate the membership of the DRB. In 1972, for example, the roster of the DRB listed four industry executives, one FDA officer, and thirteen academic physicians, ten of whom either currently or previously held affiliations with industry. "Current Membership for Drug

Research Board," National Academies Archives, Medical Sciences, folder: DRB: Membership Biographies 1972.

45. Coggeshall to Senate Subcommittee on Drug Safety, June 19, 1964.

46. NAS-NRC Division of Medical Sciences, "Appendix 7.2 of Meeting Minutes, September 29, 1963."

47. R. Keith Cannan, "The Drug Efficacy Study of the NAS-NRC: A Talk Given at the Sixth Annual Briefing in Science, Council for the Advancement of Science Writing, November 11, 1968," National Academies Archives, series 1 DES, folder: Speeches on History and Work of DES by Cannan, Gilman, and Trexler, 1966–68.

48. R. Keith Cannan, "Inter-Office Memorandum. For the Record: Conference with Dr. Goddard and Dr. Don Estes," March 28, 1966, National Academies Archives, series 1 DES, folder: Beginning of Program, 1966.

49. Dale G. Friend, "Clinical Evaluation of Drugs: Prevention and Control of Adverse Reactions," *Journal of the American Medical Association* 187, no. 5 (1964): 348–351, quotations from p. 348.

50. Clinical pharmacologists were academically appointed (or appointed in industry) and therefore did not practice as clinical pharmacologists outside of an academic institution. Because clinical pharmacologists were most often appointed (at least jointly) in basic science departments (pharmacology), their salaries were lower than the salaries of other clinical medical professors. In 1969, for example, the median salary for clinical medical school faculty at the professor level ranged from $29,000 in pediatrics and $30,000 in pathology to $37,000 in radiology. By contrast, the median salary for basic science faculty in American medical schools at the professor level was $21,200. "Medical School Salary Survey," *Journal of Medical Education* 44, no. 12 (1969): 1180–1181.

51. David G. Badman (retired director of the National Institute of Diabetes, Digestive, and Kidney Disease), interview with author, January 18, 2006. For further discussion of the NIH's reluctance to fund clinical pharmacology research and its consequences, see Dominique A. Tobbell, "Charitable Innovations: The Political Economy of Thalassemia Research and Drug Development in the United States, 1960–2000," in *Perspectives on Twentieth-Century Pharmaceuticals*, ed. Judy Slinn and Vivianne Quirke (Oxford: Peter Lang AG, 2010), pp. 301–335.

52. Albert Sjoerdsma, "Clinical Pharmacology: Present Status and Future Developments," October 4, 1965, Middleton Papers, box 25, folder: DRB Correspondence and miscellaneous data Oct–Dec 1965.

53. John H. Moyer, "Training in Clinical Pharmacology and Experimental Therapeutics," *Journal of American Medical Association* 200, no. 6 (1967): 454–456. For the history of the political economy of scientific research in American universities after World War II, see Rebecca S. Lowen, *Creating the Cold War University: The Transformation of Stanford* (Berkeley: University of California Press, 1997); Daniel L. Kleinman, *Politics on the Endless Frontier: Postwar Research Policy in the United States* (Durham, N.C.: Duke

University Press, 1995); Kleinman, *Impure Cultures: University Biology and the World of Commerce* (Madison: University of Wisconsin Press, 2003); and Henry Etzkowitz, *MIT and the Rise of Entrepreneurial Science* (New York: Routledge, 2002).

54. Harry F. Dowling, "Responsibility for Testing Drugs in Humans," *Journal of the American Medical Association* 187, no. 3 (1964): 212–215; Friend, "Clinical Evaluation of Drugs," p. 348.

55. Sjoerdsma, "Clinical Pharmacology."

56. Leon I. Goldberg, letter to all academic clinical pharmacologists, April 27, 1965, Middleton Papers, box 25, folder: DRB correspondence and miscellaneous data Jan–June 1965.

57. ASPET Council, "Statement of Council of ASPET," 1963, Harry F. Dowling Papers, National Library of Medicine (hereafter Dowling Papers), box 7, folder: Clinical evaluations—articles, reports, and notes 1954–1968. For a history of specialization in American medical practice, see Rosemary Stevens, *Medicine in the Public Interest: A History of Specialization* (Berkeley: University of California Press, 1998).

58. Harry F. Dowling, "Notes from the Pharmacology Training Committee's Discussion of Clinical Pharmacology Held at the NIH, February 3, 1964," Dowling Papers, box 7, folder: Clinical evaluations—articles, reports, and notes 1954–1968.

59. Friend, "Clinical Evaluation of Drugs," p. 348.

60. Joel Howell, *Technology in the Hospital: Transforming Patient Care in the Early Twentieth Century* (Baltimore: Johns Hopkins University Press, 1996), pp. 103–132; Stevens, *Medicine in the Public Interest*, pp. 225–231.

61. Drug Research Board, "Minutes of First Meeting of DRB," January 20, 1964, p. 33, Middleton Papers, box 27, folder: Drug Research Board minutes Jan–June 1964.

62. Ibid.

63. Drug Research Board, "Minutes of Third Meeting of DRB," October 21, 1964, p. 5, Middleton Papers, box 27, folder: Drug Research Board minutes June 1964–April 1965.

64. Jean K. Weston to Hugh Hussey, March 17, 1965, Middleton Papers, box 25, folder: DRB correspondence and miscellaneous data Jan–June 1965.

65. Drug Research Board, "Minutes of Third Meeting of DRB," pp. 5–6.

66. Ibid.

67. William S. Middleton, "Address," in *Pharmaceutical Manufacturers Association Yearbook, 1965–1966*, p. 227. Middleton's address was delivered at the Pharmaceutical Manufacturers Association's midyear meeting, December 7, 1964.

68. William Middleton to Duke C. Trexler, September 5, 1964, National Academies Archives, series 5: DES Name Files, folder: Middleton W.S.: DRB correspondence 1963–1964.

69. Gifford E. Upjohn, "Address of the Chairman of the Board," in *Pharmaceutical Manufacturers Association Year Book, 1965–1966*, p. 9. Upjohn's

address was delivered at the Pharmaceutical Manufacturers Association's annual meeting, May 24–26, 1965.

70. Drug Research Board, *Report on the Conference on Clinical Pharmacology, December 3–4, 1970* (Washington, D.C.: National Academies of Science, 1971).

71. "Kalman C. Mezey: An Interview for the Merck Archives Conducted by Louis Galambos and Robert Lewis of the Business History Group, Inc., March 6 and 7, 1990," Merck Archives, Whitehouse Station, N.J., pp. 42–46.

72. Drug Research Board, *Report on the Conference*, p. 5.

73. Ibid., p. 6.

74. Ibid., pp. 12–13.

75. Leo E. Hollister to Duke C. Trexler, January 21, 1969, National Academies Archives, series 2: DES Panels, folder: Membership: Comments on topics for Final Report 1969.

76. Drug Research Board, *Report on the Conference on Clinical Pharmacology, December 3–4, 1970*, pp. 12–13.

77. Note that Kennedy had introduced a similar bill calling for a National Center of Clinical Pharmacology the year before, although the mandate for the center was less than that in the 1975 bill. See *Congressional Record* 120, pt. 10 (1974): 13133–13161.

78. Examples of physician testimony during the Kefauver hearings include that by Haskell Weinstein, in U.S. Senate, Committee of the Judiciary, Subcommittee on Antitrust and Monopoly, *Administered Prices: General: Physicians and Other Professional Authorities* (Washington, D.C.: Government Printing Office, 1961), February 25, 1960, pp. 10239–10280; and James E. Bowes, in *Administered Prices: General: Physicians and Other Professional Authorities*, April 14, 1960, pp. 10452–10473. Studies that examined physicians' prescribing practices in relation to pharmaceutical promotion include Theodore Caplow, "Market Attitudes: A Research Report from the Medical Field," *Harvard Business Review* 30 (1952): 105–112; and "Report on a Study of Advertising and the American Physician," in *Drug Industry Antitrust Act*, hearings before the Subcommittee on Antitrust and Monopoly, United States Senate Committee on the Judiciary, 1961, pp. 490–520.

79. In 1967, the American drug industry earned $3,226 million in U.S. sales and spent $645 million on promotion. See Milton Silverman and Philip R. Lee, *Pills, Profits, and Politics* (Berkeley: University of California Press, 1974), pp. 327–328.

80. U.S. Senate, Committee of the Judiciary, Subcommittee on Antitrust and Monopoly, *Administered Prices, Drugs: Report of the Committee of the Judiciary, Subcommittee on Antitrust and Monopoly* (Washington, D.C.: Government Printing Office, 1961), p. 190.

81. For a detailed analysis of the history of continuing medical education in the United States and the role of pharmaceutical marketing in physician education, see Jeremy A. Greene and Scott H. Podolsky, "Keeping Modern

in Medicine: Pharmaceutical Promotion and Physician Education in Postwar America," *Bulletin of the History of Medicine* 83, no. 2 (2009): 331–377.

82. Drug Research Board, "Minutes of First Meeting of DRB," p. 28.

83. Ibid.

84. Ibid.

85. Jerry Avorn and Stephen B. Soumerai, "Improving Drug-Therapy Decisions through Educational Outreach: A Randomized Controlled Trial of Academically Based 'Detailing,'" *New England Journal of Medicine* 308 (1983): 1457–1463; David Siegel, Julio Lopez, Jon Meier, Mary K. Goldstein, Samuel Lee, Bradley J. Brazill, and Mazen S. Matalka, "Academic Detailing to Improve Antihypertensive Prescribing Patterns," *American Journal of Hypertension* 16 (2003): 508–511; S. R. Simon, H. P. Rodriguez, S. R. Majumdar, K. Kleinman, C. Warner, S. Salem-Schatz, I. Miroshnik, S. B. Soumerai, and L. A. Prosser, "Economic Analysis of a Randomized Trial of Academic Detailing Interventions to Improve Use of Antihypertensive Medications," *Journal of Clinical Hypertension* 9 (2007): 15–20.

86. Notes on meeting of Committee on Continuing Education, February 18, 1966, Middleton Papers, box 28, folder: Committee on Continuing Education Apr–Nov 1966.

87. Ibid.

88. Philip R. Lee, "Foreword," in *The History of Regional Medical Programs: The Life and Death of a Small Initiative of the Great Society*, by Stephen Strickland (New York: University Press of America, 2000), n.p.

89. Duke C. Trexler, "Memorandum to the Record: Discussion with Dr. Robert Marston, Associate Director, National Institutes of Health," September 5, 1967, Middleton Papers, box 28, folder: Committee on Continuing Education Apr–Nov 1966; Ad Hoc Committee on Continuing Education, "Therapeutic Consultant Program," box 28, folder: Committee on Continuing Education Apr–Nov 1966.

90. For information on the controversial history of the RMP, see Strickland, *The History of Regional Medical Programs*. Strickland's account, however, has been strongly criticized for its inaccuracies. See Daniel M. Fox's book review in *Bulletin of the History of Medicine* 77 (2003): 220–221. Fox provides important context for understanding the failure of the RMP, a manifestation of hierarchical regionalism, as an aspect of the decades-old conflicts between nonacademic practicing physicians (represented primarily by the AMA) and academic physicians. See Daniel M. Fox, *Health Policies, Health Politics: The British and American Experience, 1911–1965* (Princeton, N.J.: Princeton University Press, 1986), especially pp. 188–212.

91. Avorn and Soumerai, "Improving Drug-Therapy Decisions through Educational Outreach"; Siegel et al., "Academic Detailing to Improve Antihypertensive Prescribing Patterns"; Simon et al., "Economic Analysis of a Randomized Trial of Academic Detailing Interventions to Improve Use of Antihypertensive Medications."

92. *Federal Register* 26, no. 1 (January 14, 1961): 294.

93. Cannan, "The Drug Efficacy Study of the NAS-NRC"; Duke C. Trexler to Committee on Drug Compendium, "Memorandum: Compendium Critique by Dr. James E. Weston, Director, Department of Drugs, AMA," February 8, 1965, Middleton Papers, box 28, folder: Drug compendium 1964–1965.

94. Trexler to Committee on Drug Compendium, "Memorandum."

95. Ibid.

96. Ibid.

97. Ibid.

98. Ibid. Although the *Physicians' Desk Reference* had been published since 1947 and contained annually updated information about prescription drugs, it was not regarded by the AMA, the FDA, the PMA, or the DRB as providing sufficient drug information to serve as a national drug compendium. As Chester Keefer noted, "it contains the description of many but not *all* drugs manufactured and distributed by the companies that make and sell drugs.... The manufacturers pay for the insertions of material on a page basis. The manufacturers are discriminating in what they choose to insert in this book, which is revised every year." Chester S. Keefer to Duke C. Trexler, "Memorandum: Drug Compendium," March 8, 1965, Middleton Papers, box 28, folder: Drug compendium 1964–1965.

99. Duke C. Trexler to Chester S. Keefer, July 27, 1964, Middleton Papers, box 28, folder: Drug compendium 1964–1965.

100. Duke C. Trexler to William Middleton, September 22, 1965, and Trexler to Middleton, November 24, 1965, both in Middleton Papers, box 28, folder: Drug compendium 1964–1965.

101. R. Keith Cannan to Joseph F. Sadusk, December 30, 1965, Middleton Papers, box 28, folder: Drug compendium 1964–1965.

102. American Medical Association to Drug Research Board, "Memorandum: A Proposal: AMA Drug Information Program," May 10, 1966, Middleton Papers, box 28, folder: Drug compendium 1966.

103. Duke C. Trexler to members of the DRB, "Memorandum: Complimentary Drug Compendium," January 4, 1967, Middleton Papers, box 28, folder: Drug compendium 1967.

104. For example, Commissioner Larrick delayed undertaking the efficacy review of all drugs marketed between 1938 and 1962, as mandated by the 1962 Drug Amendments.

105. On criticisms of Larrick, see Carpenter, *Reputation and Power*, p. 267; on Goddard's reorientation of the FDA, see ibid., pp. 347–368.

106. "Notes: Meeting with FDA Representatives, 16 December 1966," National Academies Archives, series 1 DES, folder: Memoranda to PAC 1966–1968.

107. Duke C. Trexler to members of the DRB, "Memorandum: Complimentary Drug Compendium," January 4, 1967, Middleton Papers, box 28, folder: Drug compendium 1967.

108. For a detailed account of how the FDA used the findings of the DES panels, and of subsequent lawsuits filed by pharmaceutical companies that

challenged the FDA's authority to remove drugs from the market based on the DES findings, see Carpenter, *Reputation and Power*, pp. 345–357.

109. Minutes of compendium meeting with representatives of the Drug Research Board and the AMA, January 12, 1968, John Adriani Papers, National Library of Medicine (hereafter, Adriani Papers), box 27, folder 27–9.

110. Duke C. Trexler to Drug Research Board, "Memorandum: Complimentary Drug Compendium," February 10, 1967, Middleton Papers, box 28, folder: Drug compendium 1967.

111. Minutes of compendium meeting with representatives of the Drug Research Board and the AMA, January 12, 1968, Adriani Papers, box 27, folder 27–9.

112. Ibid.; Council on Drugs, "Meeting Minutes: Towards Improving Council-Staff Working Relationships," January 12, 1968, Adriani Papers, box 27, folder 27–9.

113. Minutes of compendium meeting with representatives of the Drug Research Board and the AMA, January 12, 1968, Adriani Papers, box 27, folder 27–9.

114. Ibid.

115. Walter Modell, "Editorial: FDA Censorship," *Clinical Pharmacology and Therapeutics* 8, no. 3 (1967): 359–361; Modell, "Editorial: How to HEW the FDA into Shape," *Clinical Pharmacology and Therapeutics* 9, no. 3 (1968): 285–289; Modell, "Editorial: On Speech and Silence and the FDA," *Clinical Pharmacology and Therapeutics* 9, no. 2 (1968): 139–141.

116. Modell, "Editorial: FDA Censorship," pp. 359–360.

117. Ibid., pp. 359–360.

118. John Adriani to Herbert Ley, January 29, 1968, Adriani Papers, box 31, folder 31–3. For discussion of Modell's attitude toward the FDA and his subsequent standing among other leading academic physicians, see Carpenter, *Reputation and Power*, pp. 320–324.

119. Cannan, "The Drug Efficacy Study of the NAS-NRC."

120. "Drug Label Compendium," *Congressional Record* 113, pt. 2 (1967): 1884.

121. Representative Carleton J. King, "The Proposed Drug Compendium," *Congressional Record* 114, pt. 24 (1968): 32145.

122. C. Joseph Stetler, "Statement of C. Joseph Stetler, President, PMA," in Nelson hearings, November 16, 1967, p. 1362.

123. By the early 1970s, the American Medical Political Action Committee had more than sixty thousand members and an annual budget of $3.5 million. See Gordon, *Dead on Arrival*, pp. 245–246.

124. Duke C. Trexler to the record, "Memorandum: Joint AMA-DRB Compendium Committee Meeting," January 18, 1968, Middleton Papers, box 28, folder: Drug compendium 1967–1968; Duke C. Trexler "Memorandum to Committee on Drug Compendium," December 14, 1967, Middleton Papers, box 28, folder: Drug compendium 1967–1968.

125. Cannan, "The Drug Efficacy Study of the NAS-NRC."

126. Harry F. Dowling, "A Compendium as Part of the Information System," paper presented at a meeting of the United States Pharmacopeia Convention, April 8, 1970, Dowling Papers, box 3, folder: Talks 1970–1973.

127. "S. 950—Introduction of a Compendium of Prescription Drugs," *Congressional Record* 115, pt. 3 (1969): 3134.

128. Those experts were the AMA's own Council of Drugs until the Council on Drugs was terminated in 1972, after which time the AMA relied on leading academic physicians for that expertise. For information on the final stages of completion of the *AMA Drug Evaluations,* see John Adriani to Senator Gaylord Nelson, November 8, 1971, Adriani Papers, box 40, folder: 40–5.

129. David J. Rothman, *Strangers at the Bedside: A History of How Law and Bioethics Transformed Medical Decision Making* (New York: Basic Books, 1991), pp. 51–69.

130. Ibid., pp. 85–100. As Rothman details, at the same time that the FDA introduced informed consent regulations, the NIH introduced new rules regarding patient consent, which included the requirement that all federally funded research projects must first be subject to peer review and approved by an institutional review board.

131. Carpenter, *Reputation and Power,* pp. 319, 546–549.

132. Henry K. Beecher, "Ethics and Clinical Research," *New England Journal of Medicine* 74 (1966): 1354–1360.

133. Jon Harkness, Susan Lederer, and Daniel Wikler, "Laying Ethical Foundations for Clinical Research," *Bulletin of the World Health Organization* 79, no. 4 (2001): 365–366.

134. Food and Drug Administration, "Consent for Use of Investigational New Drugs on Humans: Statement of Policy," *Federal Register* 31, no. 168 (August 30, 1966): 11415.

135. Morton Hamburger to Ray E. Bersiles, November 8, 1966, Middleton Papers, box 28, folder: Patient consent and clinical trials Nov–Dec 1966.

136. See Richard W. Vilter to Maxwell Finland, November 7, 1966, and Maxwell Finland to Duke C. Trexler, November 14, 1966, both in Middleton Papers, box 28, folder: Patient consent and clinical trials Nov–Dec 1966.

137. See, for example, James D. Hardy to Maxwell Finland, November 11, 1966, John W.P. to Maxwell Finland, November 17, 1966, and Alvin Davis and Sydney M. Finbold to William Middleton, November 25, 1966, all in Middleton Papers, box 28, folder: Patient consent and clinical trials Nov–Dec 1966.

138. William B. Castle to William Middleton, September 30, 1966, and Chester S. Keefer to William Middleton, September 30, 1966, both in Middleton Papers, box 28, folder: Patient consent and clinical trials 1964–1966.

139. Chester S. Keefer to William Middleton, November 6, 1966, Middleton Papers, box 28, folder: Patient consent and clinical trials Nov–Dec 1966.

140. Ibid.

141. Ibid.

142. C. Joseph Stetler to William Middleton, October 5, 1966, Middleton Papers, box 28, folder: Patient consent and clinical trials Oct 1966.

143. Duke C. Trexler to Ad Hoc Committee on Patient Consent, "Memorandum: Proposed Statement of Policy," October 23, 1966, Middleton Papers, box 28, folder: Patient consent and clinical trials Oct 1966.

144. R. Keith Cannan to James Goddard, November 10, 1966, Middleton Papers, box 28, folder: Patient consent and clinical trials Nov–Dec 1966.

145. Duke C. Trexler to DRB, "Memorandum: Revision of the FDA Patient Consent Regulation," January 15, 1967, Middleton Papers, box 28, folder: Patient consent and clinical trials Jan 1967.

146. Ibid.

147. Watkins, *On the Pill;* Helen Marieskind, "The Women's Health Movement," *International Journal of Health Services* 5, no. 2 (1975): 217–223; Sheryl Burt Ruzek, *The Women's Health Movement: Feminist Alternatives to Medical Control* (New York: Praeger, 1978); Mary K. Zimmerman, "The Women's Health Movement: A Critique of Medical Enterprise and the Position of Women," in *Analyzing Gender: A Handbook of Social Science Research,* ed. Beth B. Hess and Myra Marx Ferree (Newbury Park, Calif.: Sage Publications, 1987), pp. 442–472; Carol S. Weisman, *Women's Healthcare: Activist Traditions and Institutional Change* (Baltimore: Johns Hopkins University Press, 1998); Wendy Kline, "The Making of *Our Bodies, Ourselves:* Re-thinking Women's Health and Second-Wave Feminism," in *Feminist Coalitions: Historical Perspectives on Second-Wave Feminism in the United States,* ed. Stephanie Gilmore (Urbana: University of Illinois Press, 2008), pp. 63–83; Kline, *Bodies of Knowledge: Sexuality, Reproduction, and Women's Health in the Second Wave* (Chicago: University of Chicago Press, 2010).

148. James Jones, *Bad Blood: The Tuskegee Syphilis Experiment,* rev. ed. (New York: Free Press, 1993); Susan Reverby, ed., *Tuskegee's Truths: Rethinking the Tuskegee Syphilis Study* (Chapel Hill: University of North Carolina Press, 2000); Reverby, *Examining Tuskegee: The Infamous Syphilis Study and Its Legacy* (Chapel Hill: University of North Carolina Press, 2009).

149. For another example of the cooperative role of academic physicians, drug firms, and the FDA in constructing drug regulations, see Harry M. Marks, "Making Risks Visible: The Science and Politics of Adverse Drug Reactions," in *Ways of Regulating: Therapeutic Agents between Plants, Shops and Consulting Rooms,* ed. Jean Paul Gaudillière and Volker Hess (Berlin: Max-Planck-Institut für Wissenschaftsgeschichte, 2009), pp. 105–122.

150. Cannan, "The Drug Efficacy Study of the NAS-NRC."

151. Ibid.

152. Sheila Jasanoff, *The Fifth Branch: Science Advisors as Policymakers* (Cambridge, Mass.: Harvard University Press, 1990).

CHAPTER 6

1. Excerpts from this chapter have been previously published in Dominique A. Tobbell, "Allied against Reform: Pharmaceutical Industry–Academic Physician Relations in the United States, 1945–1970," *Bulletin of the History of the Medicine* 82, no. 4 (2008): 878–912, copyright © 2008, The Johns Hopkins University Press.

2. Sam Peltzman, *Regulation of Pharmaceutical Innovation: The 1962 Amendments* (Washington, D.C.: American Enterprise Institute for Public Policy Research, 1974); William M. Wardell and Louis Lasagna, *Regulation and Drug Development* (Washington, D.C.: American Enterprise Institute for Public Policy Research, 1975); Arthur Daemmrich, "Invisible Moments and the Costs of Pharmaceutical Regulation: Twenty-Five Years of Drug Lag Debate," *Pharmacy in History* 45, no. 1 (2003): 3–17.

3. See, for example, Leslie Alderman, "Patient Money: A New Disquiet about Generic Drugs," *New York Times*, December 18, 2009; on the *Times's* website, the article also carried the title "Not All Drugs Are the Same after All," www.nytimes.com/2009/12/19/health/19patient.html?ref=health (accessed December 23, 2009).

4. *Competitive Problems in the Drug Industry*, hearings before the Senate Select Committee on Small Business, Monopoly Subcommittee, 1967–1977 (Washington, D.C.: Government Printing Office, 1967–1977). Hereafter referred to as the Nelson hearings.

5. See also Tobbell, "Allied against Reform."

6. Office of the Secretary, U.S. Department of Health, Education, and Welfare, *Final Report of the Task Force on Prescription Drugs* (Washington D.C.: Government Printing Office, 1969), p. x; Milton Silverman, Philip Lee, and Mia Lydecker, *Pills and the Public Purse: The Routes to National Drug Insurance* (Berkeley: University of California Press, 1981), p. 152.

7. D.G. Chapman, L.G. Chatten, and J.A. Campbell, "Physiological Availability of Drugs in Tablets," *Canadian Medical Association Journal* 76 (1957): 102–105, quotation from p. 103; A.B. Morrison, D.G. Chapman, and J.A. Campbell, "Further Studies on the Relation between *In Vitro* Disintegration Time of Tablets and Urinary Excretion Rates of Riboflavin," *Journal of the American Pharmaceutical Association* 48, no. 11 (1959): 634–637; A.B. Morrison and J.A. Campbell, "The Relationship between Physiological Availability of Salicylates and Riboflavin and *In Vitro* Disintegration of Enteric Coated Tablets," *Journal of the American Pharmaceutical Association* 49, no. 7 (1960): 473–478; A.B. Morrison and J.A. Campbell, "Physiologic Availability of Riboflavin and Thiamine in 'Chewable' Vitamin Products," *American Journal of Clinical Nutrition* 10, no. 3 (1962): 212–216; A.B. Morrison, C.B. Perusse, and J.A. Campbell, "The Relationship between *In Vitro* Disintegration Time and *In Vivo* Release of Vitamins from a Triple-Dose Spaced-Release Preparation," *Journal of Pharmaceutical Sciences* 51, no. 7 (1962): 623–626; Denys Cook, "History of Bioavailability Testing at

the Food and Drug Directorate," *Revue Canadienne de Biologie* 32, supp. (1973): 157–162.

8. Lloyd Miller, "Physiological Availability and Homogeneity in U.S.P. Dosage Forms," Circular 30, U.S.P. Committee of Revision, September 28, 1961, p. 108, in USP Records, B82, F 11, Wisconsin State Historical Society. Cited in Daniel P. Carpenter and Dominique A. Tobbell, "Bioequivalence: The Regulatory Career of a Pharmaceutical Concept," *Bulletin of the History of Medicine* 85, no. 1 (2011): 93–131.

9. "Kalman C. Mezel: An Interview Conducted by Louis Galambos and Robert Lewis," March 6 and 7, 1990, Merck Archives, Whitehouse Station, N.J., pp. 55–58. The capsule form of Indocin (generic name indomethacin) was approved for marketing by the FDA in 1965.

10. "Statement of C. Joseph Stetler, President, PMA," in Nelson hearings, November 16, 1967, pp. 1367–1400, quotation from p. 1367.

11. "Statement of Charles T. Silloway, President, Ciba Pharmaceutical Co.," in Nelson hearings, September 14, 1967, pp. 896–922, quotation from p. 907.

12. Ibid., p. 908; Gaylord Nelson, "Therapeutic Equivalency of Drugs," *Congressional Record* 115, pt. 5 (1969): 6427.

13. "Statement of William F. Haddad," in Nelson hearings, May 15, 1967, pp. 22–26.

14. "Statement of C. Joseph Stetler, President, PMA," in Nelson hearings, November 16, 1967, p. 1367.

15. For a discussion of the economics of patent expiration and competition in the prescription drug field, see Peter Temin, *Taking Your Medicine: Drug Regulation in the United States* (Cambridge, Mass.: Harvard University Press, 1980), pp. 151–161.

16. Louis C. Lasagna, "What We Don't Know about Drugs," letter to editor of undisclosed newspaper, 1968, University of Rochester Archives, Louis Lasagna Papers, d302, box 4:1.

17. "Statement of Dr. Walter Modell, Director of Clinical Pharmacology, Cornell University Medical College, New York," in Nelson hearings, June 7, 1967, p. 304.

18. Alfred Gilman, "Therapeutic Equivalence of Generic Drugs and Problems of Drug Formulation," appendix A, minutes, Policy Advisory Committee of the Drug Efficacy Study, no. 3, March 27, 1968, National Academies Archives, series 3 DES PAC 1968, folder: Meetings: Third: 27 Mar.

19. Ibid. For more on this point, see Harry C. Shirkey, "Generic versus Therapeutic Equivalency of Drugs," 1968, National Academies Archives, series 1 Drug Efficacy Study 1967–1969, folder: Problems: Therapeutic Equivalence of Generic Drugs.

20. "Minutes, Policy Advisory Committee of the Drug Efficacy Study, no. 3, March 27, 1968," National Academies Archives, series 3 DES PAC 1968, folder: Meetings: Third: 27 Mar.

21. Drug Efficacy Study, "White Paper on the Therapeutic Equivalence of Generic Drugs: Draft for the Policy Advisory Committee," minutes of Policy Advisory Committee of DES, appendix B, March 6, 1969, National Academies Archives, series 3, DES PAC 1969, folder: Meetings: Fourth: March 6, 1969.

22. Statement submitted by Alfred Gilman to Senator Nelson, in *Congressional Record* 113, pt. 19 (1967): 25146–25148.

23. Office of the Secretary, U.S. Department of Health, Education, and Welfare, *Final Report of the Task Force on Prescription Drugs*, p. iii.

24. Ibid., p. 31.

25. Office of the Secretary, U.S. Department of Health, Education, and Welfare, *Report of the Secretary's Review Committee of the Task Force on Prescription Drugs* (Washington, D.C.: Government Printing Office, 1969).

26. The title of this section is drawn from an editorial written in 1973 by a member of the AMA's Department of Drugs: Donald O. Schiffman, "Editorial: Eroding the Physician's Control of Therapy," *Journal of the American Medical Association* 225, no. 2 (1973): 552.

27. Dale G. Friend to Duke C. Trexler, February 17, 1969, National Academies Archives, Drug Efficacy Study Collection, series 2, DES Panels, folder: Membership: Comments on Topics of Final Report 1969.

28. Edward F. Skinner, "Generic Prescribing," *Journal of the American Medical Association* 198, no. 7 (1966): 792–297. See also Charles A. Ragan, "Editorial: Are We Headed for a Dark Age of Nondiscovery in Therapeutics?" *Journal of the American Medical Association* 202, no. 12 (1967): 1099–1100.

29. Edward F. Skinner, "Generic Prescribing."

30. Donald Janson, "AMA Says Brand-Name Drugs Do Not Always Cost More," *New York Times*, May 26, 1967, p. 24; American Medical Association, "Generic Prescribing Doesn't Guarantee Lower Drug Costs, Chicago Survey Shows," news release, May 26, 1967, John Adriani Papers, National Library of Medicine (hereafter Adriani Papers), box 32, folder 32–15.

31. "Social Security Act Amendments of 1967," *Congressional Record* 113, pt. 24 (1967): 32821–32844; "Social Security Act Amendments of 1967," *Congressional Record* 113, pt. 24 (1967): 33518–33528; Representative Multer, "A Bill to Amend the Federal Food, Drug and Cosmetic Act," *Congressional Record* 113, pt. 13 (1967): 16951–16952; Senator Joseph Montoya, "Legislation to Deal with the Catastrophic Prescription Drug Expense of the Aged," *Congressional Record* 114, pt. 2 (1968): 2220–2223; Senator Russell Long, "H.R. 17550—Social Security Amendments of 1970–Amendment no. 929," *Congressional Record* 116, pt. 24 (1970): 32837–32841; Senator Joseph Montoya, "Social Security Amendments of 1970–Amendment no. 1113," *Congressional Record* 116, pt. 31 (1970): 41480–41582.

32. John Adriani to Senator Russell Long, January 29, 1967, Adriani Papers, box 40, folder: 40–2.

33. John Adriani to Jean Weston, May 18, 1967, Adriani Papers, box 34, folder 34–3.

34. Ibid.

35. John Adriani to Jean Weston, April 2, 1969, Adriani Papers, box 34, folder 34–3.

36. See, for example, "Statement of the American Medical Association re. S. 3441 and S. 966," in *Examination of the Pharmaceutical Industry, 1973–1974*, hearings before the Senate Subcommittee on Health, Committee on Labor and Public Welfare, 93rd Congress, 1st and 2nd sessions (Washington, D.C.: Government Printing Office, 1973–1974), May 21, 1974, pp. 2561–2576.

37. Donald O. Schiffman, "Editorial: On Therapeutic Equivalency and the Antisubstitution Laws," *Journal of American Medical Association* 223, no. 5 (1973): 552–553.

38. Schiffman, "Editorial: Eroding the Physician's Control of Therapy," p. 164.

39. Pharmaceutical Manufacturers Association, *Drugs Anonymous?* (Washington, D.C.: Pharmaceutical Manufacturers Association, 1967), Archives Center, National Museum of American History, Smithsonian Institution, Parke-Davis Collection, box 1964. For information on *Compulsory Generic Prescribing—A Peril to the Health Care System*, see Senator Gaylord Nelson, "Drug Quality Standards," *Congressional Record* 113, pt. 5 (1967): 5630–5631.

40. E. W. Kenworthy, "Doctor Suggests Drug Men Denied Him Post in FDA," *New York Times*, August 26, 1969, p. 1; E. W. Kenworthy, "Nixon Criticized for Withdrawing Offer of FDA Post to Physician," *New York Times*, August 28, 1969, p. 23.

41. John Adriani, "Letter to Friends," September 17, 1969, Adriani Papers, box 37, folder 37–1.

42. Senator Morse, "Drug Industry Seeks to Defeat Senator Nelson," *Congressional Record* 114, pt. 21 (1968): 27950–27951.

43. Carpenter and Tobbell, "Bioequivalence."

44. "Statement of Senator Gaylord Nelson," *Congressional Record* 118, pt. 5 (1972): 5887–5888.

45. For health care expenditure statistics, see U.S. Department of Health, Education, and Welfare, *Health United States 1975*, DHEW Publication no. (HRA) 76–1232, pp. 65, 70–71.

46. Ibid.

47. On the public interest movement, see David Vogel, *Fluctuating Fortunes: The Political Power of Business in America* (New York: Basic Books, 1989), pp. 93–112.

48. Examples of Kennedy's legislative hearings on the pharmaceutical industry include: *Examination of the Pharmaceutical Industry, 1973–1974*, hearings before the Subcommittee on Health, Committee on Labor and

Public Welfare, U.S. Senate, 93rd Congress, 1st and 2nd sessions, December 18 and 19, 1973, February 1 and 25, March 8, 12, and 13, 1974; and *Brand Names and Generic Drugs, 1974*, hearings before the Subcommittee on Health, Committee on Labor and Public Welfare, U.S. Senate, 93rd Congress, 2nd session, July 22, 1974 (Washington, D.C.: Government Printing Office, 1974). Collectively, these hearings are referred to as the Kennedy hearings.

49. Senator Edward Kennedy, "Drug Utilization Improvement Act," *Congressional Record* 121, pt. 7 (1975): 8140–8141; Senator Edward Kennedy, in *Congressional Record* 123, pt. 18 (1977): 22263–22273; Senator Edward Kennedy, "S. 2755. Drug Regulation Reform Act of 1978," *Congressional Record* 124, pt. 6 (1978): 7203–7233, 7291–7292; Representative Paul Rogers, "Drug Regulation Reform Act," *Congressional Record* 124, pt. 12 (1978): 16340; Senator Edward Kennedy, "Drug Regulation Reform Act of 1979," *Congressional Record* 125, pt. 23 (1979): 30128.

50. Senator Edward Kennedy, in Kennedy hearings, December 18, 1973, p. 1.

51. *FDC Reports*, December 19, 1973.

52. See Harold M. Schmeck Jr., "H.E.W. Drug Plan Would Save Governments $89-Million a Year," *New York Times*, November 15, 1974, p. 10.

53. "Statement of C. Joseph Stetler," in Kennedy hearings, December 19, 1973, pp. 336–363, quotation taken from p. 336.

54. Ibid., p. 337.

55. Ibid.

56. Ibid., pp. 336, 339, 346.

57. Ibid., p. 339.

58. Carpenter and Tobbell, "Bioequivalence."

59. "Statement of Ralph Nader, Accompanied by Sidney Wolfe," in Kennedy hearings, December 18, 1973, pp. 174–177.

60. Kennedy had introduced a similar bill calling for a National Center of Clinical Pharmacology the year before, but in that bill the mandate for the center was less clear than in the 1975 bill. See Senator Edward Kennedy, in *Congressional Record* 120, pt. 10 (1974): 13133–13161.

61. Senator Edward Kennedy, "Drug Utilization Improvement Act," *Congressional Record* 121, pt. 7 (1975): 8140–8141.

62. Ibid.

63. Ibid., p. 8140.

64. Senator Edward Kennedy, in *Congressional Record* 123, pt. 18 (1977): 22262–22273.

65. Senator Edward Kennedy, "S. 2755: Drug Regulation Reform Act of 1978," *Congressional Record* 124, pt. 6 (1978): 7205.

66. Vogel, *Fluctuating Fortunes*; Kim Phillips-Fein, *Invisible Hands: The Businessmen's Crusade against the New Deal* (New York: W.W. Norton, 2009).

67. William Wardell, "Introduction of New Therapeutic Drugs in the United States and Great Britain: An International Comparison," *Clinical Pharmacology and Therapeutics* 14 (1973): 773–790.

68. Peltzman, *Regulation of Pharmaceutical Innovation.* For a critique of Peltzman's economic analysis, see Temin, *Taking Your Medicine,* pp. 146–148.

69. Wardell and Lasagna, *Regulation and Drug Development.* For a detailed analysis of the history of the drug lag debate, see Daemmrich, "Invisible Moments and the Costs of Pharmaceutical Regulation." Daniel Carpenter has analyzed the rate at which new drugs were approved at the FDA in the 1950s and 1960s. His analysis shows that the slowdown in new drug approvals occurred in the late 1950s, after the FDA implemented new rules regarding the NDA process. See Daniel P. Carpenter, *Reputation and Power: Organizational Image and Pharmaceutical Regulation at the FDA* (Princeton, N.J.: Princeton University Press, 2010), pp. 177–182, 374–380.

70. Dorothy Wardell, "Medical Maverick: Fortunately He Can't Seem to Let Well Enough Alone," *Democrat and Chronicle,* December 9, 1973, pp. 4–11.

71. "SCRIP Interview with Professor Lasagna, Interviewed by Michael E. Allen of SCRIP at the IMMPI Meeting, Held in Florence, October 1975," Louis Lasagna Collection, University of Rochester Archives, Rochester, New York, Collection d302, box 7:2. For more information on Wardell and Lasagna's policy proposals, see Wardell and Lasagna, *Regulation and Drug Development,* pp. 143–159. For analysis of different regulatory approaches in the United States and Germany, see Arthur Daemmrich, *Pharmacopolitics: Drug Regulation in the United States and Germany* (Chapel Hill: University of North Carolina Press, 2004).

72. "Statement of C. Joseph Stetler," in Kennedy hearings, December 19, 1973, pp. 360–361.

73. "Statement of C. Joseph Stetler," in Kennedy hearings, August 16, 1974, pp. 2921–2922. See also Donald Kennedy, "A Calm Look at the 'Drug Lag,'" *Journal of the American Medical Association* 239, no. 5 (1978): 423–426.

74. Jules Bergman, Michael J. Halberstam, William N. Hubbard Jr., Louis Lasagna, Gaylord Nelson, and Alexander M. Schmidt, *Reforming Federal Drug Regulation: A Round Table Held on February 23, 1976, and Sponsored by the Center for Health Policy Research of the American Enterprise Institute for Public Policy Research* (Washington, D.C.: American Enterprise Institute for Public Policy Research, 1976), p. 4.

75. Donald Kennedy, "A Calm Look at the 'Drug Lag'"; Bergman et al., *Reforming Federal Drug Regulation,* p. 6.

76. Donald Kennedy, "A Calm Look at the 'Drug Lag,'" pp. 423, 425.

77. For more details on the drug lag debate, see Daemmrich, "Invisible Moments and the Costs of Pharmaceutical Regulation"; Temin, *Taking Your Medicine,* pp. 146–148; F. Anderson, "The Drug Lag Issue: The Debate Seen from an International Perspective," *International Journal of Health Services* 22 (1992): 53–72; and Food and Drug Administration, *A Historical Look at*

Drug Introductions on a Five-Country Market: A Comparison of the United States and Four European Countries, 1960–1981 (Washington, D.C.: FDA Office of Planning and Evaluation, 1982).

78. Vogel, *Fluctuating Fortunes*, pp. 113–147; Phillips-Fein, *Invisible Hands;* Benjamin C. Waterhouse, "A Lobby for Capital: Organized Business and the Pursuit of Pro-Market Politics, 1967–1986" (Ph.D. dissertation, Harvard University, 2009).

79. Bergman et al., *Reforming Federal Drug Regulation*, p. 16.

80. American Medical Association, House of Delegates, "Draft Resolutions 58, 59, 60, 75, 85, 90, and Substitute Resolution 58," 1973, p. 17, cited in Wardell and Lasagna, *Regulation and Drug Development*, p. 15; "Medical Freedom of Choice: Testimony of the Honorable Steven Symms before the Health and Environment Subcommittee," *Congressional Record* 122, pt. 18 (1976): 23257–23261; Representative Steven Symms, "Medical Freedom of Choice Act," *Congressional Record* 123, pt. 10 (1977): 12321–12322; Representative Steven Symms, "Food and Drug Reform Critical to the Health of Americans," *Congressional Record* 125, pt. 1 (1979): 666–667.

81. "Statement of Ralph Nader, Accompanied by Sidney Wolfe," in Kennedy hearings, December 18, 1973, p. 174.

82. For details on the deal Senator Kefauver made with Tennessee pharmacists to exclude pharmacy practices from his congressional investigation, see Richard Harris, *The Real Voice* (New York: Macmillan, 1964), p. 41.

83. William S. Apple, " 'Pharmacy's Lib,' " *Journal of the American Pharmaceutical Association* N.S. 11, no. 10 (1971): 528–533, quotations from pp. 528–529. For more details on the contested roles and identities of pharmacists in the 1970s, see Dominique A. Tobbell, "Eroding the Physicians' Control," in *Prescribed: Writing, Filling, Using, and Abusing the Prescription in Modern America*, ed. Jeremy A. Greene and Elizabeth Siegel Watkins (Baltimore: Johns Hopkins University Press, 2012).

84. Beth Linker, "The Business of Ethics: Gender, Medicine, and the Professional Codification of the American Physiotherapy Association, 1918–1935," *Journal of the History of Medicine and Allied Sciences* 60 (2005): 321–354.

85. "National Pharmaceutical Counsel," *FDC Reports*, December 5, 1953, pp. W3–W4; D.G. Baird, "Why Parke, Davis Is Advertising to Build Prestige for Pharmacists," reprint from *Sales Management*, September 15, 1946, Archives Center, National Museum of American History, Smithsonian Institution, Parke-Davis Collection, NL box 31, folder NLd 1946.

86. Apple, " 'Pharmacy's Lib,' " pp. 529–533.

87. Ibid.

88. "2 Generic-Drug Bills Offered," *New York Times*, February 23, 1975, p. NJ56.

89. "Bill to Allow Drug Substitutions Advances in Assembly," *Los Angeles Times*, March 6, 1975, p. A29.

90. "Generic Drug Bill Wins Senate Approval, 30–7," *Los Angeles Times*, September 12, 1975.

91. Martin Waldron, "Generic Drugs: The Fight Continues," *New York Times*, October 3, 1976, p. 316; Martin Waldron, "Assembly Approves Generic-Drug Prescriptions," *New York Times*, February 15, 1977, p. 67. For accusations against industry and physician lobbying tactics in Illinois, see William Griffin, "Drug Firms Accused of 'Dirty' Tactics against Bill," *Chicago Tribune*, November 15, 1977, p. B12.

92. "States Moving to Allow Generic Substitution," *Internist* 20, no. 4 (1979): 12–13.

93. Donald O. Schiffman, "Editorial: On Therapeutic Equivalence and the Antisubstitution Laws," p. 552.

94. "Generic Substitution Becomes Law," *Missouri Medicine* 75, no. 9 (1978): 467.

95. Sherry L. Hall, "Attorney General Limits Generic Drug Substitution," *Michigan Medicine* 74, no. 9 (1975): 148–149.

96. "Bill to Allow Drug Substitutions Advances in Assembly," p. A29.

97. For a detailed analysis of state-based health and pharmaceutical policy reform, see Daniel M. Fox, *The Convergence of Science and Governance: Research, Health Policy, and American States* (Berkeley: University of California Press, 2010).

EPILOGUE

1. For detailed analyses of the Hatch-Waxman Act, see Gerald J. Mossinghoff, "Overview of the Hatch-Waxman Act and Its Impact on the Drug Development Process," *Food and Drug Law Journal* 54 (1999): 187–194; Allan R. Fox and Alan R. Bennett, *The Legislative History of the Drug Price Competition and Patent Term Restoration Act of 1984* (Washington, D.C.: Food and Drug Law Institute, 1987); and Daniel P. Carpenter and Dominique A. Tobbell, "Bioequivalence: The Regulatory Career of a Pharmaceutical Concept," *Bulletin of the History of Medicine* 85, no. 1 (2011): 93–131.

2. The drug lag proponent William Wardell contended that in 1981 it took as long as thirteen years to a bring a drug from synthesis to market, whereas in 1964, it had taken half that time. William Wardell, "Postmarketing Surveillance vs. Phase III," *Journal of the American Medical Association* 245, no. 24 (1981): 2485–2486.

3. Office of Technology Assessment, *Patent-Term Extension and the Pharmaceutical Industry* (Washington, D.C.: Government Printing Office, 1981).

4. "S. 255, The Patent Term Restoration Act of 1981," *Congressional Record* 127, pt. 6 (1981): 7799–7800; "Patent Term Restoration Act of 1982," *Congressional Record* 128, pt. 17 (1982): 23316–23325.

5. The PMA president Lewis A. Engman noted that "in 1960, a $3.5 billion industry with patent lives averaging 16 years produced 50 new medicines. In 1979, a $20 billion industry with effective patent lives averaging less than 10 years produced only 12 new medicines." Cited in Robert Pear, "Drug Patent Extension Draws Heavy Lobbying," *New York Times*, July 28, 1982, p. D1.

6. "Patent Term Restoration Act of 1982," p. 23318. To be sure, brand manufacturers lobbied hard for passage of the bill. As the *New York Times* reported, in the nineteen months after the bill's introduction, "the political action committees of the top 22 brand-name companies have given $400,000 to various Congressional campaigns." "Patent Bill Splits the Drug Industry," *New York Times*, August 15, 1982, p. NJ4.

7. Later in the debate, AARP would switch its support, favoring passage of the bill.

8. "Patent Bill Splits the Drug Industry."

9. "Patent Term Restoration Act of 1982," pp. 23322, 23324.

10. Pear, "Drug Patent Extension Draws Heavy Lobbying." A *New York Times* editorial also noted the common practice of "evergreening" by pharmaceutical manufacturers. This is when a company files an early patent on a potential new drug so as to prevent a competitor from doing so, and then files new applications that modify or extend the original patent, thus postponing the time when the patent life starts. See "An Unwarranted Patent Stretch," *New York Times*, August 7, 1982.

11. Mossinghoff, "Overview of the Hatch-Waxman Act and Its Impact on the Drug Development Process." In 2006, *Consumer Reports* noted that 47 percent of all prescriptions written in the United States were for generic drugs. See www.consumerreports.org/health/free-highlights/manage-your-health/safe_drug_choices.htm (accessed September 2, 2010).

12. Jeff Gerth and Sheryl Gay Stolberg, "Cultivating Alliances: With Quiet Unseen Ties, Drug Makers Sway Debate," *New York Times*, October 5, 2000.

13. For a detailed analysis of the political history of the Medicare prescription drug benefit, see Thomas R. Oliver, Philip R. Lee, and Helene L. Lipton, "A Political History of Medicare and Prescription Drug Coverage," *Milbank Quarterly* 82, no. 2 (2004): 283–354.

14. "Prescription Drug Plans," *Congressional Record* 146, pt. 16 (2000): 18638.

15. Gerth and Stolberg, "Cultivating Alliances."

16. Milt Freudenheim, "Group Seeks to Counteract Drugmakers," *New York Times*, June 30, 2000.

17. Gerth and Stolberg, "Cultivating Alliances."

18. "Prescription Drug Plans," pp. 18637, 18639.

19. "The Problem of High Prescription Drug Costs," *Congressional Record* 146, pt. 8 (2000): 11823. For similar testimony from other House Democrats, see pp. 11822–11834. See also Freudenheim, "Group Seeks to Counteract Drugmakers."

20. David Rosenbaum, "Health Insurance Provides Buffer to Rising Drug Prices for Most Americans," *New York Times,* June 1, 2000.

21. David Rosenbaum, "The Gathering Storm over Prescription Drugs," *New York Times,* November 14, 1999.

22. Robert Pear, "Drug Makers and Insurers Lock Horns over Medicare," *New York Times,* February 21, 2000. The insurance industry was, however, generally supportive of Republican proposals for modernizing other aspects of Medicare, particularly what came to be called Medicare Part C.

23. John McDonough, personal communication; Sherrod Brown and Stephen Doyle, "Op-Chart: Medicare Index," *New York Times,* January 28, 2004, www.nytimes.com/2004/01/28/opinion/op-chart-medicare-index.html?scp=1&sq=%22medicare+index%22&st=nyt; Karen Ignagni, "Letter to Editor: Medicare Law's Benefits," *New York Times,* February 4, 2004, www.nytimes.com/2004/02/04/opinion/l-medicare-law-s-benefits-229636.html?scp=2&sq=%22medicare+index%22&st=nyt (both accessed September 7, 2010).

24. See, for example, Duff Wilson, "More Cost Cuts Sought from Drug Industry," *New York Times,* July 23, 2009; Billy Tauzin, "Letter to the Editor: Health Reform and Drugs," *New York Times,* July 1, 2009.

25. "The Drug Industry Cashes In," *New York Times,* November 18, 2009; Reed Abelson, "In Health Care Overhaul, Boons for Hospitals and Drug Makers," *New York Times,* March 21, 2010. On patents and biologics, see Duff Wilson, "Drug Industry Group Threatens to Withdraw Support," *New York Times,* January 15, 2010; "Work-up: Costly Drugs Prompt Exclusivity Debate," *New York Times,* July 22, 2009; and Andrew Pollack, "Biologic Drugs May Get Less Protection," *New York Times,* January 14, 2010.

26. David D. Kirkpatrick, "Groups Back Health Reform, but Seek Cover," *New York Times,* September 12, 2009.

27. See, for example, Robert Pear, "Health Care Industry in Talks to Shape Policy," *New York Times,* February 20, 2009.

28. Robert Pear, "Drug Industry, Having Long Smiled on G.O.P., Now Splits Donations Equally," *New York Times,* October 14, 2008. For detailed figures, see Center for Responsive Politics, www.opensecrets.org/industries/totals.php?cycle=2010&ind=H04.

29. Herman Somers and Ann Somers, *Doctors, Patients, and Health Insurance: The Organization and Financing of Medical Care* (Washington, D.C.: Brookings Institution, 1961); Colin Gordon, *Dead on Arrival: The Politics of Health Care in Twentieth-Century America* (Princeton, N.J.: Princeton University Press, 2003).

30. To be sure, the health insurance industry is not monolithic. For-profit plans, for example, often have different political and economic interests in health care reform than do not-for-profit plans. Despite the heterogeneity of the industry, at root the insurance industry supports prescription drug legislation that increases generic drug competition and helps reduce prescription drug prices.

31. Between 1998 and 2010, the pharmaceutical and health products industry spent more on lobbying the U.S. Congress than any other industry ($1,955,835,643), with the insurance industry in second place ($1,428,442,637). Health professionals, by contrast, spent $761,601,518 on lobbying during the same time period, with the AMA the largest single contributor ($15,170,000), followed by the American College of Radiology ($3,026,054). See www .opensecrets.org/lobby/top.php?indexType=i (accessed August 25, 2010).

32. Daniel M. Fox, *The Convergence of Science and Governance: Research, Health Policy, and American States* (Berkeley: University of California Press, 2010), especially pp. 72–76.

33. Gardiner Harris, "Cheap Drugs from Canada: Another Political Hot Potato," *New York Times*, October 23, 2003.

34. For a detailed discussion and analysis of states' policy competence on prescription drug policy, see Fox, *The Convergence of Science and Governance*, pp. 2–5, 77–103. For information on the states that established PDLs, see Robert Pear and James Dao, "States Trying New Tactics to Reduce Spending on Drugs," *New York Times*, November 21, 2004.

35. Robert Pear, "U.S. to Compare Medical Treatments," *New York Times*, February 15, 2009, www.nytimes.com/2009/02/16/health/policy/16health .html?scp=1&sq=comparative%20effectiveness%20research%20 stimulus%20bill&st=cse (accessed December 27, 2010).

36. I thank John McDonough for this insight on the relationship between state and federal prescription drug policymaking.

37. I thank John McDonough for the observation that it is the substantial annual *increases* in prices, rather than the prices themselves, that are the major source of concern for state governments, health consumer groups, and insurance companies.

38. Stephen Zuckerman and Joshua McFeeters, *Recent Growth in Health Expenditures* (New York: Commonwealth Fund, 2006), p. 3.

39. Reforming States Group, "State Initiatives on Prescription Drugs: Creating a More Functional Market," *Health Affairs* 22, no. 4 (2003): 128–136, cited in Fox, *The Convergence of Science and Governance*, p. 76.

40. Daniel P. Carpenter, "The Political Economy of FDA Drug Review: Processing, Politics, and Lessons for Policy," *Health Affairs* 23, no. 1 (2004): 52–63. Carpenter's discussion of the increasing number of patient advocacy groups since the 1970s is on p. 56. On the history and increasing activism of patient-consumers, see Nancy Tomes, "Patients or Health-Care Consumers? Why the History of Contested Terms Matters," in *History and Health Policy in the United States: Putting the Past Back In*, ed. Rosemary A. Stevens, Charles E. Rosenberg, and Lawton R. Burns (New Brunswick, N.J.: Rutgers University Press, 2006), pp. 83–110.

41. Gerth and Stolberg, "Cultivating Alliances."

42. See, for example, Steven Epstein, *Impure Science: AIDS, Activism, and the Politics of Knowledge* (Berkeley: University of California Press, 1996); Barron H. Lerner, *Breast Cancer Wars: Hope, Fear, and the Pursuit of a*

Cure in Twentieth-Century America (Oxford: Oxford University Press, 2001); Howard I. Kushner, *A Cursing Brain? The Histories of Tourette Syndrome* (Cambridge, Mass.: Harvard University Press, 1999); Colin Talley, "The Combined Efforts of Community and Science: American Culture, Patient Activism, and the Multiple Sclerosis Movement in the United States," in *Emerging Illnesses and Society: Negotiating the Public Health Agenda*, ed. Randall M. Packard, P. J. Brown, R. L. Berkelman, and H. Frumkin (Baltimore: Johns Hopkins University Press, 2004), pp. 39–70; and Dominique A. Tobbell, "Charitable Innovations: The Political Economy of Thalassemia Research and Drug Development in the United States, 1960–2000," in *Perspectives on Twentieth-Century Pharmaceuticals*, ed. Judy Slinn and Vivianne Quirke (Oxford: Peter Lang AG, 2010), pp. 301–335.

43. The decision late in 2008 by Britain's National Institute for Health and Clinical Excellence (NICE) to refuse to pay for the expensive cancer drug Sutent because comparative effectiveness studies showed it prolonged patients' lives only for six months longer than other treatments but at an estimated cost of $54,000 launched a wave of criticism in the American media. Stories of British cancer patients dying because the government health agency rationed care on the basis of cost-effectiveness fueled Republican and conservative opposition to Obama's health care reform bill. See, for example, Gardiner Harris, "British Balance Benefit vs. Cost of Latest Drugs," *New York Times*, December 2, 2008; "Letters to the Editor; Cost of Living: Who Gets New Drugs," *New York Times*, December 8, 2008; and Peter Singer, "Why We Must Ration Health Care," *New York Times*, July 15, 2009. See also Fox, *The Convergence of Science and Governance*, pp. 77–103.

44. Psychiatrists' relationship with the pharmaceutical industry is particularly distinctive in the recent history of American medicine. David Healy has published extensively on the history of psychiatry's relationship with pharmaceutical companies; see, for example, David Healy, *Let Them Eat Prozac: The Unhealthy Relationship between the Pharmaceutical Industry and Depression* (New York: New York University Press, 2004). On Healy's controversial status in academic psychiatry, see Benedict Carey, "A Self-Effacing Scholar Is Psychiatry's Gadfly," *New York Times*, November 15, 2005, www.nytimes .com/2005/11/15/science/15prof.html?scp=8&sq=paxil+glaxosmithkline+200 4&st=nyt (accessed July 14, 2010). See also the work of Daniel Carlat, a psychiatrist who, after spending a year as a paid speaker for Wyeth, became deeply critical of the pharmaceutical industry's influence on psychiatric practice. See, for example, Daniel Carlat, *Unhinged: The Trouble with Psychiatry—A Doctor's Revelation about a Profession in Crisis* (New York: Free Press, 2010); and Carlat, "Dr. Drug Rep," *New York Times Magazine*, November 25, 2007, www.nytimes.com/2007/11/25/magazine/25memoir-t.html (accessed September 2, 2010).

45. The Center for Responsive Politics lists on its website approximately 150 physician groups and their total lobbying contributions for 2010; see www.opensecrets.org/lobby/indusclient.php?lname=H01&year=2010&filter=

S. Between 1998 and 2010, the Chamber of Commerce spent $651,035,680 on lobbying, while the AMA spent $263,012,500. PhRMA, ranked fourth, spent $185,063,920; AARP, ranked fifth, spent $183,922,064; and Blue Cross/Blue Shield, ranked ninth, spent $148,091,902. See www.opensecrets.org/lobby/top .php?indexType=s (accessed September 2, 2010).

46. Pear, "Drug Industry, Having Long Smiled on G.O.P., Now Splits Donations Equally." From 1990 to 2006, the AMA, for example, contributed significantly more to Republicans than Democrats. Since then, however, it has favored Democrats slightly; see www.opensecrets.org/orgs/summary .php?id=D000000068 (accessed September 2, 2010).

47. Association of American Medical Colleges and Association of American Universities, *Protecting Patients, Preserving Integrity, Advancing Health: Accelerating the Implementation of COI Policies in Human Subjects Research* (Washington, D.C.: American Association of Medical Colleges, 2008).

48. Gina Kolata, "Citing Ethics, Some Doctors Are Rejecting Industry Pay," *New York Times*, April 15, 2008.

49. After Senator Grassley exposed the financial conflict of interest of one of the University of Minnesota's leading surgeons posed by his ties to the Minnesota-based medical device maker Medtronic, the University of Minnesota revised its conflict of interest policy. Jenna Ross, "U Regents Approve Draft of Stricter Ethics Guidelines," *Star Tribune*, March 13, 2010, www .startribune.com/local/87533487.html?elr=KArksUUUoDEy3LGDiO7aiU (accessed July 18, 2010). Harvard Medical School and its affiliated teaching hospitals have also made changes to their conflict of interest policies after several Harvard Medical School faculty were exposed by Senator Grassley for earning significant income from pharmaceutical firms. See, for example, Duff Wilson, "Harvard Medical School in Ethics Quandary," *New York Times*, March 2, 2009, www.nytimes.com/2009/03/03/business/03medschool.html?s cp=3&sq=harvard+conflict+of+interest+pharmaceutical&st=nyt; and Wilson, "Harvard Teaching Hospitals Cap Outside Pay," *New York Times*, January 2, 2010, www.nytimes.com/2010/01/03/health/research/03hospital.html?scp =1&sq=harvard+conflict+of+interest+pharmaceutical&st=nyt (both accessed July 18, 2010).

50. Benedict Carey, "Drug Maker to Report Fees to Doctors," *New York Times*, September 25, 2008.

51. Natasha Singer, "Vermont Acts to Make Drug Makers' Gifts Public," *New York Times*, May 19, 2009, www.nytimes.com/2009/05/20/ business/20vermont.html?scp=1&sq=massachusetts+ban+pharmaceutical+gi fts&st=nyt (accessed September 2, 2010).

52. John McDonough, personal communication with author; Gardiner Harris, "Drug Industry to Announce Revised Code on Marketing," *New York Times*, July 10, 2008, www.nytimes.com/2008/07/10/business/10code. html?scp=2&sq=massachusetts+ban+pharmaceutical+gifts&st=nyt; Duff Wilson, "Data on Fees to Doctors Is Called Hard to Parse," *New York Times*, April 12, 2010, www.nytimes.com/2010/04/13/business/13docpay

.html?sq=physician%20payment%20sunshine&st=nyt&adxnnl=1&scp=1&adxnnlx=1283450408-m/sAzRtvKFKfevGnoi8iQQ (all accessed September 2, 2010); PEW Prescription Project, "Fact Sheet: Physician Payments Sunshine Provisions in Health Care Reform," March 23, 2010, available at www.prescriptionproject.org/sunshine_act (accessed September 2, 2010).

53. David D. Kirkpatrick and Duff Wilson, "One Grand Deal Too Many Costs Lobbyist His Job," *New York Times*, February 12, 2010.

54. In Australia, the pharmaceutical industry has used the same tactic of arguing that pharmaceutical reform—in this case, offering preferred coverage to only the most effective drugs in a class—will inhibit innovation and jeopardize the country's economic growth. See Fox, *The Convergence of Science and Governance*, p. 130.

Bibliography

ARCHIVAL SOURCES

Archives Center, National Museum of American History, Washington, D.C.

N.W. Ayers Advertising Agency Collection
Parke-Davis & Co. Collection
Sterling Drug, Inc., Collection
Syntex Collection of Pharmaceutical Advertising

Library of Congress, Washington, D.C.

Vannevar Bush Papers

Merck Archives, Whitehouse Station, New Jersey

Corporate Documents
Oral Histories
   John T. Connor
   Karl Folkers
   John L. Huck
   Gordon R. Klodt
   Eugene L. Kuryloski
   Kalman C. Mezey
   Lewis H. Sarett
   Max Tishler

National Academies Archives, Washington, D.C.

Medical Sciences Collections
   Commission on Drug Safety Papers
   Drug Efficacy Study Papers
   Drug Research Board Papers
National Council of Drugs Papers

National Archives II, College Park, Maryland
RG 88, Food and Drug Administration Papers

National Library of Medicine, Washington, D.C.
John Adriani Papers
Harry F. Dowling Papers
Chauncey Leake Papers
William Middleton Papers

*Othmer Library of Chemical History, Chemical Heritage
Foundation, Philadelphia, Pennsylvania*
Glenn E. Ullyot Collection
    Smith, Kline & French Papers
Oral Histories
    Karl Folkers
    Lewis H. Sarett

University Archives, University of Pennsylvania, Philadelphia
Medical Affairs Collection
    Department of Pharmacology Records
    Vice President for Medical Affairs Records
Office of the President Records
    1930–1945
    1945–1955
    1955–1970
Isidor S. Ravdin Papers
Alfred Newton Richards Papers

University of Rochester Archives, Rochester, New York
Louis Lasagna Papers

CONGRESSIONAL HEARINGS

Kefauver Hearings
    Administered Prices in the Drug Industry. Hearings before the U.S.
        Senate Committee on the Judiciary, Subcommittee on Antitrust and
        Monopoly, 1959–1961. Washington, D.C.: Government Printing Office,
        1959–1961.
    Drug Industry Antitrust Act. Hearings before the U.S. House Committee
        on the Judiciary, Subcommittee on Antitrust, 1962. Washington, D.C.:
        Government Printing Office, 1962.

Drug Industry Antitrust Act. Hearings before the U.S. Senate Committee on the Judiciary, Subcommittee on Antitrust and Monopoly, 1961–1962. Washington, D.C.: Government Printing Office, 1961–1962.

Kennedy Hearings

Brand Names and Generic Drugs, 1974. Hearing on examination of the Office of Technology Assessment report of the Drug Bioequivalence Study Panel before the U.S. Senate Committee on Labor and Public Welfare, Subcommittee on Health, 93rd Congress, 2nd session, July 22, 1974. Washington, D.C.: Government Printing Office, 1974.

Examination of the Pharmaceutical Industry, 1973–1974. Hearings on S. 3441 and S. 966 before the U.S. Senate Committee on Labor and Public Welfare, Subcommittee on Health, 93rd Congress, 1st and 2nd sessions. Washington, D.C.: Government Printing Office, 1973–1974.

Nelson Hearings

Competitive Problems in the Drug Industry. Hearings before the Senate Select Committee on Small Business, Monopoly Subcommittee, 1967–1977. Washington, D.C.: Government Printing Office, 1967–1977.

SELECTED NEWSPAPER AND JOURNAL SOURCES

American Druggist
Chicago Tribune
Clinical Pharmacology and Therapeutics
Congressional Record
FDC Reports
Food, Drug, and Cosmetic Law Journal
Journal of Medical Education
Journal of the American Medical Association
Los Angeles Times
New England Journal of Medicine
New York Times
Pharmaceutical Manufacturers Association Year Book
Wall Street Journal

SELECTED PUBLISHED SOURCES

Anderson, F. "The Drug Lag Issue: The Debate Seen from an International Perspective." *International Journal of Health Services* 22 (1992): 53–72.

Anderson, Odin W. *The Evolution of Health Services Research: Personal Reflections on Applied Social Science.* San Francisco: Jossey-Bass, 1991.

Angell, Marcia. *The Truth about the Drug Companies: How They Deceive Us and What to Do about It.* New York: Random House, 2005.

Apple, Rima D. *Vitamania: Vitamins in American Culture.* New Brunswick, N.J.: Rutgers University Press, 1996.

Avorn, Jerry. *Powerful Medicines: The Benefits, Risks, and Costs of Prescription Drugs.* New York: Alfred A. Knopf, 2004.

Balogh, Brian. *Chain Reaction: Expert Debate and Public Participation in American Commercial Nuclear Power, 1945–1975.* Cambridge: Cambridge University Press, 1991.

———. "Reorganizing the Organizational Synthesis: Federal–Professional Relations in Modern America." *Studies in American Political Development* 5 (1991): 119–172.

Bergman, Jules, Michael J. Halberstam, William N. Hubbard Jr., Louis Lasagna, Gaylord Nelson, and Alexander M. Schmidt. *Reforming Federal Drug Regulation: A Round Table Held on Feburary 23, 1976, and Sponsored by the Center for Health Policy Research of the American Enterprise Institute for Public Policy Research.* Washington, D.C.: American Enterprise Institute for Public Policy Research, 1976.

Berle, Adolf A., and Gardiner C. Means. *The Modern Corporation and Private Property.* New York: Commerce Clearing House, 1932.

Bliss, Michael. *The Discovery of Insulin.* Chicago: University of Chicago Press, 1982.

Bowers, John Z., and Elizabeth F. Purcell, eds. *Advances in American Medicine: Essays at the Bicentennial.* New York: Josiah Macy Jr. Foundation, 1976.

Brandt, Allan M. *The Cigarette Century: The Rise, Fall, and Deadly Persistence of the Product That Defined America.* New York: Basic Books, 2007.

Brody, Howard. *Hooked: Ethics, the Medical Profession, and the Pharmaceutical Industry.* Lanham, Md.: Rowman & Littlefield, 2006.

Bud, Robert. "Antibiotics, Big Business, and Consumers: The Context of Government Investigations into the Postwar American Drug Industry." *Technology and Culture* 46 (2005): 329–349.

———. *Penicillin: Triumph and Tragedy.* Oxford: Oxford University Press, 2007.

Bush, Vannevar. *Science, the Endless Frontier: A Report to the President on a Program for Postwar Scientific Research.* Washington, D.C.: Government Printing Office, 1945.

Cain, Arthur S., and Lois G. Bowen. "Role of the Postdoctoral Fellowship in Academic Medicine: Report on a Survey of National Fellowship Programs in the Medical Sciences." *Journal of Medical Education* 36 (1961): 1360–1507.

Cantor, David. "Cortisone and the Politics of Drama, 1949–1955." In *Medical Innovations in Historical Perspective,* ed. John V. Pickstone. New York: St. Martin's Press, 1992.

Carlat, Daniel. *Unhinged: The Trouble with Psychiatry—A Doctor's Revelation about a Profession in Crisis.* New York: Free Press, 2010.

Carlisle, Robert D.B. *A Century of Caring: The Upjohn Story.* Elmsford, N.Y.: Benjamin, 1987.

Carpenter, Daniel P. "The Political Economy of FDA Drug Review: Processing, Politics, and Lessons for Policy." *Health Affairs* 23, no. 1 (2004): 52–63.

————. *Reputation and Power: Organizational Image and Pharmaceutical Regulation at the FDA*. Princeton, N.J.: Princeton University Press, 2010.

Carpenter, Daniel P., and Dominique A. Tobbell. "Bioequivalence: The Regulatory Career of a Pharmaceutical Concept." *Bulletin of the History of Medicine* 85, no. 1 (2011): 93–131.

Chandler, Alfred D., Jr. *Scale and Scope: The Dynamics of Industrial Capitalism*. Cambridge, Mass.: Belknap Press, Harvard University, 1990.

————. *Shaping the Industrial Century: The Remarkable Story of the Evolution of the Modern Chemical and Pharmaceutical Industries*. Cambridge, Mass.: Harvard University Press, 2005.

————. *Strategy and Structure: Chapters in the History of the Industrial Enterprise*. Cambridge, Mass.: MIT Press, 1969.

————. *The Visible Hand: The Managerial Revolution in American Business*. Cambridge, Mass.: Belknap Press, Harvard University, 1977.

Cohen, Lizabeth. *A Consumers' Republic: The Politics of Mass Consumption in Postwar America*. Cambridge, Mass.: Harvard University Press, 2003.

Conroy, Mary Schaeffer. *Medicines for the Soviet Masses during World War II*. New York: University Press of America, 2008.

————. "The Soviet Pharmaceutical Industry and Dispensing, 1945–1953." *Europe-Asia Studies* 56, no. 7 (2004): 963–991.

————. "The Soviet Pharmaceutical Industry, Past and Present." Paper presented at "Modern Medicines: The Perspectives in Pharmaceutical History," American Institute for the History of Pharmacy, Madison, Wis., October 18, 2008.

Cray, William C. *The Pharmaceutical Manufacturers Association: The First 30 Years*. Washington, D.C.: Pharmaceutical Manufacturers Association, 1989.

Critser, Greg. *Generation Rx: How Prescription Drugs Are Altering American Lives, Minds, and Bodies*. New York: Houghton Mifflin, 2005.

Daemmrich, Arthur. "Invisible Moments and the Costs of Pharmaceutical Regulation: Twenty-Five Years of Drug Lag Debate." *Pharmacy in History* 45, no. 1 (2003): 3–17.

————. *Pharmacopolitics: Drug Regulation in the United States and Germany*. Chapel Hill: University of North Carolina Press, 2004.

————. "A Tale of Two Experts: Thalidomide and Political Engagement in the United States and West Germany." *Social History of Medicine* 15, no. 1 (2002): 137–158.

Deitrick, John E., and Robert C. Berson. *Medical Schools in the United States at Mid-Century*. New York: McGraw-Hill, 1953.

DiMasi, Joseph A., R. W. Hansen, and Henry G. Grabowski. "The Price of Innovation: New Estimates of Drug Development Costs." *Journal of Health Economics* 22, no. 2 (2003): 151–185.

Dyck, Erica. *Psychedelic Psychiatry: LSD from Clinic to Campus*. Baltimore: Johns Hopkins University Press, 2008.

Engel, Leonard. *Medicine Makers of Kalamazoo*. New York: McGraw-Hill, 1961.

Epstein, Richard. *Overdose: How Excessive Government Regulation Stifles Pharmaceutical Product Innovation*. New Haven, Conn.: Yale University Press, 2007.

Epstein, Steven. *Impure Science: AIDS, Activism, and the Politics of Knowledge*. Berkeley: University of California Press, 1996.

Etzkowitz, Henry. *MIT and the Rise of Entrepreneurial Science*. New York: Routledge, 2002.

Ewing, Oscar R. *The Nation's Health: A Ten-Year Program. Report to the President by the Federal Security Administrator*. Washington, D.C.: Government Printing Office, 1948.

Facchinetti, Neil J., and W. Michael Dickson. "Access to Generic Drugs in the 1950s: The Politics of a Social Problem." *American Journal of Public Health* 72, no. 5 (1982): 468–475.

Fones-Wolf, Elizabeth A. *Selling Free Enterprise: The Business Assault on Labor and Liberalism, 1945–1960*. Urbana: University of Illinois Press, 1994.

Food and Drug Administration. *A Historical Look at Drug Introductions on a Five-Country Market: A Comparison of the United States and Four European Countries, 1960–1981*. Washington, D.C.: FDA Office of Planning and Evaluation, 1982.

Forman, Paul. "Behind Quantum Electronics: National Security as Basis of Physical Research in the United States, 1940–1960." *Historical Studies in the Physical Sciences* 18 (1988): 149–229.

Fox, Allan R., and Alan R. Bennett. *The Legislative History of the Drug Price Competition and Patent Term Restoration Act of 1984*. Washington, D.C.: Food and Drug Law Institute, 1987.

Fox, Daniel M. *The Convergence of Science and Governance: Research, Health Policy, and American States*. Berkeley: University of California Press, 2010.

———. *Health Policies, Health Politics: The British and American Experience, 1911–1965*. Princeton, N.J.: Princeton University Press, 1986.

———. *Power and Illness: The Failure and Future of American Health Policy*. Berkeley; University of California Press, 1995.

Galambos, Louis. "The Emerging Organizational Synthesis in Modern American History." *Business History Review* 44 (1970): 279–290.

———. "Technology, Political Economy, and Professionalization: Central Themes of the Organizational Synthesis." *Business History Review* 57 (1983): 471–493.

Galambos, Louis, and Joseph Pratt. *The Rise of the Corporate Commonwealth: U.S. Business and Public Policy in the Twentieth Century*. New York: Basic Books, 1988.

Galambos, Louis, and Jane E. Sewall. *Networks of Innovation: Vaccine Development at Merck, Sharp & Dohme, and Mulford, 1895–1995*. Cambridge: Cambridge University Press, 1995.

Galambos, Louis, and Jeffrey L. Sturchio. "Pharmaceutical Firms and the Transition to Biotechnology: A Study in Strategic Innovation." *Business History Review* 72 (1998): 250–278.

Galambos, Louis, Roy P. Vagelos, Michael S. Brown, and Joseph L. Goldstein. *Values and Visions: A Merck Century.* Whitehouse Station, N.J.: Merck & Co., 1991.

Galison, Peter, and Bruce Hevly, eds. *Big Science: The Growth of Large-Scale Research.* Stanford, Calif.: Stanford University Press, 1992.

Gambardella, Alfonso. *Science and Innovation: The U.S. Pharmaceutical Industry during the 1980s.* Cambridge: Cambridge University Press, 1995.

Goozner, Merrill. *The $800 Million Pill: The Truth behind the Cost of Drugs.* Berkeley: University of California Press, 2004.

Gordon, Colin. *Dead on Arrival: The Politics of Health Care in Twentieth-Century America.* Princeton, N.J.: Princeton University Press, 2003.

Greenberg, Daniel S. *The Politics of Pure Science.* Chicago: University of Chicago Press, 1999.

———. *Science for Sale: The Perils, Rewards, and Delusions of Campus Capitalism.* Chicago: University of Chicago Press, 2007.

Greene, Jeremy A. "Attention to 'Details': Etiquette and the Pharmaceutical Salesman in Postwar America." *Social Studies of Science* 34, no. 2 (2004): 271–292.

———. *Prescribing by Numbers: Drugs and the Definition of Disease.* Baltimore: Johns Hopkins University Press 2007.

———. "Releasing the Flood Waters: Diuril and the Reshaping of Hypertension." *Bulletin of the History of Medicine* 79, no. 4 (2005): 749–794.

Greene, Jeremy A., and Scott Podolsky. "Keeping Modern in Medicine: Pharmaceutical Promotion and Physician Education in Postwar America." *Bulletin of the History of Medicine* 83, no. 2 (2009): 331–377.

Harden, Victoria A. *Inventing the NIH: Federal Biomedical Research Policy, 1887–1937.* Baltimore: Johns Hopkins University Press, 1986.

Harkness, Jon, Susan Lederer, and Daniel Wikler. "Laying Ethical Foundations for Clinical Research." *Bulletin of the World Health Organization* 79, no. 4 (2001): 365–366.

Harris, Howell J. *The Right to Manage: Industrial Relations Policies of American Business in the 1940s.* Madison: University of Wisconsin Press, 1982.

Harris, Richard. *The Real Voice.* New York: Macmillan, 1964.

Healy, David. *The Creation of Psychopharmacology.* Cambridge, Mass.: Harvard University Press, 2002.

———. *Let Them Eat Prozac: The Unhealthy Relationship Between the Pharmaceutical Industry and Depression.* New York: New York University Press, 2004.

Herzberg, David. *Happy Pills in America: From Miltown to Prozac.* Baltimore: Johns Hopkins University Press, 2008.

Higby, Gregory J., and Elaine C. Stroud, eds. *Pill Peddlers: Essays on the History of the Pharmaceutical Industry.* Madison, Wis.: American Institute of the History of Pharmacy, 1987.

Hilts, Philip J. *Protecting America's Health: The FDA, Business, and 100 Years of Regulation.* New York: Alfred A. Knopf, 2003.

Hobby, Gladys. *Penicillin: Meeting the Challenge.* New Haven, Conn.: Yale University Press, 1985.

Hounshell, David A., and John Kenly Smith. *Science and Corporate Strategy: Du Pont R&D, 1902–1980.* Cambridge: Cambridge University Press, 1988.

Howell, Joel. *Technology in the Hospital: Transforming Patient Care in the Early Twentieth Century.* Baltimore: Johns Hopkins University Press, 1996.

Hull, Callie, and Mary Timms. "Research Supported by Industry through Scholarships, Fellowships, and Grants." *Chemical and Engineering News* 24 (1946): 2346.

Jackson, Charles O. *Food and Drug Legislation in the New Deal.* Princeton, N.J.: Princeton University Press, 1970.

Jacobs, Meg. *Pocketbook Politics: Economic Citizenship in Twentieth-Century America.* Princeton, N.J.: Princeton University Press, 2005.

Jasanoff, Sheila. *The Fifth Branch: Science Advisors as Policymakers.* Cambridge, Mass.: Harvard University Press, 1990.

Jones, James. *Bad Blood: The Tuskegee Syphilis Experiment.* Rev. ed. New York: Free Press, 1993.

Kahn, E. J., Jr. *All in a Century: The First 100 Years of Eli Lilly & Company.* Indianapolis: Eli Lilly & Co., 1975.

Kaiser, David. "Cold War Requisitions, Scientific Manpower, and the Production of American Physicists after World War II." *Historical Studies in the Physical Sciences* 33 (2002): 131–159.

Kargon, Robert, and Elizabeth Hodes. "Karl Compton, Isaiah Bowman, and the Politics of Science in the Great Depression." *ISIS* 76 (1985): 301–318.

Kaser, Michael. *Health Care in the Soviet Union and Eastern Europe.* Boulder, Colo.: Westview Press, 1976.

Kefauver, Estes, with Irene Till. *In a Few Hands: Monopoly Power in America.* New York, 1965.

Klein, Jennifer. *For All These Rights: Business, Labor, and the Shaping of America's Public-Private Welfare State.* Princeton, N.J.: Princeton University Press, 2006.

Kleinman, Daniel L. *Impure Cultures: University Biology and the World of Commerce.* Madison: University of Wisconsin Press, 2003.

———. "Layers of Interests, Layers of Influence: Business and the Genesis of the National Science Foundation." *Science, Technology, and Human Values* 19, no. 3 (1994): 259–282.

———. *Politics on the Endless Frontier: Postwar Research Policy in the United States.* Durham, N.C.: Duke University Press, 1995.

Kleinman, Daniel L., and Steven P. Vallas. "Science, Capitalism and the Rise of the 'Knowledge Worker': The Changing Structure of Knowledge Production in the United States." *Theory and Society* 30 (2001): 451–492.

Kline, Wendy. *Bodies of Knowledge: Sexuality, Reproduction, and Women's Health in the Second Wave.* Chicago: University of Chicago Press, 2010.

———. "The Making of *Our Bodies, Ourselves:* Re-thinking Women's Health and Second-Wave Feminism." In *Feminist Coalitions: Historical Perspectives on Second-Wave Feminism in the United States,* ed. Stephanie Gilmore. Urbana: University of Illinois Press, 2008.

Kogan, Herman. *The Long White Line: The Story of Abbott Laboratories.* New York: Random House, 1963.

Kushner, Howard I. *A Cursing Brain? The Histories of Tourette Syndrome.* Cambridge, Mass.: Harvard University Press, 1999.

Landau, Ralph, Basil Achilladelis, and Alexander Scriabine, eds. *Pharmaceutical Innovation: Revolutionizing Human Health.* Philadelphia: Chemical Heritage Foundation Press, 1999.

Lerner, Barron H. *Breast Cancer Wars: Hope, Fear, and the Pursuit of a Cure in Twentieth-Century America.* Oxford: Oxford University Press, 2001.

Lesch, John E. *The First Miracle Drugs: How the Sulfa Drugs Transformed Medicine.* Oxford: Oxford University Press, 2006.

Leslie, Stuart W. *The Cold War and American Science: The Military-Industrial-Academic Complex at MIT and Stanford.* New York: Columbia University Press, 1993.

Lichtenberg, Frank. "The Effect of Pharmaceutical Utilization and Innovation on Hospitalisation and Mortality." In *Productivity, Technology and Economic Growth,* ed. Bart van Ark, Simon K Kuipers, and Gerard H. Kuper. Boston: Kluwer, 2000.

———. "Pharmaceutical Innovation as a Process of Creative Destruction." In *Knowledge Accumulation and Industry Evolution: The Case of Pharma-Biotech,* ed. Marianna Mazzucato and Giovani Dosi. Cambridge: Cambridge University Press, 2006.

———. "Pharmaceutical Innovation, Mortality Reduction, and Economic Growth." In *Measuring the Gains from Medical Research: An Economic Approach,* ed. Kevin M. Murphy and Robert H. Topel. Chicago: University of Chicago Press, 2003.

———. "Pharmaceutical Knowledge-Capital Accumulation and Longevity." Paper presented at the Conference on Research on Income and Wealth/ National Bureau of Economic Research Conference on Measuring Capital in a New Economy, Federal Reserve Board, Washington D.C., April 26–27, 2002.

Liebenau, Jonathan. *Medical Science and Medical Industry: The Formation of the American Pharmaceutical Industry.* Baltimore: Johns Hopkins University Press, 1987.

Linker, Beth. "The Business of Ethics: Gender, Medicine, and the Professional Codification of the American Physiotherapy Association, 1918–

1935." *Journal of the History of Medicine and Allied Sciences* 60 (2005): 321–354.

Lowen, Rebecca S. *Creating the Cold War University: The Transformation of Stanford.* Berkeley: University of California Press, 1997.

Ludmerer, Kenneth M. *Time to Heal: American Medical Education from the Turn of the Century to the Era of Managed Care.* Oxford: Oxford University Press, 1999.

Madison, James H. *Eli Lilly, A Life: 1885–1977.* Indianapolis: Indiana University Press, 1989.

Marieskind, Helen. "The Women's Health Movement." *International Journal of Health Services* 5, no. 2 (1975): 217–223.

Marion, John Francis. *The Fine Old House: SmithKline Corporation's First 150 Years.* Philadelphia: SmithKline Corporation, 1980.

Markowitz, Gerald, and David Rosner. *Deceit and Denial: The Deadly Politics of Industrial Pollution.* Berkeley: University of California Press, 2002.

Marks, Harry. "Cortisone, 1949: A Year in the Political Life of a Drug." *Bulletin of the History of Medicine* 66 (1992): 419–439.

———. "Making Risks Visible: The Science and Politics of Adverse Drug Reactions." In *Ways of Regulating: Therapeutic Agents between Plants, Shops and Consulting Rooms,* ed. Jean Paul Gaudillière and Volker Hess. Berlin: Max-Planck-Institut für Wissenschaftsgeschichte, 2009.

———. *The Progress of Experiment: Science and Therapeutic Reform in the United States, 1900–1990.* Cambridge: Cambridge University Press, 1997.

———. "Revisiting 'The Origins of Compulsory Drug Prescriptions.'" *American Journal of Public Health* 85, no. 1 (1995): 109–116.

Marks, Lara. *Sexual Chemistry: A History of the Contraceptive Pill.* New Haven, Conn.: Yale University Press, 2001.

Markusen, Ann, Peter Hall, Scott Campbell, and Sabina Deitrick. *The Rise of the Gunbelt: The Military Remapping of Industrial America.* Oxford: Oxford University Press, 1991.

Mastro, Julius J. "The Pharmaceutical Manufacturers Association, the Ethical Drug Industry and the 1962 Drug Amendments: A Case Study of Congressional Action and Interest Group Reaction." Ph.D. dissertation, New York University, 1965.

McCraw, Thomas K. *Prophets of Regulation: Charles Francis Adams, Louis D. Brandeis, James M. Landis, Alfred E. Kahn.* Cambridge, Mass.: Harvard University Press, 1984.

McFadyen, Richard E. "Estes Kefauver and the Drug Industry." Ph.D. dissertation, Emory University, 1973.

McGrath, Patrick J. *Scientists, Business, and the State, 1890–1960.* Chapel Hill: University of North Carolina Press, 2002.

Miller, Karen S. *The Voice of Business: Hill & Knowlton and Postwar Public Relations.* Chapel Hill: University of North Carolina Press, 1999.

Mines, Samuel. *Pfizer ... An Informal History.* New York: Pfizer, 1978.

Mintz, Morton. *The Therapeutic Nightmare: A Report on the Roles of the United States Food and Drug Administration, the American Medical Association, Pharmaceutical Manufacturers, and Others in Connection with the Irrational and Massive Use of Prescription Drugs That May Be Worthless, Injurious, or Even Lethal.* Boston: Houghton Mifflin, 1965.

Mossinghoff, Gerald J. "Overview of the Hatch-Waxman Act and Its Impact on the Drug Development Process." *Food and Drug Law Journal* 54 (1999): 187–194.

Moynihan, Roy, and Alan Cassels. *Selling Sickness: How the World's Biggest Pharmaceutical Companies Are Turning Us All into Patients.* New York: Nation Books, 2005.

Mukerji, Chandra. *A Fragile Power: Scientists and the State.* Princeton, N.J.: Princeton University Press, 1989.

Numbers, Ronald L. *Almost Persuaded: American Physicians and Compulsory Health Insurance, 1912–1920.* Baltimore: Johns Hopkins University Press, 1978.

Office of the Secretary, U.S. Department of Health, Education, and Welfare. *The Drug Makers and the Drug Distributors: The Task Force on Prescription Drugs Background Papers.* Washington, D.C.: Government Printing Office, 1968.

———. *Final Report of the Task Force on Prescription Drugs.* Washington D.C.: Government Printing Office, 1969.

———. *Report of the Secretary's Review Committee of the Task Force on Prescription Drugs.* Washington, D.C.: Government Printing Office, 1969.

Office of Technology Assessment. *Patent-Term Extension and the Pharmaceutical Industry.* Washington, D.C.: Government Printing Office, 1981.

Offit, Paul A. *The Cutter Incident: How America's First Polio Vaccine Led to the Growing Vaccine Crisis.* New Haven, Conn.: Yale University Press, 2005.

Oliver, Thomas R., Philip R. Lee, and Helene L. Lipton. "A Political History of Medicare and Prescription Drug Coverage." *Milbank Quarterly* 82, no. 2 (2004): 283–354.

Oshinsky, David M. *Polio: An American Story.* Oxford: Oxford University Press, 2005.

Owens, Lawrence. "The Counterproductive Management of Science in the Second World War: Vannevar Bush and the Office of Scientific Research and Development." *Business History Review* 68 (1994): 515–576.

Parascandola, John. *The Development of American Pharmacology: John J. Abel and the Shaping of a Discipline.* Baltimore: Johns Hopkins University Press, 1992.

Parke-Davis & Co. *Parke-Davis at 100.* Detroit: Parke-Davis & Co., 1966.

Peltzman, Sam. *Regulation of Pharmaceutical Innovation: The 1962 Amendments.* Washington, D.C.: American Enterprise Institute for Public Policy Research, 1974.

Petticrew, Mark P., and Kelley Lee. "The 'Father of Stress' Meets 'Big Tobacco': Hans Selye and the Tobacco Industry." *American Journal of Public Health* 101, no. 3 (2010): 411–418; online preprint, May 13, 2010.

Pharmaceutical Manufacturers Association. *Brands, Generics, Prices and Quality: The Prescribing Debate after a Decade.* Washington, D.C.: Pharmaceutical Manufacturers Association, 1971.

Phillips-Fein, Kim. *Invisible Hands: The Businessmen's Crusade against the New Deal.* New York: W.W. Norton, 2009.

Powers, Lee, Joseph F. Whiting, and K.C. Oppermann. "Trends in Medical School Faculties." *Journal of Medical Education* 37 (1962): 1065–1091.

Quirke, Viviane. *Collaboration in the Pharmaceutical Industry: Changing Relationships in Britain and France, 1935–1965.* New York: Routledge, 2007.

Rasmussen, Nicolas. "The Commercial Drug Trial in Interwar America: Three Types of Clinician Collaborator." *Bulletin of the History of Medicine* 79, no. 1 (2005): 50–80.

———. "The Forgotten Promise of Thiamin: Merck, Caltech Biologists, and Plan Hormones in a 1930s Biotechnology Project." *Journal of the History of Biology* 32 (1999): 246–261.

———. "The Moral Economy of the Drug Company–Medical Scientist Collaboration in Interwar America." *Social Studies of Science* 34, no. 2 (2004): 161–185.

———. "Of 'Small Men,' Big Science, and Bigger Business: The Second World War and Biomedical Research in the United States." *Minerva* 40 (2002): 115–146.

———. *On Speed: The Many Lives of Amphetamine.* New York: New York University Press, 2008.

———. "Steroids in Arms: Science, Government, Industry, and the Hormones of the Adrenal Cortex in the United States, 1930–1950." *Medical History* 46 (2002): 299–324.

Reverby, Susan. *Examining Tuskegee: The Infamous Syphilis Study and Its Legacy.* Chapel Hill: University of North Carolina Press, 2009.

———, ed. *Tuskegee's Truths: Rethinking the Tuskegee Syphilis Study.* Chapel Hill: University of North Carolina Press, 2000.

Rodengen, Jeffrey L. *The Legend of Pfizer.* Fort Lauderdale: Write Stuff Syndicate, 1999.

Rose, Mark H., Bruce E. Seely, and Paul F. Barrett. *The Best Transportation System in the World: Railroads, Trucks, Airlines, and American Public Policy in the Twentieth Century.* Columbus: Ohio State University Press, 2006.

Rothman, David J. *Strangers at the Bedside: A History of How Law and Bioethics Transformed Medical Decision Making.* New York: Basic Books, 1991.

Rothstein, William G. *American Medical Schools and the Practice of Medicine: A History.* Oxford: Oxford University Press, 1987.

Ruzek, Sheryl Burt. *The Women's Health Movement: Feminist Alternatives to Medical Control.* New York: Praeger, 1978.

Scroop, Daniel. "A Faded Passion? Estes Kefauver and the Senate Subcommittee on Antitrust and Monopoly." *Business and Economic History On-Line* 5 (2007).

Silverman, Milton, and Philip R. Lee. *Pills, Profits, and Politics.* Berkeley: University of California Press, 1974.

Silverman, Milton, Philip R. Lee, and Mia Lydecker. *Pills and the Public Purse: The Routes to National Drug Insurance.* Berkeley: University of California Press, 1981.

Slater, Leo B. *War and Disease: Biomedical Research on Malaria in the Twentieth Century.* New Brunswick, N.J.: Rutgers University Press, 2009.

Slinn, Judy. "Price Controls or Controls through Prices? Regulating the Cost and Consumption of Prescription Pharmaceuticals in the UK, 1948–1967." *Business History* 47, no. 3 (2005): 352–366.

———. "Research and Development in the UK Pharmaceutical Industry from the 19th Century to the 1960s." In *Drugs and Narcotics in History,* ed. Roy Porter and Mikulas Teich. Cambridge: Cambridge University Press, 1995.

Smith, Mickey C. *Small Comfort: A History of the Minor Tranquilizers.* New York: Praeger, 1985.

Sogner, Knut. "A Pharmaceutical Innovation: Business Environment and Scientific Endeavour in Nyegaard & Co." *History and Technology* 13, no. 2 (1996): 115–131.

Solberg, Carl. *Hubert Humphrey: A Biography.* New York: W. W. Norton, 1984.

Somers, Herman, and Ann Somers. *Doctors, Patients, and Health Insurance: The Organization and Financing of Medical Care.* Washington, D.C.: Brookings Institution, 1961.

Starr, Paul. *The Social Transformation of American Medicine: The Rise of a Sovereign Profession and the Making of a Vast Industry.* New York: Basic Books, 1982.

Stephens, Harrison, and Nancy Fries. *Allergan's First Fifty Years.* Lyme, Conn.: Greenwich Publication Group, 2000.

Stevens, Rosemary A. *Medicine in the Public Interest: A History of Specialization.* Berkeley: University of California Press, 1998.

Strickland, Stephen P. *The History of Regional Medical Programs: The Life and Death of a Small Initiative of the Great Society.* New York: University Press of America, 2000.

———. *Politics, Science, and Dread Disease: A Short History of United States Medical Research Policy.* Cambridge, Mass.: Harvard University Press, 1972.

Swann, John P. *Academic Scientists and the Pharmaceutical Industry: Cooperative Research in Twentieth-Century America.* Baltimore: Johns Hopkins University Press, 1988.

———. "Sure Cure: Public Policy on Drug Efficacy before 1962." In *The Inside Story of Medicines,* ed. Gregory J. Higby and Elaine C. Stroud. Madison, Wis.: American Institute for the History of Pharmacy, 1997.

Talley, Colin. "The Combined Efforts of Community and Science: American Culture, Patient Activism, and the Multiple Sclerosis Movement in the United States." In *Emerging Illnesses and Society: Negotiating the Public Health Agenda,* ed. Randall M. Packard, P. J. Brown, R. L. Berkelman, and H. Frumkin. Baltimore: Johns Hopkins University Press, 2004.

Temin, Peter. *Taking Your Medicine: Drug Regulation in the United States.* Cambridge, Mass.: Harvard University Press, 1980.

Tobbell, Dominique A. "Allied against Reform: Pharmaceutical Industry–Academic Physician Relations in the United States, 1945–1970." *Bulletin of the History of the Medicine* 82, no. 4 (2008): 878–912.

———. "Charitable Innovations: The Political Economy of Thalassemia Research and Drug Development in the United States, 1960–2000." In *Perspectives on Twentieth-Century Pharmaceuticals,* ed. Judy Slinn and Vivianne Quirke. Oxford: Peter Lang AG, 2010.

———. "Eroding the Physicians' Control." In *Prescribed: Writing, Filling, Using, and Abusing the Prescription in Modern America,* ed. Jeremy A. Greene and Elizabeth Siegel Watkins. Baltimore: Johns Hopkins University Press, 2012.

———. "Who's Winning the Human Race? Cold War as Pharmaceutical Political Strategy." *Journal of the History of Medicine and Allied Sciences* 64, no. 4 (2009): 429–473.

Tomes, Nancy. "The Fielding H. Garrison Lecture: The Great American Medicine Show Revisited." *Bulletin of the History of Medicine* 79, no. 4 (2005): 627–663.

———. "Merchants of Health: Medicine and Consumer Culture in the United States, 1900–1940." *Journal of American History* 88 (2001): 519–547.

———. "Patients or Health-Care Consumers? Why the History of Contested Terms Matters." In *History and Health Policy in the United States: Putting the Past Back In,* ed. Rosemary A. Stevens, Charles E. Rosenberg, and Lawton R. Burns. New Brunswick, N.J.: Rutgers University Press, 2006.

Tone, Andrea. *The Age of Anxiety: A History of American's Turbulent Affair with Tranquilizers.* New York: Basic Books, 2009.

Tone, Andrea, and Elizabeth S. Watkins, eds. *Medicating Modern America: Prescription Drugs in History.* New York: New York University Press, 2007.

U.S. Department of Health, Education and Welfare. *Health United States 1975.* DHEW Publication no. (HRA) 76–1232.

U.S. Senate. Committee of the Judiciary, Subcommittee on Antitrust and Monopoly. *Administered Prices, Drugs: Report of the Committee of the Judiciary, Subcommittee on Antitrust and Monopoly.* Washington, D.C.: Government Printing Office, 1961.

Vogel, David. *Fluctuating Fortunes: The Political Power of Business in America.* New York: Basic Books, 1989.

Vos, Rein. *Drugs Looking for Diseases: Innovative Drug Research and the Development of the Beta Blockers and Calcium Antagonists.* Dordrecht: Kluwer Academic Publishers, 1991.

Wailoo, Keith. *Drawing Blood: Technology and Disease Identity in Twentieth-Century America.* Baltimore: Johns Hopkins University Press, 1997.

Wang, Jessica. *American Science in an Age of Anxiety: Scientists, Anticommunism, and the Cold War.* Chapel Hill: University of North Carolina Press, 1999.

Wardell, William M., and Louis Lasagna. *Regulation and Drug Development.* Washington, D.C.: American Enterprise Institute for Public Policy Research, 1975.

Waterhouse, Benjamin C. "A Lobby for Capital: Organized Business and the Pursuit of Pro-Market Politics, 1967–1986." PhD dissertation, Harvard University, 2009.

Watkins, Elizabeth S. *The Estrogen Elixir: A History of Hormone Replacement Therapy in America.* Baltimore: Johns Hopkins University Press, 2007.

———. *On the Pill: A Social History of Oral Contraceptives, 1950–1970.* Baltimore: Johns Hopkins University Press, 1998.

Weisman, Carol S. *Women's Healthcare: Activist Traditions and Institutional Change.* Baltimore: Johns Hopkins University Press, 1998.

Young, James Harvey. *Pure Food: Securing the Federal Food and Drugs Act of 1906.* Princeton, N.J.: Princeton University Press, 1989.

———. "Sulfanilamide and Diethylene Glycol." In *Chemistry and Modern Society: Essays in Honor of Aaron J. Ihde,* ed. John Parascandola and James C. Wharton. Washington, D.C.: American Chemical Society, 1983.

———. *The Toadstool Millionaires: A Social History of Patent Medicines in America before Federal Regulation.* Princeton, N.J.: Princeton University Press, 1961.

Zelizer, Julian E. *On Capitol Hill: The Struggle to Reform Congress and Its Consequences, 1948–2000.* Cambridge: Cambridge University Press, 2004.

Zimmerman, Mary K. "The Women's Health Movement: A Critique of Medical Enterprise and the Position of Women." In *Analyzing Gender: A Handbook of Social Science Research,* ed. Beth B. Hess and Myra Marx Ferree. Newbury Park, Calif.: Sage Publications, 1987.

Zuckerman, Stephen, and Joshua McFeeters. *Recent Growth in Health Expenditures.* New York: Commonwealth Fund, 2006.

Index

Text: 10/13 Aldus
Display: Aldus
Compositor: Toppan Best-set Premedia Limited
Indexer: Ruth Elwell
Printer and binder: IBT Global